STRAIGHT TALK
ABOUT
WEIGHT

STRAIGHT TALK ABOUT WEIGHT CONTROL

Taking the Pounds Off
and
Keeping Them Off

Lynn J. Bennion, M.D.
Edwin L. Bierman, M.D.
James M. Ferguson, M.D.
and the Editors of
Consumer Reports Books

Consumers Union
Mount Vernon, New York

Library of Congress Cataloging-in-Publication Data
Bennion, Lynn J.
    Straight talk about weight control : taking the pounds off and
keeping them off / by Lynn J. Bennion, Edwin L. Bierman, James M.
Ferguson ; and [edited by] the editors of Consumer Reports Books.
    p. cm.
    Includes bibliographical references and index.
ISBN 0-89043-246-5 (pb)
    1. Obesity. 2. Reducing. I. Bierman, Edwin L., 1930–   .
II. Ferguson, James Mecham, 1941–   . III. Consumer Reports Books.
IV. Title.
RC628.B385   1991
613.2'5—dc20   90-37950
                                                                CIP

Design by GDS / Jeffrey L. Ward
First printing, January 1991
Manufactured in the United States of America

Straight Talk About Weight Control is a Consumer Reports Book published by Consumers Union, the nonprofit organization that publishes *Consumer Reports,* the monthly magazine of test reports, product Ratings, and buying guidance. Established in 1936, Consumers Union is chartered under the Not-for-Profit Corporation Law of the State of New York.

The ideas, procedures, and suggestions contained in this book are not intended to replace the services of a physician. All matters regarding your health require medical supervision, and you should consult a physician before adopting the procedures in this book. Any application of the treatments set forth herein are at the reader's discretion, and neither the authors nor the publisher assume any responsibility or liability therefor.

The cases and examples cited in this book are based on actual situations and real people. Names and identifying details have been changed to protect privacy.

Figure 3.1 (page 63) adapted from M. T. Pugliese, F. Lifshitz, G. Grad, P. Fort, and M. Marks-Katz, "Fear of Obesity: A Cause of Short Stature and Delayed Puberty," *New England Journal of Medicine* 309 (1983): 513–18.

Figure 6.1 (page 126) adapted from R. I. Gregerman and E. L. Bierman, "Aging and Hormones," in *Textbook of Endocrinology, Sixth Edition*, ed. by R. H. Williams. Philadelphia: W. B. Saunders Co., 1974.

Figure 6.2 (page 133) copyright © 1988 by George A. Bray. Reprinted by permission.

Table 6.3 (page 134) and Figure 6.3 (page 135) adapted from G. A. Bray and D. S. Gray, "Obesity: Part I—Pathogenesis," *Western Journal of Medicine* 149 (1988): 429–41.

The photographs in Figure 6.5 (page 144) are (top) courtesy of Dr. G. Aagaard, University of Washington, Seattle, and (bottom) courtesy of Jerry Gay, *Seattle Times*.

Figure 12.1 (page 263) adapted from L. W. Craighead, A. J. Stunkard, and R. M. O'Brien, "Behavior Therapy and Pharmacotherapy for Obesity," *Archives of General Psychiatry* 38 (1981): 763–68.

Figure 12.2 (page 267) adapted from L. H. Kyle, M. F. Ball, and P. D. Doolan, "Comparative Effects of Caloric Restriction and Metabolic Acceleration on Body Composition in Obesity," *Journal of Clinical Endocrinology and Metabolism* 27 5(1967): 12–17.

Figures 14.3 (page 306) and 14.5 (page 310) adapted from J. M. Ferguson, *Habits, Not Diets*. Palo Alto, Calif.: Bull Publishing Co., 1989. Reprinted by permission.

Contents

Acknowledgments

We thank Andrea Kelley for drawing the illustrations, and Melissa Hilton, R.D., M.S., for help with chapters 5 and 10 as well as for careful scrutiny of the manuscript.

Our special thanks and appreciation to Sarah Uman, executive editor of Consumer Reports Books, for encouragement, guidance, and patient prodding in the production of this work.

We thank our families for understanding and support through long days and nights of research, writing, and revisions.

STRAIGHT TALK
ABOUT
WEIGHT
CONTROL

Introduction

This book is for people who are concerned about their weight. It explains what fat is, why it is important, and what's wrong with having too much of it. It describes the various types of obesity, the causes and consequences of being overweight, and the available treatments. If you think you may be too fat, this book will help you decide whether you are and, if so, to determine what you can do about it and how to succeed at what you decide on.

Current methods for the treatment of obesity are unfortunately still rather primitive. No simple cure for obesity, such as a diet or a pill that safely and easily controls appetite and prevents weight gain, has been discovered. If decisive, effective treatment were available, quackery would flourish far less than it does.

Major advances in obesity treatment will no doubt take place in the future. When they do, they will be based in solid, scientific fact. But you will be able to judge their relative effectiveness only if you understand the fundamentals of nutrition, fat metabolism, and obesity. This book conveys those fundamentals while relating them to the methods that are currently available for weight control.

No particular product or program is promoted here. We have not discovered a new drug to dissolve fat, nor have we devised a miraculous new diet. We are not magicians with a secret cure for obesity, but physicians who specialize in the problems connected with obesity, and we treat many overweight people. This book will bring you up-to-date on the facts about fat, and about what you can do if you have too much of it.

The overweight person faces two tasks: getting the excess weight off, and keeping it off. Immense as the first of these challenges may seem, the second is even greater. Most overweight people have already lost substantial amounts of weight, only to gain it back again. And that's the rub: *maintaining* a reduced weight. It does little good to lose fifty pounds of fat if you eventually gain it back again; in fact, it may even do harm.

The perspective offered here is realistic and practical. But suppose for a moment that, instead of a book, we were presenting a magic box. For a mere $2,000, you could climb into the box, throw the switch, and instantly all excess fat would disappear. No doubt many eager customers would come forward. Yet they would end up being terribly disappointed, because sooner or later—and often sooner—they would regain their lost weight. The irony is that while they were writing out their checks for $2,000, the possibility of regaining the weight would be the last thing on their minds; they would feel certain that once the weight was off, they would be so happy and so motivated that they would never gain it back again, no matter what they had to do to keep it off. But they would regain it anyway, because they would not have acquired the habits and skills necessary to maintain their lower weight. The experiment has already been done. Thousands of people have lost weight, many of them several times, only to regain it. Only a few manage to keep it off.

Usually the reason why people regain the weight they have lost is the same reason that caused their obesity in the first place. Obesity doesn't just happen—it is caused by consuming calories in excess of the amount you are expending. And until you correct the underlying causes of obesity, it will recur.

Obesity, in fact, has many causes. Some are genetically inherited, and others are environmental. Regardless of underlying cause, however, all effective remedies for obesity boil down to two fundamental approaches: (1) fewer calories taken in, and (2) more calories expended. At present, the only practical way for most people to increase their calorie expenditure is to increase their physical activity. Eating high-calorie foods, however, can so easily overwhelm the calorie output of physical activity that some control of calorie intake is required as well. An array of strategies is available for reducing calorie intake:

- deciding on your own to eat fewer calories
- individualized nutritional counseling, once or for a few sessions
- individual and/or group support and counseling weekly or daily
- commercial programs that supply a complete diet plus group support
- physician-supervised liquid-formula fasting plus weekly group support
- residential, inpatient programs
- jaw wiring
- surgery to restrict the flow of food through the stomach
- gastrointestinal bypass surgery

Cutting across all of these categories is the need for more physical activity to increase calorie expenditure, and the need for modifying one's behavior to build new habits that will allow one to maintain the reduced body weight.

Losing weight and maintaining the loss is a personal and highly specific matter. Some people simply decide to skip doughnuts and desserts, and succeed in losing twelve pounds and keeping them off. Many people, however, need more help. Some will succeed after a few visits to a dietitian for individualized dietary counseling and education. Others may need the encouragement and support of a group program, such as Weight Watchers, or Overeaters Anonymous. Even in these programs, however, many people fail to achieve permanent control of their weight. They may wish to consider more extreme measures, and move to other treatment options. In doing so, they must be sure to measure the expected benefit against the cost in time, expense, and risk. This book describes not only the benefits of weight reduction, but the risks and expenses involved in the various treatments available.

In general, of course, it is preferable to correct obesity by employing the less extreme methods that we explore. If you can correct your weight by simply deciding on your own to eat less and exercise more, you are fortunate indeed, for you will not need to avail yourself of the riskier, more expensive, and more time-consuming alternatives. On the other hand, if you don't succeed with simple measures, and if your obesity is a serious enough problem, you may wish to consider some of the more drastic options.

Three principles are basic. First, there are individual differences in the types of obesity, its causes, its consequences, and one's responses to treatment. This means that what works for one person may not be ideal for someone else. Some people thrive in the atmosphere of a support group, while others do better with individual counseling. Some people cannot exercise much because of arthritis, while others successfully walk off 3,000 calories a week. Some people get fat gorging once a day; others do it by constant grazing.

There are also individual differences in the degree to which obesity is really a problem. One person may live in a social situation in which being substantially overweight is not a disadvantage, while another person of equal weight might suffer extreme discrimination as a result of it. One person might come down with diabetes, high blood pressure, and heart failure as a result of obesity, while another person, equally fat, may suffer few if any adverse health effects. Individual differences occur even in the distribution of excess fat within the body. Some people put the excess weight on their hips, while others carry it in the upper body. As we shall see, these individual differences have important implications for the impact of obesity on an individual, and for the mode of treatment to be selected.

The second principle is that your weight is determined by *calories in and calories out*. The balance of calories eaten and calories expended through metabolism and physical activity determines your weight. Consequently, some control of caloric intake and a practical, healthy level of physical activity are parts of any successful weight-control program.

The third principle is that lasting success in weight control consists of more than just *arriving* at a healthy weight. It also includes healthy habits and healthy attitudes, values, and ways of thinking. The scales don't tell the whole story. If you have just lost weight on a crash diet, but still gorge on high-fat foods in front of the TV every night, you are unlikely to maintain your reduced weight for long. On the other hand, if you are building lasting habits of daily physical activity, you are well on your way to successful weight control even if you are still above ideal body weight.

People whose self-esteem focuses on their weight and depends on their physical shape are liable to be bowled over by the normal variations in weight that we all experience. So if you think of eating a big meal on Thanksgiving as a failure, or of eating a piece of cake at a wedding reception as an illicit activity, you will find it difficult to live in the real world and still maintain a healthy weight. If you're going to be discouraged every time you eat something delicious with a few calories in it, you will have a hard time controlling your weight. And if every new little wrinkle, sag, or bulge depresses you, it will be difficult to maintain the morale and enthusiasm needed to cope with a weight problem. It is difficult enough to avoid gaining weight in our high-calorie, labor-saving environment without bearing the burden of such feelings of failure, guilt, and depression. We hope that an appreciation of the facts will help dispel such feelings.

When overweight people start to lose weight, they commonly become excited and delighted about the changes in their body shape, and fascinated with the readings on the scales. They tend to assume that being slim will make them happy. But if a person is fat, depressed, and anxious, the best he or she should expect from weight reduction is to become thin, depressed, and anxious. As you read, please remember that there are more important things in life than weight, and many more important things about you than your shape. Instead of focusing entirely on the scales as we lose weight, we need to direct our attention toward other issues, including the development of habits that will allow us to sustain a reduced weight, to enjoy physical activity, to enjoy nourishing, low-calorie foods, and to avoid condemning ourselves for such normal activities as eating.

PART I

Causes for Concern

1

America's Obsession with Weight

For a variety of reasons, many Americans worry about their weight and want to reduce. Some of us are concerned for health reasons. Others regard weight loss or low-weight maintenance as an important matter of fashion, personal appearance, and/or sex appeal. For still others, the ability to enjoy athletics and other physical activities depends on becoming and staying slim. Because our society discriminates against overweight people in such areas as employment, education, and social life, some people's economic advancement depends on whether their weight can be kept down. A person's weight may determine crucial social opportunities, including dating and marriage. For many of those who are trying to control their weight, personal pride and self-esteem are at stake.

Like other societies, ours has certain biases about body shape and weight. At present, a lean, athletic body build is highly valued within our culture, and the pursuit of this ideal motivates many of us to diet, to exercise, and to worry about our weight. But trying to lose weight can be difficult, discouraging, and expensive. With some popular approaches it can even be dangerous. The fact that so many of us are hell-bent on becoming thin does not necessarily mean that *you* need to lose weight. Here is a questionnaire to help you assess the degree to which popular concerns about weight may have gotten under your own skin:

1. When you look at yourself in the mirror, do you have feelings of displeasure toward the body fat you see?

2. Is the desire to lose weight your main motive for exercising?

3. Have you been on a diet in the past five years?

4. Have you bought any diet books in the past two years, or any magazines because of a new diet advertised on the cover?

5. Would you feel better about yourself if you were slimmer?

6. Do you think it's disgusting to be fat?

7. Have you ever bought a piece of exercise equipment, or purchased a club membership, primarily for the purpose of losing weight?

8. Do you wish your body had the same shape now that it did when you graduated from high school?

The attitudes reflected in "yes" answers to the above questions run very strongly in our society. They underlie major industries that promote slimness, as well as significant anxieties and even dangerous diseases that derive from overdoing the attempt to lose weight.

We Americans seem to have a national preoccupation with weight control. Surveys indicate that during any one-year period, as many as 50 percent of the people in this country start a diet for weight reduction, and that 75 percent of American women think they should lose weight, including large numbers who are slim already. Approximately 45 percent of American women are on a diet at any one time. Diet books perennially occupy our best-seller lists. Even children in elementary school are weight-conscious; teasing overweight children is commonplace, and psychological testing demonstrates widespread prejudice against obesity. By the sixth grade, as many as 40 percent of girls have already been on a diet.

A survey of the most frequent daily concerns of middle-aged American adults over a nine-month period yielded the following results, with weight concerns in first place:

Table 1.1 Adult Concerns

Rank	Daily Worries	Percentage of People
1	Concerns about weight	52.4%
2	Health of a family member	48.1%
3	Rising prices of common goods	43.7%
4	Home maintenance	42.8%
5	Too many things to do	38.6%
6	Misplacing or losing things	38.1%
7	Yard or outside home maintenance	38.1%
8	Property, investment, or taxes	37.6%
9	Crime	37.1%
10	Physical appearance	35.9%

From A. D. Kanner et al., "Comparison of Two Modes of Stress Measurement: Daily Hassles and Uplifts Versus Major Life Events," *Journal of Behavioral Medicine* 4, (1981):1–39. New York: Plenum Publishing Co.

As physicians who are consulted frequently by patients who want to lose weight, we are concerned that thinness has become an unhealthy obsession for many people. Too many take seriously the Duchess of Windsor's comment that "there is no such thing as too rich, or too thin." Despite the widespread wish for slimness, human history and current medical facts undercut the notion that very thin is the normal or proper shape for our bodies. This notion is, in fact, a rather recent phenomenon.

CHANGING IDEALS OF BEAUTY AND SEXUALITY

Many of our ancestors appreciated the human body in a fuller form than is fashionable today. You need only to look at paintings from earlier periods to see that fuller figures were considered, at the times they were produced, idyllic examples of beauty and sexuality. Today the pendulum of fashion has swung far to the look of leanness. Certainly not everyone prefers the current lean look, which has been popularized primarily by the fashion industry and the media. But an undeniable societal shift in taste has taken place in our century, much of it over the past few decades. A study of the body measurements of contestants in the Miss America Pageant since its inception showed that the contestants' weights, controlled for height, have decreased significantly since 1960. The contestants have become leaner, with smaller breasts and hips, a phenomenon that is in marked contrast to that of the population trend in the United States, where the average woman weighs five to six pounds *more* than in census surveys of 20 years ago. Even though Americans now prefer a thinner look, in general they are getting heavier.

The preference for looking lean is particularly strong in the present school-age generation. Our own medical practice provides daily evidence of this, and a recent study showed that up to 80 percent of graduating high-school senior girls wished that they could lose weight. Thirty percent were on a diet. This strong preference for thinness among modern American youth may relate to their heavy exposure to television.

THE GROWING IMPACT OF VISUAL MEDIA

If you turn on the TV, you will see that most actors, actresses, and newscasters are fashionably thin. If you thumb through this morning's paper, you will invariably notice ads for fitness centers, illustrated by photographs of very lean, muscular models. What we seldom realize is that the body image projected in these media is far indeed from the actual American norm.

Television is a powerful force in shaping the American mind and body. The average American spends up to seven hours a day in front of a television set. Consider what many of those watchers do during these hours: First, instead of being up and physically active, they sit. They may also eat snacks and meals. Instead of *doing* exercise, they *watch* it.

CHANGING VALUES

A couple of generations ago, Thorstein Veblen criticized Americans as materialistically preoccupied with "conspicuous consumption": spend more, buy more, eat more. We seem now to have shifted to a new brand of materialism, centered not so much on conspicuous consumption as on matters of body image, athletic life-style, and youth. People with extra time and money are likely now to spend it on ways to look slim and youthful. These values have generated immensely lucrative industries based on our desire for a sleek and lean physical appearance; it should not be surprising that such enterprises spend millions in perpetuating and reinforcing the needs that make them prosper.

COMMERCIAL ENTERPRISE

Many people earn their livings from our concern about keeping slim. Americans spend more than $30 billion every year on efforts to control weight or induce weight loss. Diet books, exercise videotapes, TV fitness shows, "fat farms," weight-reducing programs and gadgets, athletic equipment, health spas, low-calorie foods, surgical procedures, and pills and shots for weight reduction all generate income. In turn, advertising by these businesses continues to reinforce the values that drive customers to them. The skinny models in exercise leotards, the countless photos of people before and after their diets, the covers of popular magazines touting this month's new weight-loss program— all this advertising strengthens the notion that being slim is important, valuable, and sexy.

Even businesses injurious to health try to capitalize on our desire to be slim and fit. The Virginia Slims tennis tournament appears to be in part a commercial attempt to associate cigarette smoking with slim, young, healthy, muscular bodies. NFL scoreboards are juxtaposed with ads for beer and tobacco, so that viewers will associate these products with athletic fitness. Beer companies are often the sponsors for television broadcasts of athletic events, and their advertising frequently depicts slim, athletic figures drinking beer, associating the ostensible glamour of being lean with consuming a product that hardly promotes that idealized state.

Again and again, the many industries catering to our desire for thinness hammer away at how sexy, successful, and satisfying it is to be slim. Their commercial messages and promotions, created at great expense, teach us to value thinness. In addition, we are taught that being thin is healthy—a lesson only partially supported by medical facts.

HEALTH AWARENESS

Health concerns, both real and imagined, contribute to America's infatuation with thinness. Over the last few years, popular concerns about health and our bodies have made medical research reports into news items—especially in the areas of nutrition and obesity. Weight control and obesity have become "in" topics, scientifically and medically as well as socially. The research linking obesity to major health problems is widely publicized, and medical science and the health profession are active participants in deepening our national concern about weight.

Severe obesity increases the risk of premature death. For years, insurance companies have charged higher premiums for life insurance to people defined as obese according to their statistical tables. Heart disease, stroke, high blood pressure, low-back pain, heartburn, diabetes mellitus—all of these common afflictions, some of which touch almost every family, are caused in part by obesity. Millions have been told, by their doctors or by the media, that they really should lose weight and exercise more, and that doing so will help prevent or cure these diseases. Even certain types of cancer are linked to obesity.

All of this indicates that the pursuit of health remains a big reason why many people want to lose weight. Later, we'll examine scientific data on the health consequences of obesity, and show that obesity does indeed cause many important health problems. But in some ways obesity is also beneficial, and in others it is not so detrimental as was previously thought.

AMERICANS ARE GETTING FATTER

As we noted earlier, despite the shift in values and fashion toward leanness, the average weight of Americans is increasing. Obesity is five to eight times more common among Americans today than it was in 1900. Around 1900, about 5 percent of the population of the United States was obese. Our current prevalence of obesity, however, ranges from 20 to 40 percent, according to various estimates. Several factors contribute to this national trend toward obesity. They are all products of our becoming more wealthy and "civilized."

The amount of calories we Americans expend in physical activity has declined markedly in this century. Researchers estimate that the average American today gets about 75 percent less physical activity than our counterparts did in 1900. Technical advances in our society have brought automation, with reduced energy expenditure. Jobs previously done by manual labor are now done by machine, which enables individual workers to produce more while expending less energy.

This enhanced productivity increases wealth. With greater wealth has come increased ability to afford prepackaged and processed food, a commodity that has become enormously profitable. Television advertising in turn increases the demand for such foods, and leads to their increased sales, profits, and availability.

The availability of fast foods in our society enhances weight-gain in three ways. First, many prepackaged foods contain lots of fat. As a consequence, they are very rich in calories. Foods that pack lots of calories into a small volume are said to have *high caloric density,* and most fast foods have very high caloric density. Second, these fast foods are easily available. Fifteen years ago, to get a great cookie you had to bake it yourself. Now you just reach into the cupboard for a package. The more something so good-tasting is so easily available, the more likely you are to eat. Third, since someone else has done the work of growing, gathering, and processing the ingredients, and assembling, cooking, and packaging them, that much less work and physical activity are required of those who can afford to buy them.

In a classic children's story, the Little Red Hen had to do the work of gathering the grain, grinding it, kneading the dough, and shaping and baking it before she could sit down and eat bread. The exertion required to produce food no doubt helped her stay slim. Nowadays, if the Little Red Hen were to get hungry, she could take a store-bought pastry from her freezer and toss it in her toaster or microwave oven.

TENSION BETWEEN REAL AND IDEAL

As you probably know already from hard experience, it is very difficult to lose weight and keep it off (see chapter 8). Just as powerful societal forces egg us on to reduce, powerful psychological and physiological forces oppose permanent weight reduction. Our media extol and encourage greater thinness at the same time that our high-tech, high-calorie environment produces more obesity. This tension between what we want for our bodies and what is really happening to them can make for a lot of frustration and neurosis.

As values and reality diverge, the stage is set for many people to become desperate. Such desperation spawns fad diets, weight-loss centers, intense anxiety, anorexia, and bulimia. For some people the result is the misery of chronic self-contempt. For others it has been deadly, as we shall see when we describe anorexia nervosa, liquid-protein diets, and certain surgical operations.

Throughout this book, our purpose is to help you distinguish between the mild overweight declared unacceptable by the fashions of today, and those degrees and patterns of obesity that are truly detrimental to health. Certain people really do need to lose weight in order to preserve or restore physical health. But others, who have been blessed with normal, healthy, but more generous physiques, are torturing themselves needlessly. The trick is to be able to tell the difference and, if necessary, to act wisely to make whatever adjustments are in order.

2

What's Wrong with Being Fat?

A cold, clinical listing of the adverse effects of obesity would not convey the physical and emotional suffering of those who live with it. For some understanding of how it feels to be very obese—such as 100 pounds or more overweight—here is one patient's description of his personal experience, in his own words:

> I am 59 years old and until recently weighed approximately 500 pounds. I hadn't been able to weigh myself on any scales I knew of for years, and I did not seek out a freight scale of sufficient capacity because, frankly, I was afraid I could not handle the knowledge of my true weight.
>
> The *primary* victim of gross obesity is plagued with crippling physical handicaps which keep him or her from ever being truly comfortable. For the last several years the best place to sit was on my wife's cedar chest, as it had enough surface area to accommodate the full extent of my backside.
>
> But far worse than the physical discomfort and lack of mobility is the overwhelming guilt for the embarrassment, anger, and frightened concern generated in the lives of the *secondary* victims: the family, and especially the children, of the very obese person.
>
> Until recently I had not suffered most of the litany of medical

problems normally associated with even less profound obesity.

My lack of mobility was just what one might expect in the morbidly obese, although lately it worsened at a rate faster than the accumulation of fat. My immobility resulted from years of abuse to my knee joints due to the overload, plus leg-swelling from heart failure, and shortness of breath because of the oxygen required to transport such a big load. Running has been out of the question for years. Then I became unable to walk any appreciable distance without having to stop and catch my breath. In addition, the great weight overhanging out in front severely strained my lower back muscles, such that standing or walking for more than a couple of minutes caused unbearable pain.

My obesity has shown me how callous and inconsiderate people can be. People look, talk, and laugh in the presence of a very fat person, as if you can't hear or understand what is going on. Or a total stranger will come up and ask you how much you weigh or whether you realize you are overweight and in poor health.

Discrimination against the truly obese is pervasive. It is the last bastion for bigots who want to enjoy their bigotry uninhibited by public recrimination.

I know that my close family greatly resents having to do things for me that I could do myself if I were closer to a normal size. For example, because it is painfully difficult for me to arise from a chair, my wife frequently has to pick up or fetch things for me.

Gross obesity can be very corrosive to a marital relationship. My wife must care for me deeply to have put up with it for so many years with only rather understated complaint. For just one small example, our children have been "out of the nest" for several years, which should provide an opportunity for the traveling and sightseeing that my wife, especially, and I have always wanted to do. But the logistics of planning service stops for my limited bladder capacity, finding restaurants that have tables and sturdy armless chairs instead of booths that can't accommodate my front-to-back dimension, motels with parking close to the rooms or elevator, sitting in the car while my wife walks through a museum or to a vista point, just made the effort seem not worthwhile. If she wants to travel or sightsee, she goes with friends or alone.

Clothing poses a significant problem. Most of the "big and tall" stores are too limited in the "big" department. Only recently did just one mail-order catalogue store begin to carry a reasonable variety of clothing in my sizes, and even it could not fit me in shirts except the polo-knit type which has been my "uniform" for years.

Gross obesity will get you later if not sooner. We who are very overweight are very poor risks for major surgery. And severe injuries in an accident would likely doom us where a normal person would survive.

Over the last two years, my breathing became more labored, and I coughed a lot. Finally I couldn't walk more than 50 feet without having to stop and let my breathing catch up. I began to swell up to the point that I barely could fit behind the wheel of my car (a large, old Cadillac), and even then I was too cramped to drive safely.

When I could no longer drive to work, much less walk down the hall to my office, I sought medical help. The doctor diagnosed congestive heart failure due to morbid obesity. He changed my medication for high blood pressure and prescribed an increase in diuretic dosage to get rid of the fluid building up in my lungs, abdomen, and legs. He also referred me to a physician specializing in metabolic disorders.

The following Saturday night, before I even saw the specialist, I suffered an accident that confined me to home for two months. In getting out of bed to go to the bathroom I felt a sudden blast of excruciating pain in my right side. I had torn a muscle. For the next month I never left the bedroom except to hobble with a walker on frequent and painful trips to the bathroom. Because of this extremely tender muscle, I could not get up, turn over, or move around in bed without help. I was acutely and continually miserable. It hurt to try to lie down. I slept poorly, mostly in a sitting position against pillows on one side, which also held the electric pad in place on my tormented muscle.

For two months I was tormented by discomfort, apprehension, and depression. I had very little appetite. I ate sparingly and only the things I particularly liked. That, plus the increased diuretic dosage, resulted in loss of massive amounts of both water and fat. I experienced a gratifying reduction in body dimensions, as evidenced by the improved fit of my car and clothing I "undergrew." So when I was able to get to the specialist, I already had the incentive of a significant head start to encourage me through the rigors of dieting, and so far I have continued to lose.

Two things got me going: First, I don't *ever again* want to feel the way I did at the worst. Second, I had a misfortune that gave me a tremendous head start and thus incentive to keep going. I have a long way to go, especially when you include the all-important post-diet maintenance, and I have no illusions that I have already won. But I am better, and perhaps this public exposure of my story will help sustain my motivation by further engaging the support of my personal pride.

Each person's experience is of course unique. Others with severe obesity will have suffered differently from the person who provided this description. There is no question, however, that extreme obesity entails great suffering. Only those who experience it can fully comprehend its multifaceted misery.

The above account alludes to a number of social, physical, and medical consequences of obesity. In the life of an obese person, these adverse effects compound and complicate one another. They include increased risk of death, a number of diseases that are either caused or worsened by obesity, mechanical problems interfering with mobility, psychological and social problems, and employment discrimination. Some appear only when obesity becomes severe; others become apparent with mild obesity.

Not every overweight person suffers all of the adverse effects (see chapter 6). People whose excess fat is distributed mostly in the abdomen rather than the legs are more susceptible to many of the important health consequences of obesity. Since an abdominal pattern of obesity is more common in men than in women, men tend to be more susceptible than women to the ill effects of obesity on health. Women, on the other hand, tend to bear a heavier brunt of social and employment discrimination.

INCREASED RISK OF DEATH

The chances that any individual will die are 100 percent. Obesity, however, increases the chances of one's dying sooner than if one were not obese. This increased likelihood of dying early was not clearly understood until scientists sorted out the complex relationship between fatness and survival.

Several facts have complicated this relationship. On the one hand, obesity contributes to several diseases that shorten life, such as diabetes and high blood pressure. On the other, sick people tend to lose weight. People in the final stages of chronic diseases such as emphysema or cancer, tend to be thin. In particular, thin smokers have a very high mortality rate. Consequently, there are many thin people who have a very short life expectancy. Such unhealthy thin people tend to obscure the mortality risks of obesity in those population studies that simply examine fatness and date of subsequent death. Moreover, the older you are, the more likely you are to die soon, regardless of weight. But when the effects of age, disease, and smoking are all taken into account, and obese persons are followed up for a long enough time, studies show that obesity carries a definite risk of premature death. For example, take a few minutes to look at some interesting results from a study of 750,000 men and women.

If we look across Table 2.1 from left to right for any given age, sex, or smoking status, we see that the death rate increases with increasing obesity. We also see blanks in the chart for those categories in which there were not enough people to give reliable data. These blanks occur in categories of obese smokers, because smoking apparently interferes with weight gain. If we compare smokers with nonsmokers, however, we see that smoking shortens life much more than obesity does. Looking down each column, we note that increasing age is also a stronger risk factor than increasing degrees of obesity.

Comparing men with women of the same age and smoking status, we see that the mortality risk of obesity is greater in men. Other studies have also shown that for any given level of obesity, the risk of premature death is greater among men than among women. The higher death rates in men are, of course, reflected in the fact that there are many more elderly women than men in this country.

Women appear less susceptible than men to several of the deleterious health effects of obesity. This gender difference is probably due to the fact that men, more than women, tend to store excess fat primarily in the abdomen. (See chapter 6.) Women, on the other hand, tend to accumulate fat especially in the legs, where it causes fewer health problems.

Another large study looked at men between the ages of 15 and 39 years, and recorded whether they were still alive 15 years later. Men who at the start of the study were 25 percent overweight (i.e., 25 percent heavier for height than the average) were about 25 percent more likely to die within 15 years than were men of average weight. Men 50 percent overweight (i.e., half again heavier than average) were more than twice as liable to die within the next 15 years than were men of average weight.

To summarize the relationship between obesity and mortality,

Table 2.1
Death Rate per 1,000 People by Relative Weight*

Age	Relative Weight				
	90–109%	110–119%	120–129%	130–139%	Over 140%
Men Who Never Smoked					
40–49	4	5	7	9	11
50–59	10	13	14	16	29
60–69	25	32	32	39	54
70–79	65	72	81	86	98
Men Who Smoked One or More Packs Daily					
40–49	10	12	15	17	18
50–59	19	22	24	31	...
60–69	42	45	55	53	...
70–79	81	84	85	...	...
Women Who Never Smoked					
40–49	3	3	3	4	5
50–59	5	7	8	9	13
60–69	15	19	21	24	27
70–79	45	49	53	62	73
Women Who Smoked One or More Packs Daily					
40–49	5	6	7	7	8
50–59	10	12	12	12	20
60–69	24	25	35	45	...
70–79	53	57	...	...	...

*In this study, relative weight is defined as the percentage of average weight-for-height. Average weight-for-height is arbitrarily set at 100%. For example, if the average weight for women 5'6" tall were 140 pounds, a 5'6" tall woman weighing exactly 140 pounds would have a relative weight of 100%. If she weighed 154 pounds (an additional 14 pounds, or 10% of 140 pounds) her relative weight would be 110%. At 126 pounds (10% less than 140) her relative weight would be 90%.

obesity does increase the likelihood of early death, especially in men. Obesity is not, however, as strong a risk factor as age or smoking.

Perhaps even more important than postponing death is prolonging and promoting health while we are still alive. So let us look now at diseases that result from obesity. Figure 2.1 diagrams some of the areas of the body troubled by obesity.

DIABETES MELLITUS

The prevalence of diabetes mellitus is three or more times higher in obese than in non-obese persons. Diabetes mellitus is a chronic condition in which the blood levels of glucose, fats, and other nutrients are above normal. Over a period of many years, diabetes causes damage to the kidneys, nerves, eyes, and blood vessels, including heart attacks and strokes. It is a major cause of disability and death, and contributes to the elevated death rates seen in obese people.

Typical early symptoms of diabetes include thirst, profuse urination, blurred vision, weight loss, and vaginal itching. Diabetes may be present for a long time without any symptoms, however. The diagnosis is made by measuring the sugar content of the blood.

Diabetes can be caused by a variety of underlying conditions. The most common form is known as Type II diabetes mellitus. This is the type of diabetes that runs strongly in families and strikes adults, especially when they become obese. Obesity brings on this type of diabetes because it causes body tissues to resist the action of insulin.

Insulin is a hormone, which means that it is a chemical substance made in a gland (the pancreas, in this case), secreted into the bloodstream, and influencing the function of tissues elsewhere in the body. Insulin is the hormone that enables our bodies to store calories. It causes tissues throughout the body to take carbohydrate, fat, and protein out of the bloodstream, and store them away. In this sense, insulin is a "body builder." It helps you grow and put on weight.

When we eat, the food is digested (broken into its simple building blocks) and absorbed into the bloodstream. Simultaneously, insulin enters the bloodstream from the pancreas. The insulin signals tissues throughout the body that calories are coming in, and that it is time to start storing them away. Insulin thus acts like a dinner bell, telling the tissues to start extracting nutrients from the bloodstream. Under the influence of insulin, tissues take up calories for use and storage.

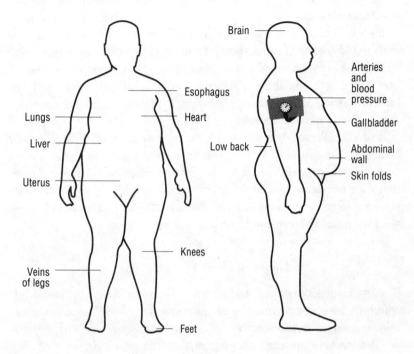

Figure 2.1 Adverse Effects of Obesity: Some Common Target Areas

Target areas for the effects of obesity on health include the brain, heart, esophagus, liver, gallbladder, stomach, blood, blood vessels, joints, skin, lungs, abdominal wall, and uterus.

When a person is obese, the tissues of his or her body are already swollen with calories, so they resist the action of insulin, unable to engorge themselves further. Sugar and fats consequently remain in the bloodstream in increased concentrations. Normally, the pancreas will compensate by secreting even more insulin, overpowering the resistance of tissues to its effect. For this reason, insulin levels are high in the bloodstreams of obese people. In people with a tendency toward diabetes, however, the pancreas fails to produce enough extra insulin to overcome the insulin resistance of their tissues. Consequently, their blood levels of sugar, amino acids, and simple fats (the building blocks of carbohydrate, protein, and fat) rise, and Type II diabetes mellitus develops. Both the presence and the duration of obesity accentuate the risk of developing Type II diabetes.

As we shall see in chapter 9, weight reduction often reverses the resistance to insulin and causes Type II diabetes to go into complete remission. This is true especially if weight reduction is accomplished early in the course of the diabetes, by means of dietary restriction and/or exercise. Uncontrolled diabetes itself can cause weight loss, however, and is *not* a healthy or beneficial way to lose weight. It leads to muscle wasting, dehydration, potassium depletion, and nerve damage, and it can be life-threatening.

If you are obese, you have an increased risk of developing diabetes. If diabetes runs in your family, you have good reason to try to reduce your weight toward normal levels. On the other hand, if you notice that your weight is coming down effortlessly, without diet or exercise, you should see a doctor to be checked for the possibility that you are already suffering from the effects of diabetes.

HIGH BLOOD PRESSURE

Obesity, insulin resistance, and high blood insulin levels are associated with high blood pressure. The medical word for high blood pressure is *hypertension*. In this instance, the words "tension" and "hyper" do not denote nervousness. They mean that the water pressure of the blood within a person's arteries is higher than normal.

Hypertension causes strokes, heart attacks, heart failure, kidney disease, and sometimes eye trouble. Because it can cause damage without showing any symptoms, it has been called "the silent killer." Hypertension is one of the causes of shortened life span in obese people.

When young adults gain considerable weight, the gain is very often followed by the development of hypertension. Weight reduction often reduces blood pressure, whether or not the blood pressure was above normal in the first place. We citizens of industrialized societies tend to gain weight with advancing age, and also tend to have lots of hypertension. Preindustrial populations that are not obese have very little hypertension. Obesity thus appears to be an important cause of high blood pressure.

How and why obesity causes hypertension are still matters of conjecture. The expanded body mass in obesity may require a higher pumping pressure for adequate blood circulation, but this does not explain why some obese people do not have hypertension. Some investigators claim that fat people eat too much salt, but studies have shown that this alone does not account for all of the hypertension associated with obesity. Other researchers theorize that the high blood insulin levels characteristic of obesity raise the blood pressure.

We do know that using a normal-sized arm cuff in the device used to measure blood pressure can give falsely elevated readings. To get a true blood-pressure measurement, people with big arms should have their blood pressure measured with a big cuff. Nevertheless, despite the use of reliable measuring techniques, obese people have been shown to have higher blood pressure than people of normal weight.

If you are obese and have high blood pressure, some of your hypertension may be due to your obesity, and may disappear with weight reduction.

ACCUMULATING FAT IN THE BLOOD AND THE LIVER

The medical term for too much fat in the bloodstream is *hyperlipidemia*. This excess blood fat may be in the form of cholesterol or of triglycerides, or both. These problems are defined and discussed in detail in chapter 5. Here we want simply to mention that obesity raises the blood levels of cholesterol and triglycerides, and that weight reduction causes a corresponding decrease in those levels. Too much cholesterol in the bloodstream leads to clogging of the arteries that supply the heart with blood and oxygen. High cholesterol levels thereby contribute to heart disease, including heart attacks, and obesity raises the level of cholesterol in the bloodstream—especially the kind of cholesterol that causes heart attacks.

Cholesterol (see chapter 5) comes in a "good" form known as HDL-cholesterol, and in a "bad" form known as LDL-cholesterol. The "good" kind is associated with freedom from heart attacks, while the "bad" kind is associated with increased risk of heart attack. Obesity lowers the blood levels of "good," or HDL-cholesterol, and raises the levels of "bad" or LDL-cholesterol. Weight reduction has the opposite effects.

The impact of obesity on HDL- and LDL-cholesterol levels is thought to contribute to the increased death rate among obese people. Some people are much more susceptible than others to the effects of obesity on blood fat levels. If you are obese, you should ask your doctor to check your blood cholesterol and triglyceride levels.

Obesity increases not only the accumulation of cholesterol in the bloodstream, but also of *triglycerides*—the other major type of blood fat. Although mild elevations of blood triglyceride levels are harmless, severe elevations can cause *pancreatitis*—a painful and dangerous inflammation of the pancreas. A medical emergency, its main symptom is severe abdominal discomfort. Reducing greatly elevated blood triglyceride levels helps a person avoid pancreatitis.

Fat builds up also in the liver of obese persons, causing *fatty liver*. When this condition occurs, the liver enlarges, and subtle abnormalities of liver function are detected on routine blood tests. So long as the diet is well balanced and excludes excessive amounts of alcohol, this fatty enlargement of the liver seldom has any serious consequences. But when too much alcohol is consumed and the diet is poorly balanced, fatty liver can progress to significant liver damage. If you are obese, and especially if blood tests indicate any liver malfunction or an excessive blood triglyceride count, your doctor will probably advise you to lose weight and to strictly curtail your alcohol intake.

HEART DISEASE

Diabetes mellitus, hypertension, and high blood cholesterol are all worsened by obesity, and they all cause heart disease. They do so by contributing to *atherosclerosis*—the fatty clogging of arteries. When the arteries supplying blood to the heart become clogged, the heart muscle is damaged, an event we call a *heart attack*. Since obesity causes or worsens diabetes, hypertension, and hyperlipidemia, it indirectly causes atherosclerosis and heart attacks.

The Nurses Health Study recently reported the results of 115,886 women, all of whom were between 30 and 55 years old and had no evidence of heart disease in 1976, when the study began. For eight years these subjects were monitored for the development of heart disease. As expected, smoking was a strong risk factor. Once the effects of smoking were taken into account, obesity was also closely linked to the development of heart disease. For example, mildly to moderately overweight women experienced 80 percent more coronary disease than slender women did. And severely overweight women were 330 percent more likely to develop heart disease than slender women were. The greater the level of obesity, the greater the occurrence of heart disease. Even a moderate weight gain of only 20 pounds or so was associated with increased rates of heart disease.

In addition to causing atherosclerosis, obesity adds to the work load on the heart. This increased work load can cause the heart to enlarge, which eventually leads to *heart failure*—failure of the heart to keep the blood circulating in a normal manner. Sometimes the term *congestive heart failure* is used to describe the fluid overload that occurs, with swelling, lung congestion, and shortness of breath. The patient whose story is recounted at the start of this chapter was suffering from congestive heart failure due to his obesity. Now that his weight is reduced, his heart failure has disappeared. His heart manages to pump sufficient blood to his current 270-pound body, but it could not do so at his previous size of 500-plus pounds. Had he not reduced his weight, he would probably have died by now of congestive heart failure.

STROKE

A stroke is a sudden loss of brain function due to loss of blood supply. Because strokes are usually caused by atherosclerosis—the same fatty clogging of the arteries that causes heart attacks—it is not surprising that obese people are subject to strokes as well as to heart attacks.

A less common form of stroke is caused not by the clogging of the arteries to the brain, but by the bursting and hemorrhaging of those arteries. High blood pressure is a major cause of this form of stroke. Since obesity worsens high blood pressure, this type of stroke is also more common in obese than in non-obese persons.

Strokes manifest themselves in many ways, ranging from sudden loss of consciousness and death to partial paralysis or clumsiness, loss of speech or memory, or loss of some other function controlled by the brain. High blood pressure, smoking, and obesity each contribute to the risk of having a stroke.

It is not obesity itself, however, that predisposes to stroke, but obesity that is predominantly in an abdominal distribution. An abdominal pattern of excess fatness also correlates strongly with the increased risks of diabetes, hypertension, high blood fats, and heart attacks seen in obesity.

CANCER

Cancer encompasses many different diseases, all of which involve the unrestrained overgrowth of abnormal tissue. Cancer invades and destroys normal tissues. Some types of cancer are readily curable, while others are usually fatal. Cancers are classified according to the type of normal tissue (such as skin or breast) from which the cancer is derived. Several different types of cancer are more common in obese than in non-obese individuals.

One type of cancer clearly linked to obesity is cancer of the endo-

metrium, or *endometrial cancer*. The endometrium is the inner lining
of the womb, or uterus. It grows under the influence of the female
sex hormone *estrogen*. Prolonged stimulation of the endometrium
by estrogen can cause it to become abnormal and eventually cancerous.

Menstruation, in which the endometrium periodically breaks down,
bleeds, and exits from the body through the vagina, interrupts this
estrogen-caused stimulation. Regular menstruation thereby prevents
abnormal endometrial tissue from building up inside the uterus and
helps prevent the development of endometrial cancer. When monthly
cycles do not occur, but estrogen is still abundant, endometrial cancer
may eventually develop.

Obesity leads to endometrial cancer because fat tissue produces
estrogen, slowly and steadily. The constantly high levels of estrogen
in obesity have two effects: the endometrium is stimulated to grow,
and the steady secretion of estrogen from fat interferes with normal
menstrual cycles. As a result, monthly cycles can cease and the endometrium continues to grow under the constant stimulus of estrogen.
Uninterrupted by menstruation, the stimulated endometrium can become cancerous.

If you are an obese woman who does not have regular periods,
we recommend regular gynecologic checkups; discussion with your
physician of the possibility of taking hormones periodically to
bring on menstrual-like bleeding and thus get rid of overgrown endometrial tissue; and prompt gynecologic evaluation in the event
of irregular vaginal bleeding, which can be a sign of endometrial
cancer.

Cancer of the gallbladder is a rare condition that is caused by a
common condition: gallstones. Since obesity causes gallstones (see
below), it indirectly increases the risk of this rare form of cancer.

Breast cancer is a common disease, striking an estimated one in ten
to eleven women. Many studies have investigated the possibility of a
link between obesity and breast cancer. Some, but not all, of these
studies have shown an association between them. The topic remains
controversial, and more scientific evidence is needed to settle the issue.

In men, *cancers of the colon, rectum, and prostate* have been associated with obesity, but as in the case of breast cancer in women,
the evidence for a causative link is not clear-cut. Further studies are
needed to clarify the possible relationship of these types of cancer to
obesity.

GALLSTONES

Gallstones are rocks that form in the gallbladder. The gallbladder is a sac connected to the liver, in the upper right-hand portion of the abdomen. It stores a cholesterol-rich digestive juice known as *bile*. When bile contains more cholesterol than can be dissolved, the cholesterol crystallizes in the bile, and these small crystals of cholesterol can grow into gallstones. Obesity causes the liver to secrete excessive amounts of cholesterol into bile, thereby overloading the bile with cholesterol and setting the stage for gallstone formation. Numerous studies have confirmed the association between obesity and the increased risk of gallstones.

Many gallstones cause no symptoms or problems at all. Sometimes, however, gallstones cause feelings of indigestion, or even severe abdominal pains. Gallstones occasionally cause the gallbladder to become acutely inflamed, a medical emergency known as *cholecystitis*. They can also cause cancer of the gallbladder, a rare condition mentioned earlier.

"HEARTBURN" AND HIATAL HERNIA

One of the problems most commonly connected with obesity is the chest discomfort that results from stomach acid getting up into the esophagus, the "food pipe" that leads from the mouth to the stomach. This discomfort is often referred to as "heartburn."

In obesity, the weight and bulk of abdominal fat presses on the stomach, just as would occur if someone sat on your abdomen as you lay down after a meal. This pressure can lead to heartburn in two ways. First, it helps force stomach contents up into the esophagus. Second, the stomach itself can be pushed partially up through the diaphragm, a condition that is called a *hiatal hernia*. It eliminates the reinforcing effect of the diaphragm on the sphincter, and facilitates regurgitation of acid into the esophagus. Unlike the stomach, however, the esophagus is not coated with acid-resisting mucus. Acid in the esophagus therefore causes pain ("heartburn"), erosions, and scarring. Although these problems can occur in people of normal weight, obesity aggravates them.

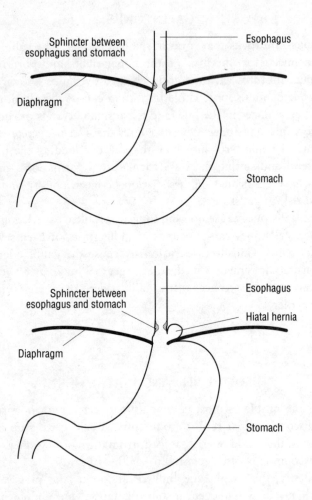

Figure 2.2 Hiatal Hernia

Anatomy of a Hiatal Hernia

The upper drawing shows the normal relationship of the stomach to the diaphragm and esophagus. The diaphragm is a thin sheet of muscle separating the chest cavity from the abdominal cavity. The esophagus passes through the diaphragm, and then opens out into the stomach. Acid from the stomach is normally kept out of the esophagus by a sphincter muscle where the esophagus and stomach meet. This sphincter muscle is reinforced by the diaphragm, a sheet of muscle that separates the chest from the abdomen.

The lower drawing shows a hiatal hernia—a bulging of the stomach up through the diaphragm into the chest cavity. When this occurs, stomach acid often gets up into the esophagus, creating a painful irritation known as "heartburn."

ARTHRITIS AND ORTHOPEDIC PROBLEMS

Arthritis means inflammation of, or damage to, the joints. There are several different types, or causes, of arthritis, and two of them are more common in obese than in non-obese persons. No matter what the original cause of arthritis, however, obesity worsens the damage to weight-bearing joints such as ankles, knees, and hips by overloading them.

One type of arthritis that is more common among people who are obese is called *gout*. The symptoms of gout are pain, swelling, and redness of joints, most commonly the joint at the base of the big toe. The pain is often excruciating. Gout results from tiny, needlelike crystals of a substance known as *uric acid*. These crystals form inside joints, causing pain and inflammation. They also form in the kidneys and urine, causing kidney damage and kidney stones. Obesity increases the levels of uric acid in the blood, and thereby increases the risk of crystal formation and gout.

The other type of arthritis associated with obesity is known as *osteoarthritis*. This is the most common type of arthritis, and its cause is not understood. Sometimes it is known as "wear-and-tear" arthritis, or *degenerative joint disease,* as the joints seem to wear out more readily than is normal. One can easily understand how excess weight would increase the wear and tear on weight-bearing joints such as the knees, hips, spine, and ankles.

In addition to arthritis, which usually strikes adults, orthopedic deformities of weight-bearing joints, especially the knees and hips, occur with increased frequency in obese children. These problems include slippage and deformity of the ball of the hip joint, and an inward-slanting deformity of the knees, producing a knock-kneed appearance.

BACK PAIN

Like the dachshund, human beings have a long and poorly supported spine and are thus susceptible to low-back problems. Obesity adds mechanical strain to the lower spine and renders persons (and dachshunds) even more prone to low-back pain.

Pain occurs in the low part of the back more commonly than higher up, between the shoulder blades. The upper part of the back is stabilized and supported by the ribs, which encircle the chest like a barrel. The lower back, on the other hand, must rely on the abdominal muscles for support and stability. When the abdominal muscles become stretched by pregnancy or obesity, low-back pains are likely to occur. Massive abdominal obesity puts a tremendous forward strain on the lower spine, distorts posture, and eliminates the protective tightness of the abdominal muscles.

SKIN PROBLEMS

Obesity often causes deep folds and creases in the skin, especially in the groin and armpits, under the breasts, and between rolls of fat on the abdomen. Subjected to constant moisture and friction, these areas develop rashes. They are also difficult to rinse well while bathing, so that soap becomes trapped there easily, increasing the irritation. Fungi and bacteria flourish in such conditions. Because these areas are so difficult to keep dry, the rashes and skin irritations can be very difficult to control, even with constant attention to hygiene.

Obesity causes another, more specific, skin condition known as *acanthosis nigricans*. This is a velvety-looking darkening and thickening of the skin, especially in such areas of skin folds as those that occur around the neck, in the armpits, and around the elbows. Sometimes it is prominent on the knuckles as a dirty-looking discoloration. Tiny tags of skin sticking up from the surface and subject to irritation are common around the base of the neck and in the armpits. The exact cause of acanthosis nigricans is unknown, but it is associated with insulin resistance and a tendency to develop diabetes.

PROBLEMS WITH BREATHING

Exertion brings on *shortness of breath* very quickly in the obese, both because oxygen requirements are high and breathing requires extra work. Breathing *is* work. It involves contracting the muscles that expand the lungs, lift the ribs, and compress the abdomen. Large quantities of fat distending the abdomen and weighing down the chest wall greatly increase the work of breathing.

Breathing, of course, provides oxygen, which is essential for energy and exertion. The greater the exertion, the greater the oxygen requirement. Activity in the obese involves transporting excess *adipose tissue* (body fat), so that for any given activity, such as climbing a flight of stairs, such persons require more oxygen than would someone who is not obese.

Even when asleep, however, obese people may have difficulty breathing. Severe obesity often is accompanied by a condition known as *sleep apnea,* in which breathing during sleep is interrupted by snoring and by periodic failure to breathe for several seconds at a time. Patients complain of feeling tired all the time. They never sleep well because of the disordered breathing pattern. Their spouses also complain, bothered by the loud snoring and the restlessness caused by sleep apnea. The saying "Laugh and the world laughs with you—snore and you sleep alone" often becomes reality in these families. Sometimes the spouse becomes terrified that one of the periods of temporary failure to breathe will become permanent. But although sleep apnea is extremely bothersome to many patients and their families, it is seldom dangerous.

More dangerous and severe, however, is *Pickwickian syndrome* (named after a fat boy in chapter 4 of Charles Dickens's *Pickwick Papers*), in which periodic failure to breathe occurs even while the patient is awake. The Pickwickian syndrome involves reduced and irregular breathing, with chronic fatigue and sleepiness. Extremely obese patients with this rare condition are barely able to breathe enough to obtain an adequate supply of oxygen and energy. Oxygen levels fall and carbon dioxide builds up from inadequate breathing, but brain and body no longer respond with sufficient respiratory effort. This is a life-threatening situation, and weight reduction is mandatory.

HERNIA

When a portion of the abdomen's contents pushes out through the abdominal wall, we call the resulting protrusion a *hernia*. Hernias occur commonly in weak spots in the abdominal walls, such as in the groin, around the navel, and at surgical incisions. Obesity stretches these weak points, and can weaken them further, to the point that hernias occur. A hernia usually shows up first as a bulge in the groin, near the navel, or at the site of a surgical scar. Some hernias may be painless and may not require medical attention. But if the defect in the abdominal wall pinches tightly on the protruding piece of bowel, it may be extremely painful and dangerous, requiring prompt surgical intervention.

VARICOSE VEINS

Varicose veins are a common affliction, and are even more common among the obese. Veins conduct blood back to the heart from other body tissues. The blood in the veins is propelled by pressure from the contraction of adjacent muscles; one-way valves within veins assure that the blood flows toward the heart instead of away from it. In obesity, the veins are surrounded by fat. Since fat doesn't contract like muscle, it doesn't compress the veins and pump the blood efficiently. The veins become distended with blood, stretching the valves to the point that they no longer function. The result is further enlargement of the veins, which can eventually be seen as wormlike bulges beneath the skin. Besides being unsightly and sometimes painful, varicose veins fail to keep blood circulating normally. Local stagnation of blood flow can then result in swelling of the ankles and/or *phlebitis,* which is the clotting of blood within the veins.

BLOOD CLOTS

When *blood clots* form within the large veins deep inside the legs, there is a temporary risk of the clots dislodging and being carried by the bloodstream to the lungs. Most blood clots do not dislodge, but simply remain in the veins where they formed, blocking circulation and causing swelling. But occasionally a large blood clot does travel to the lungs. There it can cause sudden shortness of breath, wheezing, chest pain, and even death. The stagnant circulation that characterizes the legs of many obese persons renders them more susceptible to such problems, especially when they are bedridden following surgery.

INCREASED RISKS DURING AND AFTER SURGERY

Obesity increases the dangers of major surgery, and produces frequent problems that include the following:

- difficulty taking deep enough breaths to expand the lungs thoroughly and avoid pneumonia after an operation
- increased risk of blood clots (phlebitis), which form in the veins of the legs, pelvis, or abdomen, and which sometimes dislodge and travel to the lungs, where they clog the circulation (embolism) and endanger life
- impaired healing of incisions, with occasional infection, seepage of fluid into the wound, or pulling apart of its edges, and/or subsequent hernia

PROBLEMS WITH PREGNANCY

Extreme obesity can prevent pregnancy in several ways.

First, the abdomen and thighs may become so distended with adipose tissue that sexual intercourse is physically impossible.

Second, obesity may cause a woman's monthly ovulation (egg production) cycles to become irregular, or to stop altogether. The reason appears to be that fat tissue produces estrogen hormone, which then acts like a birth-control pill.

Third, sperm production in the testicles is hindered by excessive warmth. Rolls of fat on a man's upper thighs prevent air circulation around the scrotum, keeping the testicles too warm for optimal sperm production. All of these factors reduce the likelihood of conception in extreme obesity.

Once pregnant, a markedly obese woman faces risks and problems beyond those encountered by women of normal weight. These include:

- a doubling of the risk of phlebitis
- a four- to fivefold increase in the risk of infections of the bladder and kidneys
- a severalfold increase in the incidence of developing high blood pressure during pregnancy
- a ten- to twentyfold increased risk of developing diabetes during pregnancy. Diabetes that begins during pregnancy is called *gestational diabetes*. If not properly controlled, it can have serious consequences for the health of the infant.

    Gestational diabetes that goes undetected and therefore untreated increases the likelihood of miscarriage. If the baby does survive, it is likely to be born too large, with difficulty in vaginal delivery. The newborn baby of a mother with uncontrolled gestational diabetes can also suffer from immature lungs and difficulty in breathing, as well as low blood sugar, low blood calcium, and impaired liver function.

    Gestational diabetes is easily detected by blood glucose tests ordered by a doctor. Since gestational diabetes may occur without symptoms, obese women should see a doctor early in pregnancy for diabetes testing and for close observation for the other risks of pregnancy in the obese.

    The treatment of gestational diabetes consists of proper diet, gentle exercise, and, in some cases, injections of insulin. The patient must test her blood sugar frequently throughout the remainder of the pregnancy. Gestational diabetes usually subsides as soon as the baby is born, but sometimes it persists as permanent diabetes mellitus.

- difficulties in obstetrical care. The obstetrician will need to take special care in adequately examining the very obese mother to determine the size, position, and heartbeat of her fetus. Rupture of the uterus, an unusual but life-threatening complication, is more difficult to detect when the uterus is concealed by a large layer of fat. Labor may be difficult and prolonged because, in about one-third of cases, the baby is larger than normal. This in turn can lead to damage to the baby during delivery, and to tearing of the mother's birth canal. If a very large baby or too difficult a labor necessitates cesarean section, the obese mother then runs an increased risk of infection or pulling apart of the stitched-up wound, and of postoperative pneumonia. Prolonged labor and cesarean deliveries are more common among overweight women than among women of normal weight.

IMPAIRED MOBILITY AND ATHLETIC ENJOYMENT

Most people take for granted the ability to get around easily. We climb a flight of stairs, pick up a towel from the bathroom floor, walk to the parking lot and climb into our cars, all with thoughtless ease. But if you were weighed down with a 140-pound coat of armor, or with 140 pounds of fat, these simple activities would become major exertions.

A slim teenager who goes water-skiing easily pulls him- or herself up to the standing position and glides along behind the boat for thirty minutes. Twenty years later, however, with fifty pounds more fat on his or her frame, the same person finds it hard to get up and exhausting to hang on as his or her heavier body is pulled around the same lake.

In any sport—skiing or swimming, bowling or basketball, fencing or fishing—fat gets in the way. It's difficult to win, or even to enjoy, anything athletic when you're carrying a bulky, weighty handicap.

The inconvenience of extreme obesity is enormous. People of normal weight or mild obesity don't have to worry whether the seats they will use in a restaurant or theater have armrests, or whether their abdomens will clear the steering wheel as they drive a car. They can both see and reach their shoelaces as they bend to tie them. They can get through the turnstiles of a grocery store without giving the task a second thought. Most can accept an invitation to go for a walk with a friend without being anxious about keeping up or becoming exhausted. Examples of the sheer daily bother of obesity are endless.

SOCIAL PREJUDICE

Our society almost always assumes the worst about people who are fat. "Fatty, fatty, two-by-four," and "I don't want her, you can have her, she's too fat for me" are cruel but common expressions of the prejudice against fat people that pervades our culture. What follows is a summary of extensive scientific research presented at a national conference on the implications of obesity.

In 1985 the National Institutes of Health in Bethesda, Maryland, sponsored a Consensus Development Conference of leading experts in obesity research. At that conference, Drs. Thomas Wadden and Albert Stunkard of the department of psychiatry of the University of Pennsylvania School of Medicine reported on the social and psychological consequences of obesity. Their report summarized the considerable research carried out by themselves and other experts, and stated in part:

> Research has shown that there is a strong prejudice against the obese in this country, regardless of age, sex, race or socioeconomic status. Children as young as six [years of age] describe silhouettes of the obese child as "lazy," "dirty," "stupid," "ugly," "cheats," and "lies." When shown line drawings of a child of normal weight, an obese child, and children with various handicaps, including missing hands and facial disfigurement, children and adults rate the obese child as the least likable. Not only is this prejudice relatively uniform among blacks and whites and persons from rural and urban settings, but it is also seen among obese persons. . . .
>
> Overweight is regarded not only as a sin, at odds with the Protestant ethic of self-denial and impulse control, but also a crime for which the person is held responsible. And beyond these moral and legal transgressions, obesity is an aesthetic crime: it is ugly.

DISCRIMINATION

In the same report, the researchers go on to define discrimination as "the behavioral enactment of prejudice," and to summarize extensive findings of discrimination against obese people in our society.

There is ample evidence of discrimination against the obese. Canning and Mayer found lower acceptance rates into high-ranking colleges for obese high school students, even though the two groups did not differ in high school performance, academic qualifications, or application rates to colleges. A similar study found that obese persons were underrepresented in a private college in the Northeast.

The obese are discriminated against in the work force as well. Overweight persons are thought to make less desirable employees than are persons of normal weight, even though the two groups are believed to have the same abilities. Roe and Eickwort found that 16 percent of employers surveyed said they would not hire obese women under any conditions, and an additional 44 percent would not hire them under certain circumstances. In a third study, only 9 percent of executives surveyed who earned $25,000 to $50,000 were more than ten pounds overweight, whereas 39 percent of those earning only $10,000 to $20,000 were comparably overweight. The authors estimated that each pound of fat could cost an executive $1,000 a year.

Discrimination of a similar kind may confront the obese in important social interactions such as entry into marriage. Few studies have examined whether obese persons are less likely to marry than are non-obese persons. However, for women of lower socioeconomic status, physical attractiveness is an important predictor of marrying men of higher socioeconomic status. Goldblatt and colleagues found that only 12 percent of women who moved into a higher social class were obese, whereas 22 percent who moved to a lower class were overweight.

Job discrimination against the obese takes many forms. In industry, the pre-employment physical examination may provide a convenient subterfuge to prevent the hiring of an overweight person. The armed forces and police and fire departments often have explicit rules preventing the hiring of overweight persons. Once hired, obese persons may be discriminated against in consideration for promotion, their weight being interpreted as proof that they lack the personal qualities needed for leadership.

"I don't like fat people," stated the former chairman and chief executive officer of a Fortune 500 company in a recent nationwide survey. "If I were recruiting and some guy waddled in with a big gut, he'd be dead before he opened his mouth. It just doesn't convey an impression of being dynamic and aggressive to look like that." The survey, conducted by Dr. James Rippe of the University of Massachusetts, disclosed widespread prejudice: "Not a single executive we interviewed was significantly overweight. Time and time again, they referred to their management team as 'lean and aggressive,' and admitted that carrying extra pounds can work against the careers of executives on the rise."

Discrimination appears to be lessening in some areas. The tax on obesity levied by Sweden in the 1920s—approximately one dollar per year for each pound over 200—is now unconstitutional. The clothing industry, after long neglecting the needs of obese people, is finally awakening to the commercial possibilities of supplying those needs. For years, only sacklike designs were available, with many dresses, pants, and shirts simply not available in larger sizes. Now it is becoming increasingly possible to order large sizes, but seldom at sale prices, and still too seldom from a full selection of attractive designs.

PSYCHOLOGICAL SUFFERING

We return finally to what is for many obese persons the most painful aspect of their condition: psychological suffering. The psychological consequences of obesity range from a sense of mild inferiority to severe incapacitation. The account at the outset of this chapter reflects one man's personal torture, in which his mental anguish outweighed his considerable inconvenience and physical pain. For many obese persons, contempt for their own bodies, and feelings of guilt, embarrassment, helplessness, and failure brought on by their obesity, are more painful than their physical suffering.

As medical research makes it plain that obesity is not someone's "fault," some of the guilt associated with obesity may lessen. On the other hand, until effective long-term treatment becomes available, feelings of helplessness and of the unfairness of fate and society will continue to plague many who suffer from being obese. Interestingly, surgery and behavior-modification therapy for obesity often improve mood and reduce psychological discomfort, while in many persons, dieting brings on depression, nervousness, and irritability, thus compounding their psychological distress.

HOW FAT IS TOO FAT?

The obvious and important question raised by this accounting of adverse consequences of obesity is: "How fat do I have to get before I'm vulnerable to these risks and problems?" Chapter 6 addresses that question in depth; in many instances, however, precise answers are not available, for the evidence is statistical, based on comparisons of the frequency of problems in large groups of people. This sort of population information does not define the specific risk of any one individual. Some of us are much more susceptible than others to the adverse consequences of obesity. Women appear in general to be less susceptible than men to many of the ill effects we have described. To evaluate your own personal level of risk, you will need the evaluation of your doctor, who knows your family history, your blood pressure, blood sugar, and cholesterol levels, your personality, your smoking and exercise habits, and other contributing factors. Nevertheless, it is possible to generalize about the degrees and patterns of obesity that cause certain problems.

None of the problems noted in this chapter is unique to obesity. You can get gallstones, endometrial cancer, rashes, arthritis, stroke, or back pain, suffer discrimination, or die young without ever getting fat. Obesity simply increases the likelihood that these problems will occur.

The available data suggest that risk of certain diseases climbs with even mild degrees of overweight. That is, there does not appear to be a safe "threshold" beneath which no added risk is detectable. For example, the risks of gout, osteoarthritis, menstrual disorders, and gallbladder disease appear to increase proportionally to excess fatness, even of mild degree.

Significant breathing problems and skin problems due to obesity, on the other hand, are not encountered until the degree of obesity is severe.

The degree of fatness required to raise the risk of premature death is a controversial topic. For years, life-insurance statistics showing increased risk of death starting with even mild obesity were taken as proof that mortality risk increased proportionally with weight, without any threshold effect. Then the pendulum of opinion swung the other way, as numerous studies showed that thin people had a higher death rate than average and that mild obesity carried no appreciable excess risk of mortality. Indeed, in 1983 the insurance industry changed its tables, declaring the ideal weight-for-height to be heavier than previously thought. More recently, however, careful long-term studies that take age and smoking status into account tend to show a gradual, proportional rise of mortality risk with excess weight, stronger in men than in women. The chart on page 21 shows this relationship.

The degree of obesity is not nearly so important as its pattern of distribution throughout the body with regard to the risks of diabetes, high blood pressure, high blood cholesterol, gallstones, stroke, and heart attack. Numerous scientific studies show that a person's risk of developing these conditions is strongly related to *abdominal* obesity. As chapter 6 shows, there are characteristic patterns of obesity. Some people tend to accumulate their excess fat mostly on the legs and buttocks; they have "lower segment" obesity. Others store their excess fat primarily about their abdomens and chests; their pattern has been called "abdominal" or "upper segment" obesity.

Strokes occur more frequently in people with abdominal obesity than in people whose fatness is more generalized. For example, scientists in Sweden examined 789 men in 1963, noting how fat they were and whether the obesity was mostly abdominal or not. They then monitored the health of the men for more than 18 years, during which time 57 (7.2 percent) had strokes. Statistical analysis showed that the men most likely to have strokes were those with high blood pressure and with abdominal obesity. The degree of generalized obesity showed no correlation with the risk of stroke, but excess abdominal fatness did correlate with subsequent stroke. The men were also followed for the risks of heart attack and death, and results were analyzed after 13 years of follow-up. Again, risks of heart attack and death were proportional to the degree of *abdominal* obesity.

A survey of more than 30,000 women participating in the TOPS [Take Off Pounds Sensibly] Club, Inc., showed a positive association between abdominal obesity and a history of having had gallbladder disease, diabetes, high blood pressure, and menstrual disorders.

Recent research using computerized X-ray analysis has distinguished between abdominal obesity due to lots of fat under the skin of the abdomen, versus abdominal obesity deep within the abdominal cavity, surrounding the intestines. These studies indicate that excess adipose tissue within the abdominal cavity, rather than under the skin, correlates with the tendencies to develop diabetes and high levels of cholesterol and fat in the blood.

BENEFITS OF OBESITY

Despite all the problems detailed above, there actually are a few benefits to being obese. For example, if you have plenty of fat, you are less likely to develop osteoporosis, and you are more likely to survive a famine. A person planning to lose weight may want to consider the prospect of giving up these benefits.

Survival When Food Is Scarce and/or Caloric Needs Are Great

Generous stores of adipose tissue allow a person to survive longer during periods of food scarcity. The ability of pioneer Polynesian voyagers to accomplish long migratory journeys across the Pacific may have depended on their obesity. Body fat is a very efficient, compact, and portable way to store and transport energy. In terms of calories per pound, it goes a lot farther than a canoe full of coconuts and dried fish. The tendency of some Polynesians to gain weight easily may be inherited from ancestors who survived oceanic migration partly because of their ability to store body fat abundantly before the start of a voyage.

Scientists have theorized that "thrifty genes" may have allowed prehistoric desert farmers to accumulate abundant fat at harvest time and enabled them to survive periods of drought and famine. A genetic tendency toward fatness may confer a survival advantage under conditions of unreliable food supply. Today in Africa there are starving populations who are probably undergoing genetic selection as thinner people die off sooner than those with greater stores of body fat.

In our Western society, caloric reserves can be better stored in the freezer, or on the shelves of one's basement or garage, than around one's waistline. Modern food preservation has made obsolete the advantage of storing those calories as body fat.

People with severe or chronic illness tend to lose weight because of poor food intake and/or increased metabolic demand for calories. A person's nutritional status at the outset of such an illness has an important bearing on his or her ability to survive. For example, the cancer patient with some excess fat is likely to live longer than one who is thin to begin with.

In today's affluent society, however, the most obvious benefit of obesity is not survival during long trips, famine, or illness, since alternative nutrient supplies are available. The most obvious benefit is the prevention of osteoporosis.

Osteoporosis

Osteoporosis is often referred to as "thinning of the bones." We tend to think of our skeleton as a fixed and unchanging part of our body, like the steel girders that support a building. In fact, however, our bones are living tissues that undergo constant remodeling by the tiny cells that line them. Some of these cells dig small craters in the bone, much like the divots a golfer might dig in a fairway. Other cells then come along and lay down new bone, filling in the craters and reshaping the bone. When the process of dissolving old bone outpaces the formation of new bone, there is a net loss of bone mass. Bones that have lost much of their bone structure and strength content are said to be *osteoporotic*, or "thin." Since the strength to resist breakage derives from the mass of bone, people with osteoporosis are vulnerable to fractures.

The types of fractures most common in osteoporosis are compression fractures of the spine and fractures of the wrists and hips. Compression fractures of the spine lead to loss of height, and to bowing over of the posture, with a characteristic "dowager's hump." As vertebrae in the lower spine collapse, the rib cage comes down closer to the pelvis, compressing the contents of the abdomen, which then protrudes forward in a potbellied manner. These vertebral fractures cause intense back pain, often lasting for months or more.

Hip fractures not only hurt; they usually prevent walking until they are repaired. They often require major surgery and sometimes lead to complications such as blood clots forming in the legs and going to the lungs. Hip fractures resulting from osteoporosis are a major cause of extended disability and consequent nursing-home placement among our elderly population.

Obesity helps protect a person from developing osteoporosis. One reason overweight people tend to have strong bones is that their obesity puts added load and stress on their skeleton. We know that bones respond to mechanical stress by forming more bone and becoming stronger. This is why exercise and physical activity help prevent osteoporosis. The skeleton responds to the additional mechanical strains of obesity by building more bone tissue.

A second reason why obese people avoid osteoporosis relates to the fact that fat tissue forms estrogen, the so-called female hormone. Estrogen slows the loss of bone that normally accompanies aging, and in this way prevents osteoporosis.

Risk factors for osteoporosis include aging, female gender, loss of ovarian function (such as after menopause, when the ovaries stop producing eggs and estrogen), slender body build, poor calcium intake, excess alcohol intake, smoking, and lightly pigmented skin. Blacks suffer much less osteoporosis than do whites and Orientals. The profile of a person very likely to develop osteoporosis would be a postmenopausal, fair-skinned, slender woman who smokes. The woman who decides to lose weight should protect herself against osteoporosis by not smoking, by taking in adequate amounts of calcium, by exercising regularly, and by discussing with her doctor the pros and cons of estrogen-replacement therapy if she has gone through menopause.

Social Status

Certain societies and groups have prized obesity as connoting affluence or conformity to the norms of the group. For example, members of certain Native American tribes and Polynesian groups feel pressure to remain obese, and are encouraged to regain weight should they start to look thinner than their peers. In some of these groups, a degree of obesity that is socially acceptable may nevertheless be excessive from a health viewpoint. The body-weight ideals of these groups are opposite to those of most of contemporary society.

A body that is bulky, not only with muscle, but also with some extra fat, also may provide functional advantages in certain very specialized cases, such as that of a wrestler, whose additional mass makes him more difficult to throw out of the ring.

Despite these benefits, for most people the disadvantages of obesity far outweigh the advantages.

3

Anorexia and Bulimia:
A Closet Epidemic

It seems paradoxical that while the United States is experiencing a rising tide of obesity, the health and happiness of many others are eroded by a countercurrent of self-starvation. While Americans in general are getting fatter, and are acutely aware of how miserable it is to be fat, many are learning firsthand that being too thin can be even worse. These are the people who struggle with the severe disorders *anorexia nervosa* and *bulimia nervosa*.

Most studies show that anorexia and bulimia are increasing in our society. The prevalence is especially great throughout the Sun Belt and in areas characterized by high achievement and consequent high stress. The only recent study that did not show an increase in these disorders was performed in Minnesota. Anorexia and bulimia are almost always reported to be found much more often among the middle and upper economic classes than among the less affluent, but these findings may result from sampling error, as those who seek treatment are counted most often in surveys. The fact is that cases have been reported in all social and racial groups. Although the causes of anorexia and bulimia are not completely understood, they appear to stem in part from our societal obsession with thinness.

People with anorexia nervosa and bulimia nervosa extend their concern about weight to a neurotic extreme. They overreact to the appearance of even normal amounts of body fat. Those with anorexia nervosa starve themselves intentionally. Those with bulimia, a related disorder, binge on food and then try to eliminate it through vomiting, excessive exercise, and the abuse of medications. The two conditions have many features in common and often coexist in the same individual.

The same abundance of food that sets the stage for widespread obesity probably also prepares the way for anorexia and bulimia. These disorders are rare in developing countries, where money and food are scarce, but they occur widely in wealthy, well-fed Western societies. An abundance of food and leisure helps create obesity, which, in turn, generates widespread concern about overweight. This concern, especially among the young, can become an obsession, and this obsession leads some people into relentless dieting, exercising, self-induced vomiting, and abuse of drugs to control weight. These activities often dominate the lives of people with anorexia and bulimia. While they experience severe guilt and shame, menstrual disorders, weakness, bone mineral loss, chemical imbalances, malnutrition, and illness—and even, for some, death—most of those who suffer from these disorders deny having any eating problems and usually refuse to acknowledge the damage they are inflicting on themselves.

ANOREXIA NERVOSA

Anorexia nervosa is primarily a disorder of adolescent females. Although it affects only about one out of 100,000 American women in general, approximately 1 percent of adolescent girls develop it in some degree of severity. Females with the condition outnumber males ten to twenty times. Most studies show a two- to fourfold increase in prevalence since the 1930s.

People with anorexia nervosa starve themselves to below normal weight. In a growing girl, anorexia may appear as a failure to gain weight despite a gain in height. Although she may not actually lose weight, as she gets taller she becomes thinner.

The following are the official criteria for the diagnosis of anorexia nervosa:

1. Refusal to maintain body weight over a minimal normal weight for age and height—for example, weight loss leading to maintenance of body weight 15 percent below that expected; or failure to make expected weight gain during a period of growth, leading to a body

weight 15 percent below that expected from the height-weight tables.

2. An intense fear of gaining weight or of becoming fat, even when underweight.

3. A disturbance in the way one experiences one's body weight, size, or shape. For example, the person may claim to feel fat even when she or he is emaciated, or believe that one area of the body is too fat even when she or he is obviously underweight.

4. In females, the absence of at least three consecutive menstrual cycles when these are otherwise expected to occur.

Along with these diagnostic criteria are associated symptoms, such as a distorted attitude or behavior toward food, eating, or weight, including an extreme fear of fatness, a desire for extreme thinness, enjoyment of losing weight, and a denial of hunger, nutritional needs, and of the illness itself. Unusual eating behaviors, hoarding food, and bizarre food selections are also typical. Patients also typically grow fine peach-fuzz hair all over their faces and bodies, have a slow heartbeat and low body temperature, and may vomit, purge, binge-eat, and/or be overactive.

Although it is increasing in frequency, and is now better understood, anorexia is not a new disease. At the turn of the century it was called "chlorosis" and was thought to be a blood disease of young women. In 1684, Richard Morton, a London physician, described a young woman with what he called "nervous phthisis"—thinness caused by nervousness. He wrote, "I do not remember that I did ever in all my Practice see one that was conversant with the Living so much wasted, like a skeleton clad only with Skin, yet there was no Fever, but on the contrary a coldness of the whole Body; no cough, or difficulty of Breathing, nor an appearance of any other distemper of the Lungs or of any other Entrail. Only her Appetite was diminished and her Digestion uneasy with Fainting Fitts, which did frequently return upon her."

Perhaps the earliest recorded case of probable anorexia was that of Saint Wilgefortis, the daughter of the King of Portugal, around 700 A.D. As a child she had been promised in marriage to the King of Sicily. As the year of her wedding approached, she became increasingly anxious and began to fast and lose weight to the point that her menstrual periods stopped. When the king came to claim his bride he

found an emaciated, hyperactive woman with facial hair—probably
a victim of anorexia nervosa.

A CASE HISTORY

Consider the case of Nancy. She was 16 when she first consulted a
psychiatrist, at the insistence of her parents. Although she was five
feet four inches tall, Nancy weighed only 80 pounds. The psychiatrist
noticed that she was quiet, observant, and suspicious. Among her first
words to him were, "Please don't make me eat. I'm already too fat."

Nancy had grown up in an upper-middle-class neighborhood in a
prosperous West Coast city. Her birth weight was normal, and her
history of eating and weight had been normal until junior high school.
She had always been bright, one of the best students in her class, and
at the same time was shy. She began to develop physically at about
the time of her first menstrual period, at age 12. In the seventh and
eighth grades she became increasingly weight-conscious, and frightened of social interactions. Nancy had been active in ballet since she
was five, and she as well as both of her parents were quite devoted
to the dance; she hid her fears beneath a front of bravado, and often
used her ballet practice as an excuse not to join in when other kids
went off to do things together after school.

Nancy spent several hours each day in ballet workouts. By the ninth
grade her weight had dropped from a previous high of 115 pounds
to only 100 pounds, even though she had grown taller. The loss of
weight occurred through a combination of exercise and holding back
from eating foods she felt were "bad." She became more and more
obsessed with the size and shape of her body, and often examined
herself critically before a mirror, harshly criticizing any perceived bulge
or accumulation of fat. The thought of womanly hips and breasts
horrified her.

By her 15th year, Nancy had ceased to menstruate, much to her
pleasure, and her friends at school envied her thinness and athletic
prowess. She enjoyed being very thin. Halfway through the tenth
grade, her weight reached 90 pounds. At this weight she looked too
thin and felt cold much of the time. Often she stayed up at night,
tensing her muscles while studying in order to make sure she didn't
accumulate any fat.

Nancy's diet was strange. She totally eliminated red meats and
chicken, and ate only small amounts of fish in addition to vegetables,
complex carbohydrates, and vitamin pills. Her cheeks developed a

downy fuzz, and the hair on her scalp became thin and sparse. Her skin took on an orange hue and a rough, dirty appearance. She had periods of weakness and fits of depression, alternating with anger when anyone suggested she should gain weight.

Her parents, both professionals, and proud of her ballet accomplishments and her generally achieving life-style, had a difficult time at first accepting that anything was wrong. While there was a family history of depression, they hadn't expected it to afflict their daughter. Once they realized that she was far too thin, they tried to restrict her privileges unless she ate more. When this failed, they canceled her ballet lessons and issued threats and bribes, but still to no avail. When they finally took her to the doctor—an internist—all that could be diagnosed was thinness, the lack of menstruation, and the slight thyroid abnormality that goes along with starvation from any cause. Despite the doctor's insistence, she refused to gain weight. She offered the doctor a deal: if he would let her lose five more pounds, she would stabilize her weight. In private, she shared her intense fear of gaining weight, of losing control of her appetite, and of becoming fat. The doctor diagnosed anorexia nervosa, and referred Nancy for psychiatric care.

Nancy's treatment was difficult and typical. After continuing to refuse to gain weight, she was admitted to a hospital so that weight gain could be enforced with 24-hour-a-day monitoring. She was placed on a behavioral contract for weight gain, with such rewards as hospital privileges of visiting other patients and walking around the grounds when she gained weight. When she did not meet a daily weight-gain quota, Nancy was restricted to her room. In the supportive atmosphere of the hospital, she was able to increase her food intake. She gained twenty pounds in the hospital and tolerated the weight gain emotionally as she began psychotherapy.

The psychotherapy continued long after Nancy left the hospital. She became aware of her great anxiety about growing up, her fears of sexuality, of leaving home, and of becoming independent without the protection of her powerful parents. Gradually she learned that it was not losing control of her weight that frightened her most; it was losing control of her life. Her therapist helped her learn some of the basic interpersonal skills she had missed while being sick and while practicing ballet so much, particularly how to get along with her peers, how to go on a date, how to talk with boys—in effect, how to be a normal teenager. By the time she graduated from high school, Nancy was doing quite well. Leaving her parents to go to college was difficult, and it led to a brief relapse. She came back to her therapist for a few visits during Christmas vacation, and together they looked at how her unspoken fears of being alone in college, lost among thousands of students, in some ways represented what she had feared all along. Her therapist helped her see that in fact she was coping with this as well as, or better than, most college students of her age. She went on to finish college and marry. When her therapist saw her last, she had two children.

TREATING ANOREXIA

Nancy's story is typical in many ways, including the intense conflict with parents over the refusal to maintain normal weight, the great fear of becoming fat, the mistaken notion of feeling fat despite actually being very thin, the peculiar eating patterns, the use of additional measures (exercise, in Nancy's case) to maintain thinness, and the eventual recovery. Fortunately, most cases of anorexia nervosa occur as a single episode, with a return to normal weight within two to three years.

The treatment of anorexia may involve hospitalization, forced feeding through a tube into the stomach, behavior-modification therapy, nutrition education, individual psychotherapy, and group counseling. Medications affecting mood, sleep, and bowel function are often prescribed, usually on a symptom-by-symptom basis; they often alleviate such symptoms but do not "cure" the anorexia. Social skills, sex education, and family interactions often need therapeutic attention. Therapy is thus often broad-ranging, depending on the needs of the patient and the perceptions of the therapist. Its goals include the following:

1. The patient's realizing that he or she is a competent individual who does not have to use weight control to cope with the stresses and fears of life.

2. Normalizing the patient's body image.

3. Overcoming excessive fear of being fat.

4. Correcting nutritional misconceptions, such as one patient's notion that a single pat of butter contained 1,000 calories and turned into cellulite immediately.

5. Achieving normal competence and confidence in interpersonal relationships, including establishing a healthy, mature, independent identity. (In short, psychotherapy for anorexia addresses many of the issues of maturation normally faced by adolescents and young adults.)

About 75 percent of anorexic patients eventually do well with treatment. Repeated hospitalizations are frequent, but they do not necessarily predict poor outcome. Around age 18, when patients are about to leave home, flare-ups are common.

Factors affecting the likelihood of complete recovery from anorexia nervosa are similar to those affecting the outcome of many illnesses. The prognosis is generally better in females than in males; in patients from middle and upper rather than from lower socioeconomic classes; in patients who have not been chronically ill; in patients with stable, supportive families and friends; in patients with less severe symptoms; in patients whose problems did not begin when they were very young; and in patients who were not more than 20 percent overweight before becoming anorexic.

Many people with anorexia recover spontaneously, without formal therapy. Typically, a high school or college student with a mild case of anorexia will fall in love and stop worrying about dieting as her new relationship consumes her time, attention, and energies. Or a college student will become "fed up" with the amount of time and effort going into dieting and fasting, and, in order to save her college career, will put her anorectic behaviors aside. In other cases, maturity seems to provide the cure. On the other hand, anorexia can be unremitting, and despite intensive treatment, it can result in death.

Mortality Rates

The mortality rates for anorexia nervosa are not known, since mild cases are rarely counted in statistics. A series of patients studied for twenty years in Sweden had a mortality rate of one in five, or 20 percent. The causes of death ranged from actual starvation to medical complications of anorexia, including heart problems, kidney failure, seizures, and suicide. Extreme weight loss from anorexia affects the functioning of all organ systems, including the brain, the infection-fighting cells of the body, the muscles that provide heart and lung function, and the gastrointestinal tract. The malnourished patient is in a precarious position, given the ensuing weakness, decreased resistance to infection, loss of appetite, and impaired intestinal absorption. An acute illness such as pneumonia or influenza can propel her or him into a fatal tailspin.

Most studies suggest a mortality rate of between 5 and 15 percent—far higher than the percentage of recovered anorexics who ever realize their ultimate fear of becoming overweight. About two-thirds of patients return to normal weight, but only half of these are considered to be free of psychological problems. About 15 percent of patients have a very low body weight for the rest of their lives without being overtly anorexic, while 20 percent go on to repeated cycles of relapse and recovery throughout their lives.

Social Consequences

The adverse effects of anorexia are educational and economic as well as social, psychological, and medical. It is difficult to study or to hold down a job when you are very weak and excessively thin. Anorexic people also often become isolated socially, both because of their skeletal appearance and because of their neurotically narrowed focus of interests. Delayed puberty due to anorexia can also reinforce the social isolation.

Delayed Puberty

Anorexia nervosa is a major cause of delayed sexual maturation. Puberty, or sexual maturation, occurs normally in the early teens. In females, it usually begins with enlargement of the breasts, as the ovaries begin to secrete the "female hormone" estrogen. Not long thereafter, pubic and armpit hair make their appearance, a growth spurt begins, and within a year or so, menstruation commences. In males, growth of the testicles is the first sign of impending puberty. Soon to follow are pubic, armpit, and facial hair growth, enlargement of muscles, deepening of the voice, and rapid growth in height. While the exact timing and sequence of these events are variable, the process is in each case triggered by control centers in the brain.

The brain initiates puberty partly in response to the amount of body fat that is present. Until a certain minimum of fat is present, the brain will not stimulate the pituitary gland to start puberty. Once adequate body fat is present, the pituitary gland stimulates the gonads—ovaries in girls and testicles in boys—to secrete the hormones (estrogens and androgens) that bring on adolescence: a normal but revolutionary upheaval in one's body, behavior, and attitudes. For many cases of delayed puberty, the only treatment needed is more calories.

Lack of Menstruation

Just as menstruation will not begin until a girl attains a certain minimal body-fat content, it will not continue unless fat content remains above that minimum. Except for pregnancy, excessive thinness is the leading cause of failure to menstruate in American women of childbearing age. Lack of menstruation due to excessive thinness is almost epidemic among ballerinas, long-distance runners, fashion models, and young women trying to look like fashion models. Many slender women spend thousands of dollars in medical evaluations, only to find that their lack of menstruation is caused by their being too thin.

THE CAUSES OF ANOREXIA

The causes of anorexia nervosa are not well understood. About one-third of patients with anorexia were definitely obese prior to the illness and went on a diet that seemed to unleash the anorexia. Many cases appear to stem simply from the usual teenage preoccupation with weight, size, dieting, and exercise that then gets carried to extremes. These tendencies, rather common in our weight-conscious society, seem to acquire in some people a power and momentum of their own, once weight loss begins. In anorexia, typically, a girl goes on a diet, starts losing weight, becomes excessively thin, stops menstruating, and becomes obsessed with food and body shape.

We do not know why some people are more susceptible to anorexia nervosa than others. The disease is more common among the sisters and mothers of anorexic women than in the general population, and relatives of girls with anorexia nervosa have a very high incidence of severe depression, manic-depressive illness, and alcoholism. Although these family tendencies suggest a possible genetic predisposition to the disease, the link could be entirely environmental.

In two-thirds of cases, there are family disturbances and conflicts. Often the mother is overly protective and the father hard-driving and emotionally detached, but it is difficult to determine whether the ensuing family disruption caused the anorexia, or whether the anorexia caused so much stress that the family became dysfunctional.

Since the causes of anorexia are poorly understood, we have no sure way to predict who will become anorexic, and no good data on how to prevent it. It is certain, however, that our nation continues to be obsessed with fatness and thinness, and that we present these obsessions to our children at very young ages. Just as moral and social values and behaviors are acquired while children grow up, and are learned largely from parents, so are dieting behaviors and nutritional habits. The best prevention we currently have is example and education. Parents who eat sensible, well-rounded diets of nutritional foods, and who are not constantly on diets or intensely concerned with their weight, size, shape, and external appearance, are likely to raise children with similar healthy nutritional attitudes and behaviors.

BULIMIA NERVOSA

Bulimia nervosa shares many features with anorexia nervosa, and sometimes coexists with anorexia in the same person. Its distinguishing feature is repeated binges of overeating followed by purging to get rid of the food consumed.

Bulimia is an old and widespread disorder. The Talmud, almost 2,000 years old, contains a good description of it, and we know that the Romans, for example, feasted and purged in sensuous displays of plenty. Bulimia, like anorexia, occurs throughout the world, but much more commonly in Western countries.

Many people in our society occasionally purge after overeating, but not frequently enough to qualify for the diagnosis of bulimia nervosa. An estimated 10 percent of adolescents occasionally binge and purge. Bulimia nervosa, in which such behavior becomes repeated and habitual, occurs in about 4 percent of the general population, and it is thus considerably more common than anorexia. Its prevalence is greatest among persons in weight-related occupations—for example, models (both male and female), ballet dancers, gymnasts, wrestlers, and jockeys.

Although there are documented cases of middle-aged women becoming bulimic in a desperate attempt to lose weight, bulimia begins most often toward the end of high school, when concerns about weight and sexuality are intense. At one high school in La Jolla, California, a study found that 20 percent of graduating females vomited regularly for weight control. Surveys of college students have shown up to 5 percent of the women, and 0.4 percent of men, binging and purging on a regular basis. One survey of college students in summer session found 19 percent of females bulimic, and 13 percent of all students.

Another study, in Nebraska, found 7.8 percent of freshman women, and 1.4 percent of freshman men, bulimic.

Diagnosing Bulimia Nervosa

The following features define the diagnosis of bulimia nervosa:

- recurrent episodes of binge-eating (the rapid consumption of a large amount of food in a short period of time)
- a feeling of lack of control over eating behavior during binges
- regular use of self-induced vomiting, strict dieting or fasting, laxatives or diuretics, or vigorous exercise to prevent weight gain
- a minimum average of two binge-eating episodes a week for at least three months
- a persistent preoccupation with body shape and weight

The eating binges are usually concentrated on high-calorie, easily ingested food, and the eating is usually done in private or kept very inconspicuous. Binge-eating episodes are terminated by abdominal pain, sleep, social interruption, or self-induced vomiting. Patients with bulimia repeatedly attempt to lose weight by severely restricting their food intake, and engage in vomiting, exercising, or use of laxatives or diuretics to get rid of calories. Their weight frequently fluctuates more than ten pounds due to their alternating binges and fasts. They are almost always aware that their eating patterns are abnormal, and fear that they will be unable to stop eating voluntarily. They usually are depressed, and have self-deprecating thoughts before and after an eating binge.

A CASE HISTORY

Bulimia nervosa is so varied and widespread that no one case history can epitomize the entire array of features of the disease, but the story of Sally is fairly typical. One of three children, Sally grew up in an upper-middle-class neighborhood. Her parents divorced when she was six, and she and her sister and brother lived with their mother. By the time she entered the sixth grade, Sally felt overweight and had begun to diet. Her mother, who was also weight-conscious, supported these efforts and suggested various diets to her. By the time of her first menstrual period, at age thirteen, Sally had been on and off six diets, none of which had been successful. Although she felt fat, her height and weight were normal for her age. She was particularly concerned about the fullness in her hips and breasts, normal aspects of maturation, which she referred to as "baby fat."

In junior high school, Sally became more and more concerned with her appearance, and began trying every fad diet that came along. She bought diet pills at the local drugstore, but they didn't seem to work, either. In senior high school she began dating, and became increasingly aware of her appearance. On one date, her boyfriend commented that she was "a bit chunky." Sally felt as though a knife had been plunged into her heart.

At Thanksgiving that year, she ate the normal dinner and felt stuffed and a little nauseated. She remembered a friend who had talked about throwing up when she had eaten too much, and after dinner she went into the bathroom and made herself vomit by sticking her fingers down her throat. She was disgusted, but at the same time she felt the power of this new-found control over her weight. Now she wouldn't have to worry about eating, partying, or getting fat; all she had to do was vomit.

In the next few months, Sally purged only once in a while when she ate too much. After six months she began to crave foods rich in carbohydrates: breads, pastas, candies, and other sweets. A vicious cycle began of craving food, binging (always in secret), and purging to get rid of it—well before any was absorbed into her body, she hoped. Her obsession with weight became more constant, and she measured everything in calories. Her sense of self-worth revolved around her size and weight. Her schoolwork and even her relationships with boyfriends began to fail. When she was elected queen of a local beauty pageant, she felt that the officials were fools, because she knew she was "too fat." Soon she began taking laxatives to purge what little food was left in her intestines after binges—one or two tablets at first, and eventually as many as 25 to 50 at a time. The violent cramps scared her until she became used to them.

In her second year of college, a friend in nursing school told Sally about diuretics. With one or two pills, she could urinate quarts of fluid, and the scale would go down from two to six pounds! It didn't matter that it came right back with the first drink of water. What was important to her was the fact that her weight went down.

She began dating regularly as a junior in college. By this time she was vomiting and using diuretics and laxatives regularly. None of the young men she dated seemed interested in a lasting relationship with her, she thought. They always ended up rejecting her—because of her weight, she felt. Much later, she realized that it was her singleminded obsession with food, calories, and weight that made her seem superficial and boring to men.

Sally's menstrual periods were irregular and infrequent. Her muscles were weak and often cramped painfully. In an effort to get rid of more food, she began using an emetic, ipecac, to vomit, but the side effects frightened her: terrible nausea, muscle twitching, and severe weakness. She gave this up and soon learned to vomit at will by simply thinking about it and pushing on her abdomen with one finger.

Sally neglected her schoolwork and began to steal, laxatives at first, and later food from grocery stores, in order to supply her habit of gorging and purging. Her feelings of guilt and depression grew, and now she began to have frequent thoughts of suicide. When she attempted to kill herself by cutting her wrists, she was taken to a hospital emergency room.

In the emergency room she denied any problems other than depression, but the laboratory test results indicated a more complicated story. The amount of potassium in her blood was dangerously low, and her heart rhythm was abnormal and irregular. She was admitted to the hospital, first to a medical floor for treatment of her cardiac and biochemical problems, and then to the psychiatric ward.

In the hospital, Sally was confronted with her false beliefs about food. Her treatment plan specified that she be forced to eat three meals a day so she could realize that she could eat with control, without purging, and that her body would not react by gaining huge amounts of weight. She hated it at first, but as she became aware of many of the issues behind her bulimia, she became resigned to the fact that she was an attractive but very lonely, extremely empty young woman. During psychotherapy in the hospital, she was able to remember that she had been molested as a child—something she had never told her parents. Medication helped her depressed mood and helped her control the "pressure" of her appetite. As she stopped binging, the fear of being fat lessened and she stopped purging. After a month in the hospital she was released to outpatient care, where she met individually with a therapist; she also joined a therapy group for women with eating disorders.

Sally's weight remained normal, and she gradually came to accept her shape. She learned to deal with stress without binge-eating or purging. Holidays presented some of the greatest stresses, when she, along with the rest of America, gained a few pounds. But with group and individual therapy support, she seldom vomited, and she did not resume use of laxatives or diuretics.

Gradually, Sally learned to interact with men in ways more meaningful than her previous series of superficial sexual relationships. A year after leaving the hospital, she met and began dating a man with whom she developed a close and satisfying friendship. The closeness frightened her at first, but with the help of her therapist she stuck it out, and did not turn to food as a refuge from intimacy. A year later they were engaged and subsequently married. Sally is no longer in therapy, and at last contact with her therapist she was coping well with marriage and with normal body weight.

THE CAUSES OF BULIMIA

As with anorexia, the causes of bulimia are not well understood, but many cases seem to be triggered by dieting. Also like anorexia, bulimia is a reason why dieting is not an entirely benign endeavor. Certain people seem to respond to dieting with a loss of normal satiety (feeling of fullness) in response to food. They then start to binge-eat, and then to purge, usually by vomiting.

Current theories of bulimia nervosa hold that low levels in the brain of a certain chemical substance known as *serotonin* may cause uninhibited binge-eating. Eating carbohydrates tends to raise brain serotonin levels, and many bulimics appear to crave carbohydrates specifically. Moreover, certain drugs helpful in the treatment of bulimia, such as *fluoxetine,* increase the levels of serotonin in the brain. Doctors cannot measure the level of serotonin in the brains of their patients. No single diagnostic test can predict who is susceptible to bulimia.

Often the detection of bulimia depends on recognizing signs, such as a bag of vomit in the trashcan, or other characteristic symptoms or behaviors. For example, people with bulimia nervosa frequently

- compare themselves with other underweight people, yet see themselves as overweight
- are fanatically concerned with weight and body shape
- become overinvolved with food and calories, even to the point of hoarding food
- deny hunger, yet eat in ravenous binges, usually in private, often consuming prodigious quantities of high-calorie "junk" foods

- interrupt the process of binging by self-induced vomiting, often augmented by laxatives (to produce diarrhea), diuretics (to stimulate urination), enemas, and at times strict dieting or fasting or overexercising
- develop physical signs such as the erosion of tooth enamel (from the acid in vomit), abrasions of the backs of the hands (from putting the hands down the throat to induce vomiting), and sunken eyes (from fluid loss)
- feel a lack of control over eating behavior and appetite
- were obese prior to the onset of the bulimia, had a history of repeated dieting, and have a strong family history of obesity, often involving the mother
- periodically suffer symptoms of depression (about 80 percent)

In extreme cases of bulimia, the person's entire life is dominated by binging and purging, thoughts of dieting, worries about calories, and fears of being fat and sexually unattractive. Studies have shown that as many as 50 percent of bulimic women abuse drugs or are dependent on alcohol. Approximately one-third steal food, laxatives, or money to support their binge-eating and vomiting habits, and are referred to treatment by courts of law.

Bulimia nervosa is an embarrassing disease, but rarely debilitating if the binging and purging are infrequent, such as once or twice a week. When individuals vomit five to ten times per day, dental problems are common, along with swelling of the saliva glands. When enemas, laxatives, diuretics, alcohol, or other drugs are added to the binging and vomiting, the stage is set for disaster.

Drastic means for controlling body weight carry serious consequences. Large doses of over-the-counter diet pills cause dangerous elevations of blood pressure, hallucinations, and even psychosis. Large quantities of laxatives produce dangerous chemical imbalances and painful abdominal cramps. The acute abdominal distress can be severe enough to mimic a ruptured appendix. Chronic dependence on laxatives leads to a lazy, enlarged bowel that works only when stimulated by more laxatives. Diuretics can cause many metabolic complications, including depletion of potassium and magnesium, leading to fatigue, muscle weakness, cramps, irregular heartbeat, and even fatal cardiac arrest. Syrup of ipecac, used to induce vomiting, acts as a poison when used in chronic excess, and can damage the heart and other muscles. There have been many cases of ruptured stomach and esophagus from severe binge-eating and vomiting. Several girls have died as a result of using baking soda to induce vomiting; when the baking soda mixed with their stomach acid, carbon dioxide gas was released and expanded their already bloated stomachs like a balloon. Tragedies like these demonstrate that our societal obsession with slimness is as dangerous as it is distressing.

TREATING BULIMIA

Fortunately, most cases of bulimia are not severe, and may resolve without formal treatment. Many young girls experiment with vomiting and fasting, along with food fads, in the course of adolescent exploration and development, only to discard the behavior after a few months. In some cases, bulimia may resurface only in times of emotional stress. All too often, however, the behavior becomes fixed and chronic.

The treatment of bulimia depends on the specific features of each case. Medical, metabolic, or psychiatric problems may require emergency hospitalization. Often the vomiting and abuse of laxatives, diuretics, and ipecac can be arrested only in the hospital. Inpatient treatment for concurrent drug or alcohol dependency is sometimes necessary. As in the treatment of anorexia, therapy may encompass psychotherapy (group and individual), nutrition education, and training in social skills, assertiveness, and self-esteem. Support groups and "buddy" systems provide continuing help for many patients. Several medications that influence bowel function, mood, and anxiety are used in the treatment of bulimia, as they are in anorexia nervosa. In addition, however, research is showing certain antidepressant medications to be helpful in diminishing the desire to binge and purge. As we have noted, these drugs may work by altering levels in the brain of certain natural chemical substances, such as serotonin.

Recovery rates from bulimia nervosa mirror the severity of the underlying disorder. The situation is analogous to that of drug-abusing teenagers: Some children who experiment with drugs discard the habit easily and quickly; others are eventually classified as addicts when the behavioral pattern becomes so integrated into their lives that they cannot function without it. The prognosis is poor for bulimic patients who feel constantly lonely, with rapid mood swings and an overwhelming sense of emptiness that is satisfied only by eating and vomiting, and in those who engage in other self-destructive acts, such as self-mutilation. In these difficult cases, prolonged psychotherapy may be needed to help the patient cope with life in more positive ways. For the majority of high school and college students with bulimic behavior, however, bulimia may be brought under control by peer counseling, self-help groups, and a stern warning in the form of candid information about the medical and psychological consequences.

As with anorexia, the most important avenue of prevention is education and example. There is no way to predict who will become bulimic. We do know that all teenagers go through a period in their maturation when they are unsure of their identities. Their bodies are developing and changing rapidly. They face concerns and unaddressed fears about sexuality and becoming independent adults while at the same time remaining dependent (at least financially) into their twenties, as schooling continues. As if these tasks were not difficult enough, adolescents of today are bombarded by advertisements that highlight both the quick fix from high-calorie foods and the virtues of a very lean body. As a society, we must begin to question some of these values taught and learned at so early an age. As individuals and parents, we can become role models who are less confusing and more psychologically sound for the adolescents of the future.

While teaching proper nutrition and physical activity, especially by example, parents should avoid focusing attention on weight and dieting. Children need to be helped to feel that their moral, intellectual, social, and spiritual qualities are of more importance and of greater worth than their physiques.

WHAT'S WRONG WITH BEING VERY THIN?

Given that most people eventually recover from anorexia and bulimia, one might fairly ask what lasting adverse effects are incurred by going through this "phase" of starvation and/or excessive thinness. The principal medical problems that sometimes persist after temporary starvation are impaired growth and brittle bones.

Short Stature

The earlier the age at which anorexia starts, the more likely it is to impair growth. Calories are necessary to grow upward as well as to grow outward. Undernourished children wind up being shorter than well-nourished children. Figure 3.1 illustrates the risk of growth retardation from undernutrition. It shows the doctor's growth chart for a six-year-old child who expressed fear of becoming fat and therefore stopped eating normally.

Osteoporosis

As we noted in chapter 2, excessive fatness helps prevent the development of osteoporosis, a brittleness of the bones that often devastates the elderly. Excessive thinness, on the other hand, *causes* osteoporosis. It does so in part through the body's inadequate intake of calcium and protein. In addition, excessive thinness induces a deficiency of hormones—such as estrogen—which are essential for strong bones.

Estrogen is a so-called sex hormone produced by fat tissue and also by the ovaries during menstrual cycles. Excessive thinness causes estrogen deficiency in two ways: by the absence of fat, which normally produces some estrogen; and because the ovaries, the major source of estrogen, stop functioning as menstrual cycles cease. Estrogen deficiency, whether due to menopause (the normal cessation of menstruation that occurs around age 50) or to excess thinness, weakens the bones and renders a person vulnerable to fractures. But what about someone who becomes thin because she exercises all the time? Doesn't exercise strengthen bone? While it is true that it does, exercising to the point of the loss of one's menstrual periods causes a decreased bone mineral content.

The benefits of exercise do not make up for the lack of estrogen. Women who are too thin to menstruate because they starve themselves, whether through anorexia or bulimia, are particularly vulnerable to osteoporosis. Their bones have the benefits neither of exercise nor of estrogen. Next worse off are those women who have exercised to the point of being too thin to menstruate. Their bones are stronger than those of equally thin women who do not exercise, but they still become osteoporotic. In terms of osteoporosis alone, anorexia or bulimia should never be dismissed as a conventional phase of development or a normal response to stress. Given the severe physical consequences, being "too thin" is not a matter of fashion, but of life and death and health.

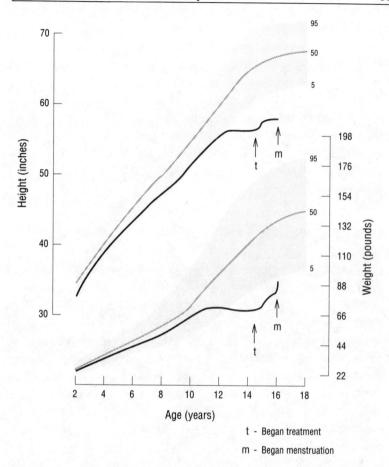

t - Began treatment

m - Began menstruation

Figure 3.1 Growth Data for Patient Whose Growth Was Stunted by Inadequate Nutrition

Growth chart of a girl whose growth was stunted by anorexia. Her height is plotted on the upper curve, and weight on the lower curve. The shaded areas indicate the normal ranges of height and weight for girls from age two to age 18 years. The ranges include 90% of children with normal growth, extending from the fifth percentile at the lower edge of the shaded area to the ninety-fifth percentile at the top edge. The dashed line in the center of each normal range represents the fiftieth percentile—at which half of normal children are higher, and half are lower. Note that this girl was growing normally until age 10, at about the tenth percentile for height, and the twenty-fifth percentile for weight. Then she became very concerned about her weight, cut down her eating, and stopped gaining weight. She continued to gain height for two more years, however, thereby becoming thinner. By age 13 she was very thin, and she stopped growing in height. At age 15½, anorexia was diagnosed, counseling was begun, and her calorie intake finally improved. She then gained some weight and height, but she remained shorter than normal. Her menstrual periods finally began at age 16.

PART II

Understanding Fat, Cholesterol, and Obesity

4

Fat: What It Is
and What It Does

Many people think of fat as something that is bad for them. In fact, fat is a great blessing, indispensable to the survival of the human race. In appropriate amounts, it is extremely beneficial.

Fat is a major source of energy in our diet, containing more than twice as many calories as either of the two other main classes of food, protein and carbohydrate. Fats are essential for proper nutrition. Although the body itself can manufacture certain types of fat, it cannot produce other types that are necessary to our health; these we must acquire by eating.

Fats that are liquid at room temperatures are called *oils*. Thus, vegetable oil is a type of fat. Cream is also mostly fat. While we can see fat in many cuts of meat, there are also invisible fats, such as those that are finely dispersed through apparently lean meat, and in nuts and fish. But fats and oils are more than just part of our diet. They are part of our bodies—part of us.

The fat in our bodies provides us with a portable storehouse of energy. To understand fat, therefore, one must comprehend energy and its importance to life and health.

ENERGY AND CALORIES

Our bodies require a constant supply of energy for working, thinking, eating, reading this book, and even for breathing and the pumping of the heart. Basal metabolism (the chemical reactions that keep our tissues alive and warm) requires energy. The energy used in all of our activities and bodily processes derives from food.

The amount of energy contained in food can be measured and expressed as *calories*. Calories are units of energy. They are released from food as it combines with oxygen, a process called *oxidation*. We commonly speak of "burning up calories," a phrase that refers to how our bodies oxidize fuel and release the stored energy.

Like a rocket engine, we derive energy from a constant supply of oxygen and a constant supply of fuel. As oxygen combines with the fuel, energy is generated. Food provides our fuel, and air provides the oxygen necessary to oxidize it and release energy. Our bodies can store fuel, especially in the form of fat, but they cannot store oxygen.

Think how wonderful it would be if our bodies *could* store oxygen. Like whales, we could take a few deep breaths in the morning at breakfast time, a few more at noon, and then some more deep breaths in the evening to replenish our oxygen stores. The rest of the time we wouldn't have to bother breathing or maintaining a constant air supply.

Although we do not have a system for storing significant amounts of oxygen, we do have a marvelous mechanism for storing fuel. Instead of having to eat constantly, as we must breathe constantly, we eat only intermittently. We can even go for days without eating. Unlike machines, which must be plugged in or supplied with fuel at all times while running, we don't have to keep eating in order to continue functioning. For this freedom and practical convenience, we can thank our fat.

Because we eat only intermittently, at meals, we require a means of transforming our irregular, sporadic intake of fuel into a steady supply for our tissues and organs—muscles, liver, heart, brain, and all our living tissues.

We have two ways of storing the food energy (calories) we eat. The first is to store carbohydrate in the form of *glycogen*. Glycogen is manufactured from simple sugar units (glucose) derived from the carbohydrates we eat. Sometimes glycogen is called "animal starch," since, like vegetable starch, it consists of chains of simple sugar molecules. Our muscles make and store glycogen, then break it down quickly into glucose when it is needed as a fuel. The liver also manufactures and stores glycogen, and breaks it down and releases it into the bloodstream as glucose when it is needed elsewhere, such as in the brain.

The body's ability to store fuel in the form of glycogen is very limited. For example, if we stop eating for just one day, our glycogen stores will be completely used up. If we had no fat, we would then have to break down muscle protein rapidly to provide the fuel needed for life.

The body's second mechanism for fuel storage is fat. Our capacity for storing energy in the form of fat, unlike glycogen, is virtually unlimited. Fat is a much more efficient way to store energy than carbohydrate (glycogen) because it contains more energy and is lighter and more compact. To grasp the relative importance of the different kinds of energy storage, consider these figures: Upon awakening in the morning, the normal adult usually has stored in his or her body less than 2,000 calories as glycogen, but more than a hundred thousand calories as fat. A pound of pure fat contains a little over 4,000 calories, while a pound of protein or carbohydrate contains only about 1,800 calories.

Body fat, or adipose tissue, contains some blood vessels, nerves, and fluid, as well as pure fat, and consequently contains a little less than 4,000 calories per pound—about 3,500. Lighter than water, fat is a very lightweight, compact energy source. Since water and fat do not dissolve in each other, fat tissue contains very little water. It is a naturally dehydrated depot of energy. Glycogen, on the other hand, tends to hold water, and is already partially oxidized; it is therefore much less efficient than fat, per pound of tissue, in storing energy.

Figure 4.1 shows the basic chemical structures of fat and of carbohydrate.

Because fat is an efficient means of storing calories, it enables us to get through periods of food scarcity. The ability to store fuel during periods of plenty has allowed humans to survive periods of famine. Cycles of "feast and famine" have characterized most of human history.

Probably in the interests of survival, our bodies are very well engineered for fat accumulation. Unfortunately, the normal mechanisms for fat storage, indispensable in scarce times, can go awry and cause obesity when food availability is unlimited (see chapter 7).

Those of us who live in Westernized societies now rarely face famine.

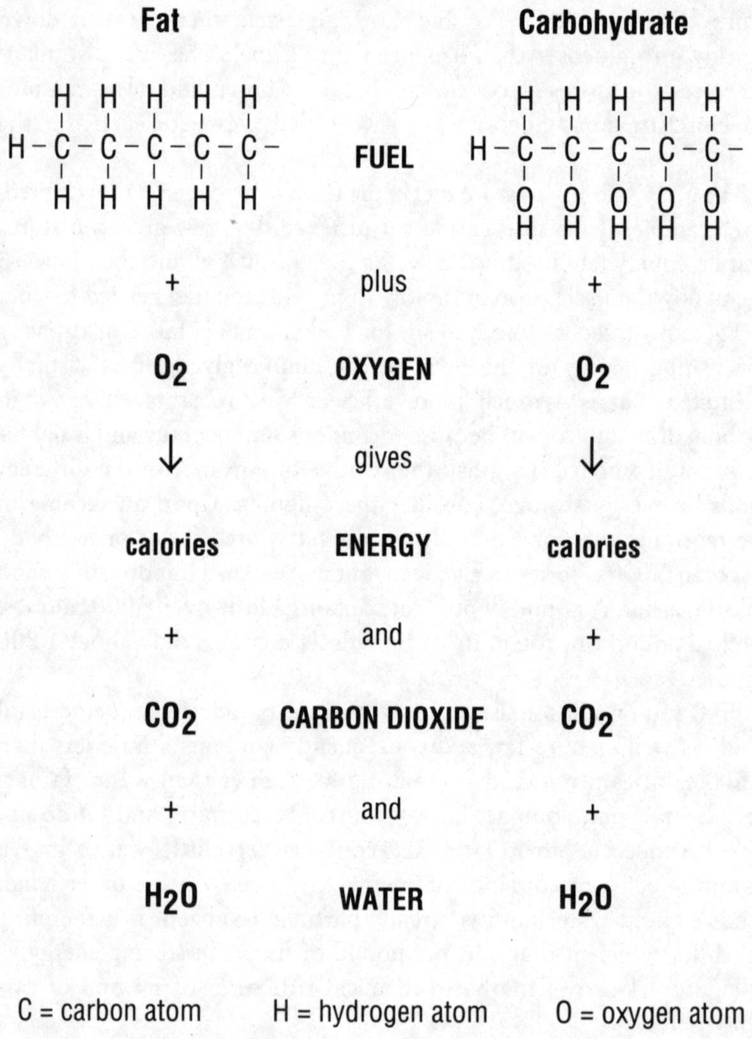

Fat		**Carbohydrate**
$\begin{array}{ccccc} H & H & H & H & H \\ | & | & | & | & | \\ H-C & -C & -C & -C & -C- \\ | & | & | & | & | \\ H & H & H & H & H \end{array}$	**FUEL**	$\begin{array}{ccccc} H & H & H & H & H \\ | & | & | & | & | \\ H-C & -C & -C & -C & -C- \\ | & | & | & | & | \\ O & O & O & O & O \\ | & | & | & | & | \\ H & H & H & H & H \end{array}$
+	plus	+
O_2	**OXYGEN**	O_2
↓	gives	↓
calories	**ENERGY**	calories
+	and	+
CO_2	**CARBON DIOXIDE**	CO_2
+	and	+
H_2O	**WATER**	H_2O

C = carbon atom   H = hydrogen atom   O = oxygen atom

Figure 4.1 The Molecular Structures of Fat and Carbohydrate and Their Combustion to Calories, Water, and Carbon Dioxide

As you can see, the main basic difference between fat and carbohydrate is that carbohydrate contains oxygen. In fact, most of the carbon atoms in carbohydrate have two hydrogen and one oxygen atom. Two hydrogen and one oxygen make H_2O, or water. (*Hydrate* means "water," and *carbo-* is the prefix for carbon—hence the term *carbohydrate*.) Fat, on the other hand, has not yet combined with oxygen. Consequently, fat can accept more oxygen than can carbohydrate, and can release more energy (calories) during oxidation to CO_2 (carbon dioxide) and H_2O (water). This is why fat contains more calories than does carbohydrate.

So long as we can rely on society for a constant food supply, we have no need to store large amounts of fat for survival. In fact, too much fat is detrimental to health and survival—too much of a good thing.

ADIPOSE TISSUE

Storing energy as fat takes place in one of the most sophisticated tissues in the body: adipose tissue. Commonly called fat, adipose tissue is virtually everywhere in the body, not only where we can see it under the skin and around the waist and buttocks, but inside the cavities of the body, particularly the abdomen. Fat also insulates and provides a cushion around major body organs. One of the few places in the body where fat is sparse is within the skull, a bony compartment reserved almost entirely for brain tissue.

Adipose tissue consists of very specialized cells that have the capacity to store large amounts of fat. When viewed under a microscope, these tiny cells look like signet rings with fat in the center and a tiny rim of the working tissue of the cell surrounding the fat droplet within. The cell's nucleus, or control center, forms the signet part of the ring, as shown in Figure 4.2.

Each of us has billions of fat cells like this in the body, containing variable quantities of fat. When we take in more calories than we expend through activity and basal metabolism, the excess calories are stored as fat within our fat cells. The little fat droplets in our fat cells enlarge. When we ingest fewer calories than we burn up, the fat cells shrink as they give up some of their fat to supply the needed fuel to the rest of the body. If we exercise without eating, we are simply burning the fuel (oxidizing the fat) stored up from previous meals.

The visible fat that we see on meat is the adipose tissue of the animal and consists of these tiny fat cells, just as it does in humans. In addition to fat cells, adipose tissue also contains blood vessels and fibrous strands. The blood vessels carry calories to and from the tissue; the fibrous strands hold the adipose tissue together, keeping it compact.

CELLULITE

Sometimes the fibrous strands within adipose tissue become stretched, producing a dimpling effect on the overlying skin. This dimpled look has been given the name *cellulite*, which is nothing more than ordinary adipose tissue. It is often seen on the legs and buttocks, but contrary to the implications of much current advertising, there is nothing unique

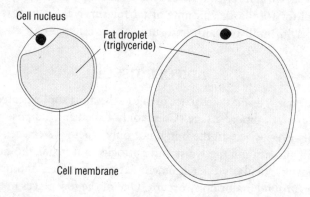

Figure 4.2 Fat Cells

Fat cells, greatly magnified. Under the microscope, fat cells look like little signet rings. Most of the volume of each fat cell is comprised of a tiny droplet of triglyceride. This is surrounded by the cell membrane. Enzymes controlling fat storage and fat breakdown are associated with the cell membrane. When fat cells take on more triglyceride, they enlarge as the triglyercide droplet expands. When fat cells give up trigylceride, such as during weight reduction, they become smaller.

or special about this kind of fat. Apart from removing this sort of adipose tissue surgically, no special tricks, such as specific foods, diets, drugs, machines, or exercises, will selectively remove this so-called cellulite.

BROWN FAT VS. WHITE FAT

Besides storing energy, fat helps us to maintain our body temperature. It is a portable heating blanket and provides insulation against extreme changes in temperature. While we humans have very little of it, some animals have a specialized kind of adipose tissue—brown fat—which is much better at providing heat than is the usual kind of fat we have been describing: white fat. Brown fat functions specifically to break down triglyceride—the chemical form of fat stored in adipose tissue— to generate heat, a process called *thermogenesis*. Brown fat takes its name from the fact that when this tissue is dissected, it looks reddish brown because of its rich blood supply. Blood vessels winding in and out of these very specialized fat cells carry heat to the rest of the body.

Animals that hibernate have extensive brown-fat stores to keep them warm and cozy during the long winter months without food. Claims to the contrary notwithstanding, it is very unlikely that abnormalities in brown fat metabolism play any role in human obesity. Claims that you can lose weight by taking something to activate your brown fat, and thereby burn more calories, are misleading.

TRIGLYCERIDES AND FATTY ACIDS

Triglyceride, the chemical form of fat stored in adipose tissue, is the most abundant form of fat. This is the kind of fat that we can actually see in such foods as cream, oil, shortening, and meat. Each molecule of triglyceride is made of three ("tri") chains of carbon and hydrogen called *fatty acids,* attached to a short backbone composed of *glycerol* ("glyceride").

When you have a meal consisting of a hamburger with mayonnaise, french fries or potato chips, and ice cream, you are eating a lot of triglyceride. After you swallow the food, it passes into your stomach and intestines, where the triglyceride is broken down (digested) into fatty acids and glycerol. These are absorbed in the intestine, and are eventually reassembled into triglycerides and made available to the body through the bloodstream. In chapter 5 we shall review the transport of triglycerides in the blood as we examine another important type of fat: cholesterol. Suffice it to say here that the fat we eat is mainly triglyceride, and after digestion, absorption, and transport, it is ultimately stored in tiny adipose cells as triglyceride.

The glycerol portions of triglycerides are all alike, but there are very important differences among the various types of fatty acids. We noted earlier that the body can produce many types of fatty acids, but that certain ones essential for health cannot be manufactured by our bodies, and therefore must be acquired by eating. These are called *essential fatty acids.* To remain healthy, we must have these essential fatty acids in our diet; no long-term diet plan, therefore, should be totally free of fat. The essential fatty acids are mostly of the unsaturated type.

SATURATED AND UNSATURATED FATS

An important aspect of fat and fatty acids is whether or not they are *saturated.* You have no doubt heard about "saturated fats" and "unsaturated fats." Have you ever wondered what these fats were saturated with? The answer is *hydrogen.* Saturated and unsaturated fats

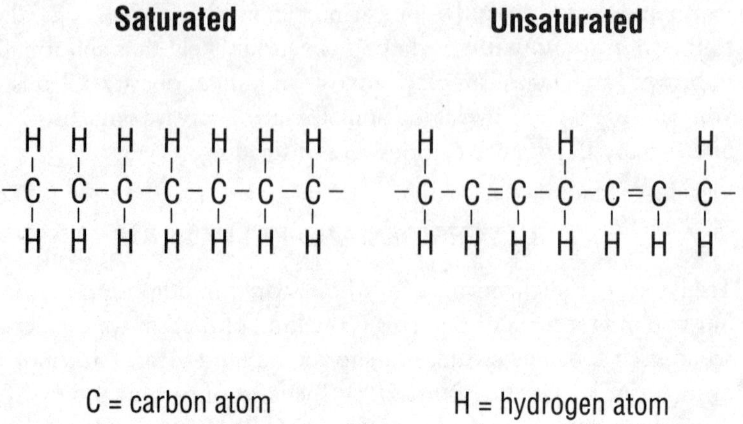

Saturated   **Unsaturated**

$$\begin{array}{c} \overset{H}{|} \ \overset{H}{|} \ \overset{H}{|} \ \overset{H}{|} \ \overset{H}{|} \ \overset{H}{|} \ \overset{H}{|} \\ -C-C-C-C-C-C-C- \\ \underset{H}{|} \ \underset{H}{|} \ \underset{H}{|} \ \underset{H}{|} \ \underset{H}{|} \ \underset{H}{|} \ \underset{H}{|} \end{array}$$

$$\begin{array}{c} \overset{H}{|} \qquad\quad \overset{H}{|} \qquad\quad \overset{H}{|} \\ -C-C=C-C-C=C-C- \\ \underset{H}{|} \ \underset{H}{|} \ \underset{H}{|} \ \underset{H}{|} \ \underset{H}{|} \ \underset{H}{|} \ \underset{H}{|} \end{array}$$

C = carbon atom   H = hydrogen atom

Figure 4.3 The Molecular Structures of Saturated and Unsaturated Fat

Saturated fatty acids contain as much hydrogen as the carbon atoms are capable
of binding. In unsaturated fatty acids, some of the hydrogen atoms are absent.

differ in their effects on blood cholesterol levels, and in their degree
of physical firmness. Saturated fats tend to raise blood cholesterol,
and tend to be solid at room temperature. Unsaturated fats tend to
be softer, or even liquid, and tend to lower blood cholesterol. Saturated
and unsaturated fats are approximately equal in calorie content. '

Please glance back at Figure 4.1 on page 70, where you will see that
fat consists of chains of carbon and hydrogen. These are the fatty acid
chains. Carbon atoms in the middle of a chain are connected to two
adjacent carbon atoms, and also to two hydrogen atoms. Such a fatty
acid chain is "saturated" because each carbon atom is connected to
as many hydrogen atoms as it can hold. It is saturated with hydrogen,
and we therefore call it a *saturated fatty acid*. When it is incorporated
into triglyceride, it becomes saturated fat.

Other fatty acid chains, however, do not have this much hydrogen,
as shown in Figure 4.3. They are capable of taking on some more
hydrogen, and they are therefore not saturated with it.

These are the *unsaturated fats*. If a fatty acid chain has just *one* pair
of carbon atoms without a full complement of hydrogen, we call it a
monounsaturated fat. Olive oil, for example, has lots of monoun-

saturated fatty acids. Fatty acids having many pairs of unsaturated carbon atoms are called *polyunsaturated*. When you hear vegetable oils being advertised as "rich in polyunsaturates," this is what they are talking about: lots of polyunsaturated fatty acids.

The issue of saturated versus unsaturated fats is important because the two types of fat have very different effects on your blood cholesterol level (see chapter 5). In brief, dietary intake of monounsaturated and polyunsaturated fat tends to *reduce* your serum cholesterol, while taking in saturated fat tends to raise it.

Another term for saturated fat is *hydrogenated fat*. Because of what we noted earlier, you can see why the two terms are interchangeable: it is possible to add hydrogen to unsaturated fat, and make it saturated. This is a regular practice in the food-processing industry. But why would anyone want to take unsaturated fat, which lowers cholesterol, and hydrogenate it to saturated fat, which raises cholesterol? The reason is that saturated fats are firmer, more solid, and have a longer shelf life. Fat doesn't go rancid as rapidly if it is saturated. If you want people to be able to spread margarine on their bread, instead of to pour it on, you have to take the unsaturated vegetable oil and hydro-genate (saturate) it, at least partially. This will make it firm enough to spread. Likewise, to firm up the texture of peanut butter and prevent separation of a liquid oil layer, manufacturers often hydrogenate the oil in peanut butter. If you go to your refrigerator, find some margarine, and read its ingredients, you will see that the vegetable oils have been partially saturated, or hydrogenated. Likewise, the labels on your pea-nut-butter jar and your vegetable shortening will explain that the oil has been hydrogenated. In general, the more hydrogenated the fat product, the firmer it will be—and the more it will raise your choles-terol count.

Regardless of whether they have been hydrogenated, oil and mar-garine are still fat—triglycerides—and are very rich in calories. That is, they contain a lot of energy, and lots of exercise will be required to burn off those calories.

You cannot lose weight by eating lots of unsaturated fats, even though they may be good for your cholesterol level. Many people with high cholesterol levels are obese and therefore need to lose weight. They should reduce their intake of all types of fat so they can start burning up their own excess adipose tissue. (See chapter 5.)

OMEGA-UNSATURATED FATTY ACIDS

So-called "omega-3 fatty acids" are enjoying a current popularity. These are fatty acids with unsaturated carbon atoms whose placement along the chain is designated as the omega-3 position. They are the subject of intense medical research and advertising hype, and the advertising hype has gotten way ahead of the medical research. Intake of oils rich in these fatty acids, such as fish oils, tends to reduce the blood concentration of triglycerides. It has little effect on blood cholesterol. It may also have other important effects, such as possible interference with certain blood elements necessary for clotting, but until further medical research clarifies their impact on health, we do not recommend supplementing your diet with extra doses of this rather expensive form of fat.

BODY FAT AND ITS RELATION TO DIET

Body fat accumulates whenever caloric intake exceeds caloric expenditure. Caloric intake, of course, consists of the calories we eat— our diet—plus whatever might be administered intravenously. From the point of view of putting on body fat, it matters extremely little whether the caloric intake is in the form of fat, protein, or carbohydrate. Our bodies can convert protein and carbohydrate calories to fat. Just as a steer can get fat by eating only grass, a human can get fat by eating only fruits and vegetables. If you eat an average of 2,600 calories a day, but expend an average of only 2,400 calories, you will accumulate fat at the rate of 200 calories per day. At that rate, since each pound of fat stores about 3,500 calories, you will gain a pound of fat every 17 to 18 days, or approximately one and a half pounds per month, or 18 pounds per year. The arithmetic of the body is inexorable, and a calorie is a calorie, whether consumed as lettuce or as lamb chop.

Energy expenditure is, of course, the other half of the equation. Our bodies expend energy in three ways. First, there is the process of *basal metabolism,* also known as *resting energy expenditure.* Basal metabolism comprises all the chemical reactions that keep our tissues warm and alive and functioning, even at rest. It includes the thermogenesis (heat production) noted earlier. It also includes the work of breathing, the beating of the heart at rest, the function of the kidneys, and the constant repair work needed to keep our muscles, intestines, and other tissues in working order. Basal metabolism also includes the pumping of sodium out of body cells and of potassium into body cells—a process essential for keeping them alive. It involves the consumption of oxygen and the release of energy (calories) and of carbon dioxide.

The second way our bodies expend energy is through the *thermic effect of food,* formerly called "specific dynamic action," which is the energy expended in absorbing and processing the food we have eaten. Some of the warmth experienced after eating a large meal may result from this release of energy, which occurs as the body absorbs, transports, and processes nutrients for storage. Although there are small differences in the amounts of energy required for the body to process different kinds of food, these differences are of no practical importance and play no part in rational attempts to control weight through diet.

The third means of expending energy is, of course, *exercise,* or physical activity. It is the only means of energy expenditure over which we have safe and conscious control, and plays an indispensable part in the prevention and treatment of obesity for most people.

When total energy expended exceeds calories eaten, energy stores—fat and glycogen—are consumed and temporarily depleted. Fat stores shrink. When caloric intake exceeds expenditure, fat stores expand. This tide of energy in and energy out rises and falls continually in each of us. Fat stores, and weight, increase with meals, and then decrease with exercise. You can think of your current average weight range as your "tidal zone." The encouraging fact is that a relatively small change in dietary intake, or in exercise, *if habitually maintained,* can in the long run make a significant difference in the amount of fat that your body stores. A habit of regular exercise, or of choosing low-calorie foods instead of high-calorie ones, can have a big influence on your body fat level.

Beware of claims that certain foods "burn fat" or flush it out of your system. Such claims have been made for many nutrients, including lecithin, vitamin C, pectin, garlic, and substances with diuretic or laxative actions. Lecithin contains calories, and is absorbed like any other food. Although diuretics do cause the kidneys to release water, they do not thereby expend calories or decrease body fat stores. Laxatives increase the frequency and fluid content of stools, and thereby temporarily reduce body weight, but not body fat. *Starch-blockers* are substances that interfere with carbohydrate absorption. They occur naturally in beans, and account for the flatulence associated with eating beans, since the carbohydrate that is not absorbed by the intestine is converted to gas by bacteria in the colon. These substances are not, however, an effective prevention of obesity, or a treatment for it.

LET'S GO TO LUNCH

By following a meal from your plate to your waistline, we can see the process of fat accumulation. Figure 4.4 diagrams the flow of nutrients into your mouth, down to the stomach, and then to the intestines where absorption into the bloodstream takes place.

Let's suppose you are at a fast-food restaurant for lunch, about to devour a salad, a hamburger, and a chocolate shake.

As you put food into your mouth, chew, and swallow, you commence the process of digestion. Digestion is the breaking down of food into its simple components, or building blocks, and must occur before food can enter the bloodstream. Only individual molecules—the very smallest particles of any substance—can be absorbed through the lining of the intestines. Once digested into simple molecules, food is absorbed through the walls of the intestines into the bloodstream. The blood then carries the food to the rest of the body.

Fat travels in the bloodstream in little particles known as *lipoproteins,* which derive their name from the fact that they are composed of both fat (lipid) and protein. Some of these lipoproteins are formed in the intestine when food is absorbed, and others are made in the liver from excess dietary calories, especially alcohol. As lipoproteins reach the adipose tissue, an enzyme known as *lipoprotein lipase* (LPL) helps transfer the triglyceride into fat cells.

All of these steps—eating, digestion, absorption, processing, transportation, and transfer into fat cells for storage—are necessary for calories to journey from your plate to your waistline. If even one of these steps is impaired, it is difficult to gain weight. If these steps are very efficient, on the other hand, weight gain may be facilitated.

Having taken this brief overview of the flow of nutrients from your plate into your body, let's look more closely at each of the major types of nutrients in your meal, and how they function. Remember that food comes in three major forms: carbohydrate, fat, and protein.

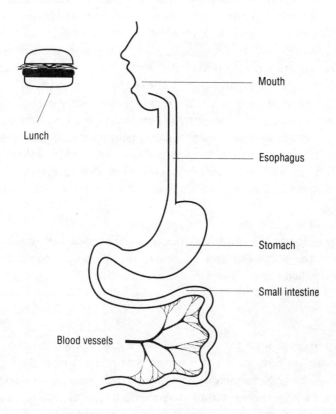

Figure 4.4 Food Pathway

Digestion begins in the mouth as enzymes in saliva start to break down starch into its simple building blocks of sugar. Powerful acids and enzymes added in the stomach and intestine continue the process of digestion. Once digested into simple molecules, food is absorbed through the intestinal walls and into the bloodstream for transportation to the rest of the body.

Carbohydrate

Carbohydrates in food are either "simple" or "complex." *Simple carbohydrates* are sugars—the individual building blocks of all carbohydrates. *Complex carbohydrates* are the starches in vegetable foods and the glycogen in animal foods. They are composed of long, branching chains of sugar molecules joined together. During digestion, starches and glycogen are broken down into simple sugars before they are absorbed into the bloodstream.

Sugars are found in many foods, particularly fruit and sweeteners. Pure sugars are virtually never eaten alone except as a component of soft drinks and honey, and as an additive to hot beverages. When you eat simple sugars, they enter the bloodstream quickly because no digestion is needed prior to their absorption. On the other hand, it takes some time to digest complex carbohydrates into individual sugar molecules. Consequently, starches are not absorbed into the bloodstream as rapidly as are simple sugars. They therefore hang around longer in the gastrointestinal tract and cause more of a sensation of fullness.

When carbohydrate calories are consumed in excess of need, the liver transforms the excess calories into triglyceride—the main form of fat in the body. The liver secretes the lipoproteins into the bloodstream, which carries it to fat tissue for storage.

Fat

Fat contains more than twice as many calories per ounce as carbohydrate or protein. Fat is thus the type of food with the highest *caloric density*. Nevertheless, we know that a calorie is a calorie is a calorie, whether it comes from fat, protein, or carbohydrate. All these calories count, and can be stored as fat or expended as energy. The fat in your food is mainly in the form of triglyceride, whether the fat is of animal origin (as in the meat in your burger) or of plant origin (as in the mayonnaise on your burger and the oil in your salad dressing). Fat is the nutrient that usually provides the highest taste satisfaction, particularly when combined with sweeteners. (Ice cream and pastries are prime examples of this attractive fat/sugar combination.) Fat is also the nutrient that gives the greatest feeling of fullness; fatty foods tend to linger in the intestinal tract, prolonging the period of nutrient absorption. Once absorbed, dietary fat is packaged into lipoproteins for transportation by the bloodstream to body tissues, including adipose tissue.

Fats, including oils, contain nine calories per gram, as compared with seven calories per gram for alcohol and only four calories per gram for protein and carbohydrate. A diet high in fats and oils will therefore be a high-calorie diet.

Protein

Protein is found in most foods of both animal and plant origin, and consists of chains of amino-acid molecules linked together. Many of these amino acids can be made by the body, but a number of them cannot. Those that are necessary for health but cannot be made in the body are called *essential amino acids*. Like essential fatty acids, they must be included in the diet for good nutrition.

Some of the storage forms of nutrients are related to the original food eaten. For example, muscle protein comes from dietary protein, and glycogen comes from dietary carbohydrate. But when we eat more of any type of nutrient than we need, the excess calories end up as triglyceride in our fat tissue, because the liver converts them to glucose and fatty acids, and eventually ships them to our fat tissue as lipo-proteins. Adipose-tissue triglyceride is thus derived from any of the foodstuffs—protein, fat, or carbohydrate. The conversion of fat in food to fat in adipose tissue is more efficient than is the conversion of carbohydrate or protein to body fat. In terms of fat accumulation, however, there are no "free calories" and no types of foods that "burn up" calories rather than contribute to caloric intake and fat accumulation. You can even get fat from eating too much grapefruit!

HOW MUCH FAT IS IT HEALTHY TO EAT?

United States government health experts recently advised that most Americans should reduce their dietary intake of fat. This is good advice for people who need to lose weight or to stop gaining weight, since fats are the form of food highest in calories. On the other hand, growing children need lots of calories, and fat provides them efficiently. Everyone, of course, needs *some* fat intake to obtain the essential fatty acids. Recent reports of malnourished children whose well-intentioned parents removed fat from their diets point up the need for well-balanced nutrition, rather than simple restriction of fat intake.

The exact amount of fat that should be in a person's diet is a subject of controversy. Current scientific data do not justify a rigid prescription of any certain amount or percentage of fat intake for everyone. Nevertheless, important illnesses have been linked statistically to the generous consumption of dietary fat, and it may be possible to help prevent these diseases by reducing fat intake. Coronary heart disease, breast cancer, colon cancer, and prostate cancer have been associated with high-fat diets in various populations. Although it has not been proven that reducing fat intake will reduce your chances of getting these diseases, it would appear reasonable to do so within the guidelines of balanced nutrition. Consequently, the United States Surgeon General, the Diet and Health Report of the National Academy of Sciences, the American Heart Association, the National Cancer Institute, and the American Cancer Society have recommended that not more than 30 percent of calories be taken in the form of fat—as opposed to the current American average of 37 to 40 percent. Substituting fruits, vegetables, grains, and fish for foods high in fat, such as lard, meat, and cream, appears to be prudent for persons with a high fat intake and no need to gain weight.

The role of excess dietary fat in coronary heart disease appears to be twofold. First, it contributes to obesity, which increases the risk of heart disease. Second, saturated fats raise the blood cholesterol level, and high blood cholesterol levels cause clogging of the coronary arteries (see chapter 5). Ridding oneself of obesity and lowering blood cholesterol are positive steps toward avoiding a heart attack, and reducing dietary fat should help on both counts.

SHERLOCK HOLMES AT THE SUPERMARKET

Deciding to reduce fat intake may be far easier than doing the kind of detective work that is often necessary to execute the decision. U.S. government regulations require that food labels contain information on the fat content of foods, and that all ingredients be listed in the order of their abundance in the product. Thus, the product contains more of the first-listed ingredient than of the second, more of the second than the third, and so on. Many crackers and cookies, for example, list fat as their second ingredient, but its position in the list may be mildly camouflaged by a lengthy description of the first ingredient. And the relative amount of animal fat may be obscured by a statement that a particular vegetable fat is used. A typical list from the side of a box of crackers reads as follows: "Ingredients: Enriched wheat flour containing niacin, reduced iron, thiamine mononitrate (vitamin B$_1$) and riboflavin (vitamin B$_2$), animal and/or vegetable shortening (lard and/or coconut oil and/or partially hydrogenated soybean oil), sugar, salt, corn syrup and leavening (sodium bicarbonate, sodium acid pyrophosphate, monocalcium phosphate)." This means that flour (enriched with vitamins) is the product's most abundant ingredient, and that fat is the next most abundant, in the form of lard (animal fat) or vegetable oil. Since lard and coconut oil are highly saturated, and since the soybean oil is hydrogenated (saturated), the fats in these particular crackers are of a type that tends to raise serum cholesterol levels. (For more about label reading, see chapter 5.) Not only virtue but patience is required for this kind of tedious but vital on-the-spot research. But the results in terms of good health are well worth the effort.

5

Cholesterol:
Bad News and Good News

A NATIONAL EPIDEMIC

The U.S. government has launched a national crusade to educate physicians and the public about the dangers of high blood levels of cholesterol, and to motivate them to lower those levels. Should you be concerned about your cholesterol level? For many people, the answer is yes.

The current crusade derives from solid evidence that high levels of cholesterol in the bloodstream greatly increase the risk of having a heart attack, the leading cause of death in this country. More than 500,000 people die of heart attacks in the United States every year. Reducing the blood cholesterol concentration reduces the risk of having a heart attack.

Heart attacks result from the thickening, or "hardening," of the arteries, the muscular tubes that carry blood throughout the body. Our body tissues depend on the flow of blood for a constant supply of oxygen and nutrients. When the arteries to any area of the body thicken, they can eventually clog completely, and blood will no longer flow to that area. The tissue that was supplied with blood by that artery then dies for lack of oxygen. For example, when the arteries supplying blood to the heart become blocked, part of the heart muscle dies, an event we refer to as a heart attack. When an artery supplying the brain becomes blocked, part of the brain may die. We call this a stroke. When the same process involves another part of the body, such as a foot, a leg, or part of the bowel, and the tissues involved die, we call it gangrene. In each case, tissues die because the arteries have clogged and that part of the body lacks oxygen.

The medical term for this "hardening" of the arteries is *atherosclerosis*. It is the leading killer of Americans. The process is thought to begin when blood-vessel walls are damaged. Causes of such damage to blood-vessel walls include trauma, high blood pressure, smoking, and diabetes. Once the blood-vessel wall is damaged, specialized cells congregate at the area of damage. Although their function is to repair the damage, they also tend to take up cholesterol from the bloodstream, especially if blood concentrations of cholesterol are high. Thus begin the cholesterol deposits in the arteries that are known as atherosclerosis. The process continues until the opening in the artery is so narrow that a blood clot forms, completely blocking blood flow.

Of the more than one-half million Americans that atherosclerosis kills each year, many die in their forties, fifties, and sixties, and could have enjoyed many more years of healthy life if their arteries had not closed off. Not only death but tremendous disabilities result from heart attacks and strokes. If we add up the cost of medical care for these maladies (including hospital and nursing-home care, special cardiology procedures, heart bypass surgery, and extensive X rays and other tests), plus the disability and loss of earnings they produce, the financial costs rise into the billions of dollars each year. The human cost in terms of suffering due to premature death and disability is beyond estimation.

Atherosclerosis is largely preventable. It is virtually nonexistent in certain parts of the world, such as rural Japan and parts of Greece and Yugoslavia. Yet when Japanese people whose families have been free of atherosclerosis for centuries move to the United States, and adopt much of our diet and life-style, their blood cholesterol levels rise, they develop atherosclerosis, and they start having heart attacks.

Blood concentrations of cholesterol are measured in metric units: milligrams per deciliter, abbreviated as "mg/dl." (A milligram is one-thousandth of a gram. To give you an idea of how small a milligram is, a nickel weighs 5,000 milligrams. A deciliter is one-tenth of a liter, or a little over three ounces.) Average levels of cholesterol for American adults are over 200 mg/dl. On the other hand, in those areas of rural Japan, Greece, and Yugoslavia where heart attacks are almost unknown, the average levels of cholesterol in the blood are between 160 and 180 mg/dl. There is abundant evidence that the higher levels of cholesterol prevalent in America are a major reason why heart attacks are so much more common in our country.

High levels of cholesterol in the blood, smoking, high blood pressure, physical inactivity, diabetes, and obesity (especially abdominal obesity) all promote atherosclerosis. That is why they are called "risk factors." *Each of these risk factors is reversible.*

You can do a great deal to reduce your own risk of heart attack and stroke by acting to reduce those risk factors that apply to you. The national campaign against high blood pressure appears to have increased awareness about the necessity to control blood pressure, and seems to have helped reduce the numbers of strokes and heart attacks. Stopping smoking also helps prevent atherosclerosis, and increased physical activity helps prevent heart attacks. We encourage you not simply to focus on cholesterol alone, but to take steps to correct all coronary risk factors that apply to you.

Your own personal prevention program should include the complete cessation of all smoking (yes, it's difficult, but it's essential); blood pressure control; regular exercise, unless some medical problem contraindicates it; and weight control, especially if you have abdominal obesity. If you have diabetes, you should work with your doctor to control it. And if your cholesterol is high, what follows will show you the appropriate steps to bring it down to a healthy level. If you follow the complete program, you *can* significantly reduce your chance of heart attack by reducing your blood cholesterol concentration.

WHAT IS CHOLESTEROL?

Cholesterol is a fatty substance or *lipid* that is a natural, necessary part of every cell in our bodies. It is a building block within our cells and tissues, and is used for the production of hormones and other important natural substances. Cholesterol is therefore not in itself detrimental to health. What is detrimental is to have excessive amounts of cholesterol in the bloodstream, since this promotes atherosclerosis.

Cholesterol is present in our food and is also produced within our bodies. Certain tissues, such as the liver, export cholesterol into the bloodstream for delivery to other tissues that need it. Cholesterol absorbed in the diet, as well as that secreted by the liver, enters the bloodstream. The flowing blood then transports it to tissues that extract it from the blood. En route, however, the cholesterol can enter the walls of blood vessels, contributing to atherosclerosis.

Cholesterol is not the only lipid in our bloodstream. As noted earlier, the other major form of blood lipid is called *triglyceride*. Triglyceride is fat—the same kind found in adipose tissue. That roll of fat that typically appears around the midsection of overfed persons is almost all triglyceride; it got there by being transported through the blood-stream.

The medical term for too much cholesterol in the bloodstream is *hypercholesterolemia*. Breaking the word down, you can see that "hyper" means "too much," or "too high," and "emia" means "in the blood." Likewise, *hypertriglyceridemia* denotes too much triglyc-eride in the blood. A more general term, encompassing both of these problems, is *hyperlipidemia*.

Hyperlipidemia is a subject of tremendous scientific and medical progress. If you take advantage of this progress and reverse those risk factors that apply to you, you will greatly reduce your chances of heart attack and stroke.

"GOOD" AND "BAD" CHOLESTEROL

Since cholesterol and triglyceride are fatty substances (lipids), they do not dissolve by themselves in watery solutions, such as blood. Our body manages to dissolve these lipids in blood by encasing them in proteins and emulsifier-type lipids such as lecithin. These little clusters of fat, protein, and lecithin are called *lipoproteins*. The cholesterol in our bloodstream is virtually all contained in these tiny lipoprotein particles.

Lipoproteins come in four major classes, or types:

1. High-density lipoproteins (HDL)

2. Low-density lipoproteins (LDL)

3. Very-low-density lipoproteins (VLDL)

4. Chylomicrons

The classification derives from the density, or weight, of the lipo-proteins. Since fat is lighter than protein, those particles with lots of triglyceride are very light (of very low density), while those with less fat are heavier (of high density). It is important for you to understand these four types of lipoproteins, because intelligent treatment of hy-perlipidemia is based on knowing which types are present in excess.

Having lots of cholesterol in LDL form leads to atherosclerosis, because it is LDL that carries cholesterol into the damaged areas of arteries. LDL has therefore been called the "bad" kind of cholesterol, and an important goal of treatment is to reduce the amount of LDL in the bloodstream.

Having lots of HDL-cholesterol, on the other hand, is associated with *not* getting atherosclerosis, so HDL has been called "good" cholesterol. A brief description of each type of lipoprotein follows.

High-Density Lipoproteins (HDL)

When the liquid portion of blood (called plasma or serum) is put into a centrifuge, the heavier particles that had been suspended in the serum will settle to the bottom, while the lighter-weight particles will float. All the lipoprotein particles that sink to the bottom are called high-density lipoproteins. They are not all alike. Several different types of lipoprotein particles have high density, and are all lumped together as HDL because together they form the heavy sediment at the bottom of a centrifuge tube.

Some of these HDL particles are beneficial in preventing heart attacks. This is because they are involved in *removing* cholesterol from body tissues. Other HDL particles, however, do not affect your cardiovascular risk. This is probably why scientists have not been able to show that you can prevent heart attacks by raising your HDL-cholesterol levels. For example, drinking alcohol raises your HDL-cholesterol levels, but not in that subspecies of HDL involved in preventing heart attacks. Moreover, estrogens given to men will raise their HDL-cholesterol levels, but actually worsen their risk of heart attack. In the future, better diagnostic tests, probably measuring the individual proteins in HDL, will give us means to follow the beneficial effects of manipulating the amounts of the individual species of high-density lipoproteins.

A patient whom we shall call Stella reported that she felt well when she visited her doctor for a routine physical examination and Pap smear just after her forty-sixth birthday. She had no family history of relatives with heart attack or stroke at an early age (such as before age sixty). During her examination, the doctor found no symptoms or signs of disease, but did order some routine laboratory tests, including blood cholesterol. Stella was greatly alarmed a week later when her doctor called and told her that she had a high level of cholesterol in her blood: 282 mg/dl.

According to the doctor, the first step in evaluating this abnormal laboratory value was to repeat the test. This time the doctor also ordered a measurement of the LDL and HDL levels in order to find out whether the high cholesterol count was due to increased amounts of the "good" (HDL) or the "bad" (LDL) cholesterol. The doctor also ordered a "fasting" triglyceride count (performed after Stella had not eaten for twelve to fourteen hours), a fasting blood-sugar test, and a test of her thyroid gland function. The purpose of the thyroid test and the blood-sugar test was to make sure that Stella didn't have hypothyroidism (an underactive thyroid gland) or diabetes—diseases that can cause high blood cholesterol.

A week later the doctor called back with the test results. The cholesterol was indeed high on the repeat test—267 mg/dl. The LDL-cholesterol value, however, was normal, at 116 mg/dl. The HDL-cholesterol level was markedly elevated at 125 mg/dl; normal for that particular laboratory was a level of 40–50 mg/dl. The triglyceride count was normal at 130 mg/dl, and the blood-sugar and thyroid tests were also normal. The doctor reassured Stella that although her blood cholesterol level was quite high, the elevation was due to HDL, the "good" kind of cholesterol. No futher evaluation or treatment was needed. In fact, consistent with her family history of longevity and freedom from heart attacks, her pattern of blood lipoproteins was one that would probably help protect her from getting atherosclerosis.

If your total cholesterol count is elevated, you should have your HDL-cholesterol measured to find out whether the excess cholesterol in your blood is due entirely to HDL-cholesterol. If your high cholesterol count is explainable by an elevation of HDL-cholesterol, you do not need to take steps to change your cholesterol level. On the other hand, if your high cholesterol is due to excess LDL, you are at increased risk for atherosclerosis.

Low-Density Lipoproteins (LDL)

Having some LDL-cholesterol in your bloodstream is normal and healthy. For example, LDL carries cholesterol to the adrenal glands, which use it to make important hormones.

High levels of LDL-cholesterol are a major risk factor for atherosclerosis. When LDL-cholesterol levels get much over 130 mg/dl, atherosclerosis is more likely to occur. Population studies suggest that levels under 100 are probably even healthier than the 120–130 mg/ dl that most experts now adopt as their target for therapy.

Reducing the level of LDL-cholesterol reduces the risk of heart attack. Therefore, if your total cholesterol level is elevated, and the elevation is due to increased amounts of LDL, you should consider taking corrective measures. Effective, safe treatment is available, and it does prevent cardiovascular disease. (See page 100.)

Several underlying causes contribute to high levels of LDL-cholesterol, including a diet rich in saturated fats and cholesterol, hypothyroidism (an underactive thyroid gland), diabetes mellitus, liver disease, and inherited defects in cholesterol metabolism.

About one in 500 Americans have inherited a genetic deficiency in the ability to remove LDL-cholesterol from the bloodstream. This deficiency is known as *familial hypercholesterolemia,* and the affected individuals are highly susceptible to heart attacks at a young age. An even more prevalent genetic disorder is known as *familial combined hyperlipidemia.* It usually involves elevations of both cholesterol and triglycerides in family members. Genetic conditions such as these contribute to the tendency for coronary disease to run in families. If you have a relative who has had a heart attack or a stroke before age 60, you should have your own cholesterol level measured.

George was 32 years old when he suddenly noticed severe pressure in his chest and a feeling of indigestion. The discomfort seemed to spread into his left arm, and he remembered that his father had experienced similar symptoms during a heart attack at age 41. His wife dialed 911, and George was rushed by ambulance to the hospital emergency room. The diagnosis of heart attack was made, and he was hospitalized. Fortunately, he made a smooth recovery. The specialist who took care of George waited three months before ordering a cholesterol count, because he knew that heart attacks caused a temporary lowering of blood cholesterol, and that a normal count right after a heart attack could be deceptively reassuring.

When George's cholesterol was measured three months later, it was abnormally high, at 310 mg/dl. He had already quit smoking as of the day he was hospitalized, and was on a low-saturated-fat, low-cholesterol diet; he was also walking two miles every day for exercise. His weight and blood pressure were normal. George wanted to do everything he could to avoid any further atherosclerosis, and the first step, according to his doctor, was to repeat the measurement of his blood cholesterol to make certain of the level. The repeat test result was 326 mg/dl. The doctor reassured George that his cholesterol was not skyrocketing upward—that much difference between two tests was to be expected on the basis of normal, day-to-day variations. He informed George, however, that this level of cholesterol, especially in so young a man, who had a proven propensity to heart attack, demanded intervention.

George's LDL-cholesterol was measured, and was 238 mg/dl. Repeat values were 247 and 226 mg/dl, both very high levels. His triglyceride counts were normal. Tests for underlying conditions, such as hypothyroidism, diabetes, and liver and kidney disease were negative. The doctor concluded that George probably had the inherited disease known as familial hypercholesterolemia, and therefore ordered measurements of blood cholesterol in George's children and in all of his siblings. Two of George's four children did have elevated cholesterol elevations, in the high 200s. George and his two affected children are all now taking medication (see page 114) that successfully keeps their LDL-cholesterol levels under 130 mg/dl. They know that they must never smoke, and they stay physically active. George has had no further cardiac symptoms, and his children have had none. They are examples of the appropriate diagnosis and treatment of familial hypercholesterolemia.

Very-Low-Density Lipoproteins (VLDL)

Manufactured in the liver, very-low-density lipoproteins are vehicles that transport excess dietary carbohydrate and alcohol calories to our fat tissue for storage. When we eat, our food is digested and absorbed into the bloodstream, and the carbohydrate, alcohol, and protein are taken directly to the liver. The liver then processes these calories, storing some and secreting excess calories back into the bloodstream in the form of VLDL. These VLDL particles carry the calories, in the form of triglyceride, to adipose tissue, which extracts the triglyceride and stores it.

We've noted that you don't have to *eat* fat in order to *get* fat. If you consume excess calories, as alcohol or carbohydrates, for example, the liver will convert these excess calories into triglyceride, package them into very-low-density lipoproteins (VLDL), and secrete them into the bloodstream. The triglyceride in the VLDL will be extracted by your fat tissue, and *voilà*, your fat stores have grown.

After most of the triglyceride has been extracted from VLDL, the remaining lipoprotein particles, smaller and heavier because most of their triglyceride has been removed, are low-density lipoprotein (LDL) particles. Thus you can see that LDL derives from VLDL, and that certain factors, such as overeating, will increase *both* your VLDL- *and* LDL-cholesterol levels. Conversely, measures taken to reduce your VLDL production, such as losing weight or taking certain medications, may also reduce your LDL levels.

Roger, a carpenter, came to the doctor because of an itching rash on his buttocks. Although he was not dieting, he had been losing weight gradually, had mildly blurred vision, and had been quite thirsty for the past two months. Four or five beers helped assuage his thirst every night after work, he said. He had been overweight for some time.

When the doctor examined Roger, he saw that the rash looked like little red pimples with yellowish-white centers. Similar lesions were scattered over much of Roger's body. The doctor also noted that Roger was about 35 pounds overweight, had a severe infection of his gums, and also had an infected ingrown toenail. Looking into the back of Roger's eyes with an ophthalmoscope, the doctor detected an orangish hue in the blood vessels there, as though they contained cream of tomato soup instead of normal, red-looking blood. The doctor suspected that Roger had very high levels of triglyceride in his blood, and that the rash was actually the triglyceride-rich lipoprotein particles accumulating in the skin. He also suspected that the reason for Roger's high triglyceride level was that Roger had come down with diabetes mellitus.

Laboratory tests proved the doctor's hunch to be correct. The triglyceride level was over 16,000 mg/dl, and the cholesterol level was over 2,000 mg/dl. Diabetes plus obesity, plus beer intake, were combining to raise Roger's triglyceride-rich lipoprotein levels to astronomical heights. The gum and toe infections were making the diabetes worse.

Treatment was instituted immediately, and was directed toward the underlying problems. The doctor gave Roger a low-calorie, low-fat, no-alcohol diet as initial treatment of the diabetes. Since infections of any kind worsen diabetes, penicillin was prescribed, and a podiatrist performed a minor operation later that same day to relieve the infected ingrown toenail. The next day, a dentist treated the gum problems.

Roger's diabetes responded promptly to this treatment. His blood sugar, which had been twice normal, was down to normal within a week. By then his triglycerides had come down to 725 mg/dl, and his cholesterol to 268 mg/dl. His vision had improved, and the rash was subsiding. Roger was no longer thirsty, and his energy was much better. Two weeks later the triglycerides were only 335 mg/dl, and the cholesterol was normal at 198 mg/dl. Since then, Roger's triglyceride and cholesterol levels have remained stable, on diet and exercise. Even though his levels of triglyceride and cholesterol were extremely high when he first sought medical attention, he requires no medications.

In retrospect, Roger's severe hyperlipidemia appears to have been due to a combination of underlying factors including diabetes, alcohol intake, overeating, obesity, and a genetic defect causing the mild overproduction, or the decreased removal, of VLDL particles. Once the first four problems were corrected, the remaining mild hypertriglyceridemia probably could be attributed to the inherited defect, without which the levels of VLDL would probably never have gotten so high. The mild hypertriglyceridemia is not severe enough to endanger Roger's health, and requires no additional treatment.

Roger's case illustrates the important point that correcting underlying conditions can often correct hyperlipidemia, even without the need for drug therapy. Unlike George, Roger did not need medications to correct his blood lipids. Rational treatment of Roger's hyperlipidemia consisted simply of treating the underlying disorders that were causing the massive elevation of VLDL levels.

Chylomicrons

Chylomicrons, the other form of lipoprotein, are made in the intestine and are the means of transporting dietary fat through the bloodstream. Chylomicrons are similar to VLDL in that they are mostly triglyceride; they function to carry triglyceride (fat) to our adipose tissue for storage; and, after the triglyceride has been removed, the remaining particles can contribute to atherosclerosis.

When you eat lots of fat—such as the typical American meal of a hamburger, french fries, and a milkshake—the fat is absorbed and packaged into chylomicrons, which flow into the bloodstream. For several hours thereafter, high levels of triglycerides, in the form of chylomicrons, will be present in your bloodstream. Normally, within twelve hours all the triglycerides in chylomicrons will have been cleared out of your bloodstream. This is why measurements of your triglyceride levels are usually done after a 12-to-14-hour fast.

Fasting triglyceride levels of over 500–700 mg/dl put a person at risk for a very dangerous and painful condition known as *pancreatitis,* or inflammation of the pancreas. Such levels should be treated in order to prevent pancreatitis. The treatment usually involves reducing intake of fat and total calories, eliminating alcohol intake, and exercising regularly. It may also involve correcting an underlying problem, such as diabetes or alcoholism. Drugs that reduce VLDL and chylomicron levels, such as *gemfibrozil* (see page 118), may also be needed, at the discretion of your physician.

THE LIPID HYPOTHESIS: ONLY A THEORY?

As shown in Figure 5.1, the chances of your having a heart attack correlate directly with your cholesterol level. Likewise, LDL-cholesterol levels correlate with the risk of having a heart attack. HDL-cholesterol, on the other hand, shows an *inverse* correlation with coronary risk: The lower your HDL levels, the higher your coronary risk.

For many years, doctors and scientists were aware of the statistical correlation between cholesterol levels and heart attacks. But they were uncertain whether lowering the cholesterol levels would prevent heart attacks. Based on the correlation, they devised a theory known as "the lipid hypothesis."

The lipid hypothesis states that if you take steps to lower blood cholesterol levels, the incidence of heart attacks will drop. Testing this theory was a gigantic task because so many other factors, besides cholesterol, influence coronary risk. What was required for valid statistical analysis was to follow large numbers of individuals over several years' time. In some of the most expensive medical research projects ever conducted, the lipid hypothesis was resoundingly confirmed in middle-aged males; it is still being tested in other groups.

It is no longer a theory but a proven fact that, in at least some groups of people, lowering one's levels of cholesterol really does reduce the risk of heart attack. The benefits are quite remarkable: A 1-percent reduction in cholesterol concentration reduces heart-attack risk by about 2 percent. This is true over a wide range of blood cholesterol concentrations, down to at least 180 mg/dl. As expected, the benefit appears to be due to a drop in LDL-cholesterol levels.

What has not yet been proven, however, is that taking steps to raise your HDL-cholesterol level provides any cardiovascular protection. It appears likely that further research, looking at the individual types of particles or proteins within the HDL category, will be required to show which ones can and should be raised to produce a therapeutic benefit. At present, repeated measurements of HDL-cholesterol as a guide to medical therapy are not warranted. It's best to focus instead

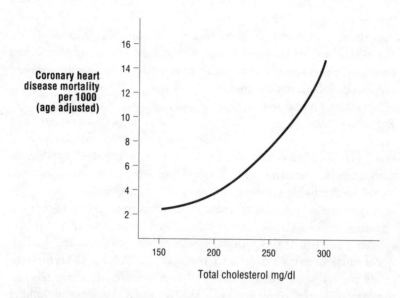

Figure 5.1 Coronary Risk vs. Blood Cholesterol

The relationship between blood cholesterol levels and the death rate from heart attack among 361,662 men, age 35–57 years, during six years of follow-up. In general, the higher the blood cholesterol, the higher the coronary death rate. The death rate for men with cholesterol levels about 260 mg/dl was three times higher than for men with levels around 200. Below 200 the curve starts to flatten out; for this reason, doctors seldom push patients to reduce total cholesterol level much below 200 mg/dl.

A curve depicting the relationship between LDL-cholesterol and coronary risk would look very similar to this one, except that the LDL-cholesterol levels would be about 70 points lower, so that the curve would flatten out around 130 mg/dl. For this reason, doctors tend to push for LDL-cholesterol levels around 130 mg/dl. A graph of HDL-cholesterol versus coronary risk, on the other hand, would look very different from this one, with high HDL-cholesterol levels corresponding to low levels of coronary risk, and lesser amounts of HDL corresponding to higher risk.

on your total cholesterol and LDL-cholesterol levels, and on bringing them down into a safe range.

MEASURING BLOOD CHOLESTEROL: SOME PRECAUTIONS

The national campaign to control cholesterol has generated so much awareness and concern that entrepreneurs have recognized the commercial possibilities it offers them. Many new products are competing for the resulting market in easily obtaining a measurement of one's cholesterol level. Some of the newest entrants into this field use a drop of blood, obtained by simply pricking the fingertip, to measure blood cholesterol. As such products continue to evolve, the consumer should keep several cautions in mind:

Cholesterol measurements are subject to human and technical error, and different methods of measurement give different answers. The degree of quality control varies widely among commercial laboratories, and state laws governing the quality of lab work are variable. In particular, the measurement of HDL-cholesterol levels has been notoriously unreliable in many commercial laboratories.

Proper quality control of cholesterol measurement involves using reference materials that have been certified and standardized to the reference method at the national Centers for Disease Control (CDC). A National Reference Method Laboratory Network has been established to help standardize cholesterol measurements, and the lab you use for cholesterol measurements should validate its work by linking into this reference network. Ideally, a laboratory would periodically split samples by sending one portion to the reference lab and doing its own measurement on the other portion. The lab's own measurement should be within 3 percent of that done at the reference lab. Good labs also ensure the quality of their work by participating in a proficiency-testing program, such as those provided by the American Association of Bioanalysts or the College of American Pathologists.

Unless the laboratory you use is adhering to these quality-control guidelines, we would be suspicious that its cholesterol measurements, especially for HDL-cholesterol, may be unreliable. As we shall see, if HDL-cholesterol measurements are unreliable, so are estimates of LDL-cholesterol, because they are based in part on the HDL-cholesterol result.

The measurement of LDL-cholesterol is indirect. What is actually measured is total cholesterol, HDL-cholesterol, and triglyceride, and these results are then used to calculate the estimated LDL-cholesterol.

Here, for example, is how the LDL-cholesterol results were obtained in the case of Stella, whose high blood cholesterol was due to high levels of HDL. Because tests were taken while Stella was fasting and did not have elevated triglycerides, it was assumed that no chylomicrons were present, and that therefore all of the cholesterol was present as VLDL, LDL, and HDL. The total cholesterol was measured directly at 267 mg/dl. VLDL-cholesterol was estimated by dividing the fasting triglyceride level by 5. This is the standard way of estimating VLDL-cholesterol, and is fairly reliable. In this instance, triglycerides were measured at 130 mg/dl, so the calculated VLDL-cholesterol was obtained by dividing 130 by 5. That gave an estimated VLDL-cholesterol of 26 mg/dl. HDL-cholesterol was measured at 125 mg/dl. Subtracting 26 for VLDL and 125 for HDL from the total cholesterol of 267 yields a difference of 116 mg/dl for the estimate of LDL-cholesterol.

As you can see from this example, errors in any of the three values actually measured—total cholesterol, total triglycerides, and HDL-cholesterol—will throw off the estimated LDL value.

Eating raises the cholesterol level relatively little (10 percent or less) in most people, but much more in some others. If the cholesterol level is elevated after a meal, the measurement should be repeated after a 12- to 14-hour fast (water and usual medications allowed, but no food).

HDL-cholesterol values may be misleading when triglyceride concentrations are high. Elevated triglyceride levels are usually associated with low HDL-cholesterol measurements. This is because VLDL and chylomicrons, the two types of lipoprotein particles that contain lots of triglyceride, take up cholesterol from HDL. When the VLDL and/or chylomicron levels are excessively high, therefore, HDL-cholesterol tends to be low, and may not be representative of cardiovascular risk. As noted earlier, while we measure HDL-cholesterol, we suspect that specific protein levels *within* HDL may be the components that are actually pertinent to cardiovascular risk. For these reasons, we tend to disregard HDL-cholesterol measurements when triglyceride levels are very high.

Acute illnesses, and also pregnancy, alter the cholesterol concentration. Consequently, readings taken during these circumstances are not representative of one's usual cholesterol level. Nevertheless, these are the times when patients are most likely to consult a doctor and have blood tests done. Make sure that decisions about your cholesterol management are based on measurements made when you are not acutely ill, not pregnant, and have not had a heart attack, a stroke, or surgery within the prior two months.

HOW HIGH IS TOO HIGH?

Since the relationship between blood cholesterol concentration and cardiovascular risk is continuous over a wide range, as shown in Table 5.1, there is no single desirable level of cholesterol that can be logically recommended for everyone. The cardiovascular risk associated with any particular level of cholesterol also depends on age, sex, smoking habits, activity level, family history, and other risk factors. We would not be concerned about a cholesterol level of 240 in a man 85 years of age with a family history of longevity free of coronary disease. On the other hand, a cholesterol level of 220 in a young smoker with a strong family history of heart disease would be of grave concern.

To get a feel for the numbers, and where you stand, you probably will want to have your own blood cholesterol level measured, and then see where you fit on the following table, adapted from data accumulated by the Lipid Research Clinics and published in the *Journal of the American Medical Association:*

Table 5.1   Plasma Cholesterol Concentrations (mg/dl) Associated with Increased Risk of Cardiovascular Disease

Age	High Risk (90th percentile)		Moderately High Risk (75th percentile)	
	Total Cholesterol	LDL-Cholesterol	Total Cholesterol	LDL-Cholesterol
Men				
0–14	170	120	173	106
15–19	183	123	165	109
20–29	216	148	194	128
30–39	244	171	218	149
40–49	254	180	231	160
50+	258	188	230	166
Women				
0–14	190	126	174	113
15–19	195	135	173	115
20–29	208	148	184	127
30–39	220	163	202	143
40–49	246	177	223	155
50+	281	195	252	170

As you can see by studying the above table, there are age- and sex-related variations in blood cholesterol. A level of 195 would be considered dangerous in a teenager, and would demand intervention to prevent the development of atherosclerosis. The same level would be considered excellent for someone in middle age. It is especially important to detect and correct hypercholesterolemia in young people,

since atherosclerosis is a process that progresses silently for many years
before the patient is suddenly seized with symptoms. For this reason,
screening for high cholesterol is especially important in the young.
Once you have already reached the age of 70 or 80, you may not
regard a heart attack as the disaster it surely would have been if it
had hit you in your forties or fifties.

Having determined your cholesterol level, you should confer with
your physician about all aspects of your health and your profile of
cardiovascular risk (including your age, family history, blood pressure,
body weight, activity level, tobacco usage, tendency toward diabetes,
and cholesterol level). Then the two of you can decide whether atherosclerosis threatens your health enough to warrant preventive action.

The U.S. government's National Cholesterol Education Program
promotes simplified guidelines for desirable cholesterol levels that
apply only to adults over age 40. The purpose in giving such simplified
guidelines is to ensure ease of widespread usage. We reproduce the
guidelines below, in Table 5.2, because they are used by doctors and
laboratories throughout the country, but we prefer to base our own
treatment on the data displayed in Table 5.1.

Table 5.2   Guidelines of
the National Cholesterol Education Program

	Total Cholesterol	LDL-Cholesterol
Desirable:	under 200 mg/dl	under 130 mg/dl
Borderline-high:	200–239 mg/dl	130–159
High:	240 mg/dl or more	160 mg/dl or more

As you can see by comparing them to Table 5.1, the guidelines in
Table 5.2 are simplified, and do not apply to younger age groups, for
whom cholesterol screening is particularly important, and in whom
lower cutoff points are recommended. Moreover, these simplified
guidelines could lead to undue concern in old age groups, where resistance to atherosclerosis has already been demonstrated, and where
a heart attack might be no more severe an event than the alternatives.
We know that the human organism virtually never outlives the age of
120 years. (Isolated reports to the contrary appear to be due to faulty
record-keeping.) It is in the young that atherosclerosis is especially
devastating and needs most to be prevented.

Some people seem relatively young at 70 or 80—we don't presume
to specify any particular cutoff point for youth or middle age. The

general guidelines presented here should be adapted, with your physician, to your own specific situation. For example, if you have already suffered a heart attack, you are obviously at serious risk for atherosclerosis. In such a case, you may want to aim for a total cholesterol of under 180, and an LDL-cholesterol of under 120, as well as work on all other risk factors, including blood pressure and smoking. If you do have other risk factors, even borderline-high cholesterol values may be too high for you and may require treatment.

CORRECTING AN ELEVATED CHOLESTEROL COUNT

You don't "cure" a high cholesterol level in the same sense that you usually cure a strep throat with ten days of penicillin treatment. Neither six weeks nor six months of a "cholesterol cure" permanently corrects a high cholesterol level. Like your weight, your blood cholesterol concentration tends to return to its previous stable level unless you make some fundamental changes *on a continuing basis.*

Diet, exercise, and medications are the three major classes of treatment for elevated blood cholesterol.

Detecting and Treating Underlying Diseases

As we noted in the case of Roger, many instances of high cholesterol are due to some other, underlying disease, such as diabetes mellitus, hypothyroidism (also known as "underactive thyroid"), liver disease, certain kidney diseases, excess alcohol intake, and obesity. In those cases, and they are frequent, the blood lipid problem disappears when the underlying disease is treated. Roger's case involved very high blood levels of both cholesterol and triglyceride, and responded beautifully to treatment of underlying conditions—diabetes, obesity, and excess alcohol intake—that were causing the hyperlipidemia.

Diabetes mellitus. Diabetes is a very common condition, characterized by the presence of too much food in the bloodstream. When we eat, food is digested into simple building blocks, then absorbed into the bloodstream. The bloodstream acts as a transportation system to carry the food to various body tissues. Normally the food then leaves the bloodstream and enters the tissues under the influence of the hormone insulin. In diabetes, however, there is inadequate insulin action, due to insulin deficiency, defective insulin, or tissue resistance to the action of insulin. Consequently, food—carbohydrate, protein, and fat—remains in the bloodstream in excessive amounts, resulting in abnormally high levels of blood sugar, blood amino acids (the building blocks of protein), and blood fats (cholesterol, triglycerides, and free fatty acids). Elevated cholesterol and triglyceride, therefore, can be part and parcel of diabetes mellitus. The successful treatment of the diabetes, whether by diet, exercise, pills, or insulin shots, reduces the blood levels of cholesterol and triglyceride as well as sugar. In poorly controlled diabetes, the blood levels of VLDL- and LDL-cholesterol tend to be high, and levels of HDL-cholesterol tend to be low. Successful treatment raises HDL-cholesterol while reducing VLDL and LDL levels.

Diabetes often runs in families, especially the type of diabetes that comes on in adult life and with obesity. Typical symptoms begin with thirst, increased urination, and blurred vision, then progress to weight loss, fatigue, and sometimes even coma. Other cases, however, smolder unnoticed for years and don't come to medical attention until detected by routine blood-test screening, or until nerve damage, with numbness or pain or impotence, drives the patient to a doctor. Sometimes diabetes-induced atherosclerosis causes a heart attack before the diagnosis of diabetes is made. If you have such symptoms, you should have your doctor check you for diabetes.

Hypothyroidism. The thyroid gland is located in the neck. It produces a chemical substance known as *thyroid hormone,* which it secretes into the bloodstream. Deficiency of thyroid hormone is called *hypothyroidism.* Thyroid hormone affects virtually every tissue in the body, and its deficiency can manifest itself in many different ways, including a high blood concentration of cholesterol. The treatment of hypothyroidism consists of taking thyroid hormone orally, in pill form. In proper dosage, this treatment corrects all the manifestations of hypothyroidism, including hypercholesterolemia.

Common symptoms of hypothyroidism include fatigue, chilliness, constipation, dry skin, muscle cramps, fluid retention, and weight gain. These symptoms are obviously very common, and are experienced by all of us at one time or another. They are not conclusive in themselves, and may be due to many other conditions besides hypothyroidism. To find out whether such symptoms indicate hypothyroidism, one must measure the amount of thyroid hormone in the bloodstream. This simple lab test is readily available. An even more sensitive test for hypothyroidism is performed by measuring the blood level of *thyroid-stimulating hormone* (TSH), a hormone released from the pituitary gland in response to thyroid deficiency. An elevated TSH can detect even very mild cases of hypothyroidism. If the TSH test is above normal, treatment with thyroid hormone may correct an elevated level of blood cholesterol.

Liver disease. Certain diseases of the liver, especially those involving blockage of the flow of bile, cause elevations of blood cholesterol. The liver normally excretes cholesterol into the bile. Bile is a digestive juice made in the liver, stored in the gallbladder, and secreted into the intestine at mealtimes. When cholesterol cannot escape into bile, it backs up into the bloodstream. This is called *biliary obstruction,* and its symptoms can include itching, jaundice (a yellow discoloration of the skin and especially the whites of the eyes), nausea, and lack of appetite. Usually the liver disease has come to medical attention before cholesterol becomes an issue. But if cholesterol elevations are detected by routine screening, the doctor will often want to do some blood tests to make sure liver disease is not the underlying cause of the hypercholesterolemia.

Kidney disease. Certain types of kidney disease involve the leakage of massive amounts of protein from the blood into the urine, and are referred to as *nephrotic syndrome* or *nephrosis.* These conditions are often characterized by fluid retention and by elevated levels of triglycerides and/or cholesterol. As with obstructive liver disease, the kidney disease has usually become evident before the blood-fat problems attract attention. A urine test for the presence of protein is a simple, reliable, and inexpensive way to screen for nephrotic syndrome.

Excess alcohol intake. Especially in people with an underlying inherited defect of triglyceride metabolism, such as that manifested by Roger in the case described earlier, alcohol intake can cause remarkable rises in VLDL levels. Sometimes it causes the triglycerides to climb high enough to trigger pancreatitis. The amount of alcohol required to cause such problems varies greatly from individual to individual. For most people a beer or two per day will not make much difference in their blood lipids, and may even slightly raise their HDL-cholesterol levels. For others, especially those with genetic predisposition to hyperlipidemia, or with another underlying condition such as diabetes, even moderate alcohol intake can induce dangerous rises in blood triglyceride concentrations. If your blood triglycerides are over 500 mg/dl, you are at risk for possible pancreatitis, and you should see how much improvement in your triglyceride level will result from stopping the intake of alcohol.

Obesity. As we noted earlier, obesity—especially abdominal obesity—leads to elevations in blood triglycerides and cholesterol. It appears to do this by way of the increased production of VLDL in the liver. Weight reduction is typically accompanied by reduction in VLDL levels and, to a lesser extent, in LDL levels. HDL-cholesterol levels often rise with successful weight reduction. Since all of these effects are beneficial, the normalization of weight is a basic part of treatment for all cases of hyperlipidemia in obese persons.

Poor diet. We include diet as a cause of hyperlipidemia because dietary cholesterol raises the blood cholesterol in some people, and eating lots of saturated fats raises it in most people. Generous intake of carbohydrates or of alcohol raises VLDL (and therefore triglyceride) levels in some people. Changing the diet is, of course, a good way to treat hyperlipidemia caused by eating too much of the wrong foods. In general, improving the diet helps most people with hyperlipidemia, even if their diet was no worse than the American norm in the first place.

Medications that raise blood lipoprotein levels. A number of commonly prescribed medications can elevate your blood cholesterol. These drugs include certain heart and blood-pressure medications known as *beta-blockers,* diuretics in the thiazide category, and, for some people, birth-control pills. Some patients' high blood lipids return to normal when these medications are stopped.

Beta-blockers are an entire class of very widely used medications, and are beneficial in many cases of high blood pressure, angina (chest pain due to the blockage of arteries to the heart), heart attack, glaucoma, heart rhythm problems, migraine headache, and overactivity of the thyroid gland. The chemical names of most beta-blockers end with the suffix -*olol,* such as *propranolol* and *metoprolol.* Some people react to these medications with increased blood cholesterol and/or triglycerides, while others do not. If your blood lipids are dangerously elevated, and you take beta-blocker medication, your doctor may wish to try some other treatment to see whether your blood lipid levels improve.

Thiazide diuretics are widely used to treat high blood pressure, heart failure, and edema. They work on the kidney to induce the release of salt and water into the urine. Frequently they induce a mild to moderate elevation of VLDL levels. Now that many other medications are available for the treatment of high blood pressure and heart failure, doctors often avoid the use of thiazide diuretics when blood triglycerides or cholesterol are elevated.

Birth-control pills, also called oral contraceptives, often cause some elevation of blood cholesterol and trigylcerides. So does pregnancy, which involves hormones similar to those found in oral contraceptives. The effects of birth-control pills on atherosclerosis are still a matter of controversy and the subject of continuing medical investigation. A prudent approach would be to check the blood cholesterol and triglyceride levels of persons who take birth-control pills, especially if they have risk factors for atherosclerosis such as diabetes, high blood pressure, smoking, or a family history of heart disease at a young age.

CHANGE YOUR DIET TO LOWER YOUR CHOLESTEROL

Once you have corrected any underlying disease or drug that caused high blood cholesterol, diet is the correct starting point for any further attempt at cholesterol reduction. Many good books full of delicious low-cholesterol recipes are available. Often you can simply modify your own recipes to cut down on fat and cholesterol. The essentials of dietary treatment are as follows:

- reducing the intake of saturated fat and cholesterol
- correcting any obesity, which usually means reducing total fat intake
- using monounsaturated or polyunsaturated fat instead of saturated fat
- increasing the intake of water-soluble fiber

Keeping these objectives in mind, let's look at the main food groups and their content of fat, cholesterol, and fiber. More detailed information on cholesterol and saturated fat in foods can be obtained from your local chapter of the American Heart Association, which also offers an excellent handbook, *Dietary Treatment of Hypercholesterolemia: A Manual for Patients,* published in 1988.

Meat, Poultry, and Fish

Since cholesterol is found only in animal products, this food group is a major source of cholesterol. It also contributes saturated fat. Reducing your intake of cholesterol and saturated fat means cutting way down on "organ meats," such as liver, and red meats, such as beef, pork, and lamb.

The fat in poultry meat, such as chicken and turkey, is less saturated than that in red meat. Poultry meat and red meat, however, contain similar amounts of cholesterol. Since saturated-fat intake is even more important than cholesterol intake in its effect on blood cholesterol, poultry is preferable to red meat for those who need to reduce blood cholesterol.

Even within categories such as red meat and poultry, there are important differences in fat content. For example, the dark meat of poultry contains more fat than the white meat. Some cuts of red meat contain more fat than others. Lean cuts of meat are listed on page 223, in chapter 10. Most processed meats, such as sausage, weiners, and luncheon meat, are very high in saturated fats. So are cuts of red meat that are heavily marbled with fat.

The method of preparing meat also makes a big difference in cholesterol and saturated-fat intake. To minimize fat and cholesterol, trim away all visible fat from meat and remove skin and visible fat from poultry before cooking. After cooking meat for soup or stew, or when using juices for gravy, allow it to cool so that most of the fat can rise to the top and be skimmed off before the other ingredients are added. Cook meats by methods that use little or no added fat, such as broiling, barbecuing, stewing, or roasting. Limit frying, basting, and sautéing, since these methods tend to add fat. Breaded meats fried in fat, such as fried chicken or chicken-fried steak, are heavily laden with fats and oils. Since ground meat tends to be higher in fat than non-ground meat, limit use of the former. Buy only the leanest ground beef, turkey, and pork. Pour off fat after browning.

Most fish are relatively low in fat and cholesterol. Moreover, their fats tend to be unsaturated and to contain omega-3 fatty acids (see chapter 4). This is probably why studies in several countries have shown that people who eat more fish tend to have fewer heart attacks. Although some forms of shellfish are higher in cholesterol than other seafood, their fats tend to be unsaturated, and they are no longer on the list of foods forbidden to people with high cholesterol. They can be eaten in moderate portions.

Since even lean meat, poultry, and fish contain some saturated fat and cholesterol, those who need to reduce blood cholesterol should limit their portions of these to about six ounces per day.

Meats, poultry, and fish are good sources of zinc, iron, and protein. If intake of these foods is severely restricted, vitamin and mineral supplements, and other sources of protein such as legumes and low-fat dairy products, may be needed for balanced nutrition.

Eggs

Egg whites are a good source of protein. The yolk contains the cholesterol and saturated fat, as can be seen in Table 5.3. In a diet aimed at lowering blood cholesterol, two or three egg yolks per week may be allowed. But if cholesterol remains elevated after several months on a low-cholesterol, low-saturated-fat diet, egg yolks should be restricted to no more than one per week.

In many cases it is possible to use only the whites of eggs in cooking; for example, two egg whites can be used in place of each whole egg in muffins, cookies, and pudding. Egg substitutes provide the egg white with the yolk already removed. Some may contain vegetable oils, but they contain little saturated fat and virtually no cholesterol.

Dairy Products

The lower the amount of fat in a dairy product, the lower the content of cholesterol and saturated fat. Skim (nonfat) milk provides the nutrients needed for good nutrition without the cholesterol and saturated fat. Cheeses made with skim milk, such as mozzarella, skim-milk Swiss, low-fat cottage cheese, and farmer's cheese, are lower in saturated fat and cholesterol than are most other cheeses. Some newer varieties of low-fat cheeses are becoming available, including gammelost, sapsago, and hoop or baker's cheese. Nondairy cheese and other nondairy products contain no cholesterol, but may have significant amounts of saturated fat. Nondairy cream, sour cream, whipped topping, and nondairy coffee-cream substitutes often contain coconut oil, palm oil, palm-kernel oil, hydrogenated vegetable oils, or a combination of these undesirable, highly saturated oils. These products should not be used as substitutes for dairy products, even though the label correctly states "no cholesterol," since they lack the nutritional value of dairy products and they contain saturated fats that raise blood cholesterol. Possible healthy substitutions would include nonfat plain yogurt for sour cream, whipped skim evaporated milk for whipped cream, and skim evaporated milk for coffee creamer.

When evaluating the information on the labels of these foods, think carefully of the portion size that you are likely to use. For example, if you normally use one-quarter cup of the product, but the label portion size is two tablespoons, you would need to double the indicated fat and calories.

Table 5.3 Fat and Cholesterol Content of Some Common Foods

	Total fat (grams)	Saturated fat (grams)	Cholesterol (milligrams)
Meat/Poultry/Fish			
Beef arm, roasted lean only, 3 oz.	6	3	77
Ground beef, cooked lean, 3 oz.	15	6	80
Beef liver, fried, 3 oz.	9	2	372
Chicken, roasted without skin, 3 oz.	6	2	76
Halibut filets, broiled with margarine, 3 oz.	6	1	48
Eggs			
Egg, 1 large			
1 yolk	6	2	215
1 white	trace	0	0
Dairy Products			
Milk, whole, 1 cup	8	5	33
Milk, skim, 1 cup	1	trace	5
Cheese, cheddar, 1 oz.	9	6	30
Cheese, mozzarella, part skim milk, 1 oz.	5	3	15
Butter, 1 tablespoon	12	7	33
Fats/Oils			
Margarine, 1 tablespoon	12	2	0
Vegetable oil, 1 tablespoon (excluding palm, palm kernel and coconut oil)	14	2	0
Lard, 1 tablespoon	13	5	12
Fruits/Vegetables			
Potato, baked, 1 medium	trace	trace	0
Potato, fried, 10 strips	8	3	0
Potato chips, 2 oz.	20	5	0
Cabbage, ½ cup	trace	trace	0

	Total fat (grams)	Saturated fat (grams)	Cholesterol (milligrams)
Fruits/Vegetables (*cont.*)			
Apple, 1 medium	trace	trace	0
Banana, 1 medium	1	trace	0
Breads/Cereals/Grains			
Bread, 1 slice	1	trace	0
Bagel, 1	2	trace	0
Doughnut, yeast, 1	13	5	21
Oatmeal, ½ cup	1	trace	0
Rice, plain, ½ cup	trace	trace	0
Cookie, oatmeal, 1	2	1	1
Brownie, 1	13	4	15

Adapted from "How to Have Your Cake and Eat It Too: A Painless Guide to Low-fat, Low-cholesterol Eating," a pamphlet published in 1987 by the American Heart Association.

Fats and Oils: Some Guidelines

As mentioned earlier, saturated fats—those that tend to be solid at room temperature—tend to raise blood cholesterol. The terms *hydrogenated* or *hardened* mean the saturated fatty acid content is higher than in the original oil. This is why physicians and dietitians recommend "tub" margarines rather than the firmer, more saturated ones that come in bars and sticks. Be sure to select margarines with liquid oil as the first ingredient on the label, since ingredients are listed in order of abundance. Butter is high in saturated fats and cholesterol, and its use should be minimized. Since coconut oil, palm oil, and palm-kernel oil (the so-called "tropical" oils) contain more saturated than unsaturated fat, these should be avoided. Make it a habit to read labels on containers of commercial cookies, crackers, and candies, where these oils are often found.

Use monounsaturated and polyunsaturated fats and oils instead of saturated ones. Monounsaturated and polyunsaturated fats and oils tend to reduce blood cholesterol levels. But remember that fats and oils are high in calories, whether they are saturated or not. If you need to reduce your weight, you will have to go easy on all types of fat and oil.

Most Americans already eat a very high-fat diet, and should reduce total fat intake in order to lower their cholesterol intake. The United States Surgeon General and numerous research groups and institutions, including the American Heart Association and the Committee on Diet and Health of the National Research Council, have recommended reducing fat intake to less than 30 percent of total calories. At 1,500 total calories per day, this would mean 50 grams of fat (or oil) per day. You can verify this by remembering that each gram of fat contains 9 calories. Therefore, 50 grams of fat times 9 calories per gram equals 450 calories from fat, which is 30 percent of 1,500. For every 100 calories over or under 1,500, you can add or subtract 3 grams of fat to remain within the guideline, since 3 grams of fat times 9 calories per gram equals 27 calories as fat.

Additional guidelines indicate that saturated fats should account for only 7–10 percent of the total calories, or 11–15 grams, while the intake of monounsaturated fats should be 10–15 percent or 15–25 grams, and 10 percent of total calories, or 15 grams, should be polyunsaturated. Consulting with a registered dietitian can help ensure that your diet conforms to these guidelines.

Vegetable oils such as corn oil, cottonseed oil, and soybean oil are naturally unsaturated, and are classified as polyunsaturated. Olive oil, canola oil, and peanut oil are monounsaturated. Olive oil appears to be particularly beneficial, and may account for some of the low cholesterol levels—and low rates of heart attacks—seen in certain populations around the Mediterranean. Canola oil, made from rapeseed, has a beneficial effect similar to olive oil. Since polyunsaturated oils contain the essential fatty acids, it is important to include these in your diet, even though they tend to lower HDL-cholesterol as well as LDL-cholesterol. One way to include them is to use margarine as your source of polyunsaturated fat and to use monounsaturated oils for all other fat uses, such as salad oil and cooking.

Once again, remember that *all* fats are high in calories, and their intake should be limited by people who need to lose weight. Obese people with high cholesterol levels should severely limit both fat and calorie intake.

Breads, Cereals, and Grains

Grains contain no cholesterol and very little fat, and contribute fiber to the diet; they should be used generously. Because most breads are made with little or no fat or oil, they are good choices. Take care, however, about what gets spread on top of the bread, since this is where we find butter, margarine, peanut butter, cream cheese, and other concoctions rich in fat. When making muffins, cornbread, rolls, pancakes, or waffles, you can modify the recipes to eliminate egg yolks, as we noted earlier. When buying crackers, cookies, pastries, and other commercial snack foods made with grain, remember to read labels for the fat content, which is often considerable.

Vegetables and Fruits

This food group has little or no fat except in avocados and olives. The fats in avocados and olives are mostly mono- and polyunsaturated. How the vegetables and fruits are prepared for meals must be carefully considered, however, since adding butter, cream, or cheese adds fat. Fried vegetables contain relatively high amounts of saturated fat and cholesterol, as shown in Table 5.3.

Vegetables and fruits are good sources of fiber, as shown in Table 5.4.

Table 5.4   Soluble Fiber Content of Some Common Foods

Food, serving size	Grams of soluble fiber
Graham cracker, 2, 2½ in. square	.33
Macaroni, raw, ¼ cup	.34
Oat bran, ⅓ cup	2.01
Rolled oats, ⅓ cup	1.33
White bread, 1 slice	.28
Whole-wheat bread, 1 slice	.34
White rice, raw, ⅙ cup	.25
Garbanzo beans, canned, ⅙ cup	.16
Green beans, canned, ½ cup	.45
Kidney beans, canned, ½ cup	1.45
Lentils, dried, cooked, ½ cup	.56
Lima beans, canned, ½ cup	.79
Navy beans, dried, cooked, ½ cup	2.29
Pinto beans, canned, ½ cup	1.10
Asparagus, canned, ½ cup	.51
Broccoli, frozen, ½ cup	.98
Brussels sprouts, frozen, ½ cup	1.42
Potato, white, raw, ½ cup	.77
Apple, raw, 1 small	.97
Orange, California seedless navel, 1 small	1.13
Peach, canned, ½ cup	.78
Pear, canned, ½ cup	.79
Plum, canned, purple, ½ cup	.19

Reprinted from M. S. Lawrence and J. W. Anderson, "Dietary Fiber Content of Selected Foods," *American Journal of Clinical Nutrition* 47 (1988): 440–47.

Fiber

Grains, fruits, and vegetables contain fiber. Some of the fiber dissolves in water; this is called *water-soluble,* or simply *soluble,* fiber. Other fiber does not dissolve in water, and is referred to as *insoluble.* Our intake of insoluble fiber helps prevent and relieve constipation, but does not lower blood levels of cholesterol. Intake of soluble fiber, on the other hand, may help reduce cholesterol. In particular, oat-bran fiber and legume fibers are useful in reducing cholesterol. In choosing oat fiber, however, look closely at what else is included in any particular food product. Many "granola" preparations and some oat-bran cereals, for example, are loaded with calories from saturated oils. Bran muffins are often high in fat. The mere presence of oat bran or some other soluble fiber does not mean a product is low in fat.

The effects of soluble fiber intake on cholesterol level are modest, and require fairly generous amounts of fiber. Many products that contain oat bran don't have enough of it to make a significant difference. Read the label. At least five grams of soluble fiber per day, in conjunction with a low-fat diet, are needed to achieve a measurable benefit.

BECOME A LABEL READER

Check to see how many grams of fat are present, and what percentage is saturated. Remember that cholesterol is found only in animal products. Therefore, the fact that a vegetable product contains no cholesterol is nothing to brag about. You will see that many vegetable foods high in saturated fats, such as potato chips and granola cereal, often come in packages advertising "no cholesterol." Of course they have no cholesterol, since they are not of animal origin, but they may have lots of saturated fat, and therefore tend to raise your blood cholesterol level as well as your weight. Remember that saturated-fat content is more important than cholesterol content in terms of impact on your blood cholesterol level.

Ingredients are listed on labels in the order of their abundance *by weight* in the food product. This is important, since fat is higher in calories than are other foods, and although it may be farther down the label than other ingredients, it is still higher than those ingredients in the percentage of total calories that it contributes to the product. Because fat is light in weight but high in calories, a food can be under 30 percent fat *by weight,* but far more than 30 percent fat *in calories.*

You can easily determine the percentage of calories as fat and the grams of fat by using the following formulas:

$$\text{Percent fat} = \text{fat calories/total calories} \times 100\%$$
$$\text{Grams of fat} = \text{fat calories} \div 9$$
$$\text{Fat calories} = \text{grams of fat} \times 9$$

Consider the portion size indicated on the label, since it may not correspond to your own usual serving. Current law does not require labels to display saturated-fat content if it is less than one gram per serving, and some companies use a very small portion size to avoid having to display this information. The U.S. Food and Drug Administration is currently reviewing regulations on labeling so that the consumer is not misled in this way.

If the information you need is not indicated on the label, it's a good idea not to use the product until you can determine the content by contacting the company. This kind of encouragement from consumers may stimulate companies to provide more candid nutrition information on their labels.

BATTLING THE BULGE

Most overweight people with high blood cholesterol will benefit from weight reduction. We've noted that correcting obesity reduces the production of VLDL. Consequently, weight reduction reduces triglyceride levels. Because LDL derives from VLDL, weight reduction often also reduces LDL-cholesterol (the "bad" kind). Happily, weight reduction also raises the level of HDL-cholesterol. Because so many people with high blood cholesterol and/or triglyceride also need to lose weight, most of them need to reduce their intake of fat.

CONSULT A TRAINED PROFESSIONAL

If you are serious about reducing your cholesterol level, consulting with a registered dietitian is an excellent investment, especially if your own initial attempts at dietary reform do not succeed. Depending on your location, a typical one-hour session with such a professional might cost from $45 to $85, and would include an individualized analysis of your present diet as well as specific dietary modifications that would be reasonable for your particular life-style. As you implement these changes in your transition to a better way of eating, follow-up sessions with the dietitian can be especially important. Many health-insurance policies cover this service if you are referred by your physician (see chapter 10).

To summarize the dietary therapy for high blood cholesterol:

Reduce your intake of saturated fats and oils. This means cutting down on animal fats, such as cream, butter, whole milk, most cheeses, sausages, cold cuts and lunch meats, and red meat such as beef, pork, and lamb. It also means reducing the intake of coconut, palm-kernel, and palm oil, and of vegetable oils that have been artificially saturated or hydrogenated. It means choosing softer margarines and low-fat cheeses, and eating a diet in which the greater percentage of the calories is derived from grains, vegetables, and fruits.

Reduce your intake of cholesterol. In practical terms, this means eliminating egg yolks, organ meats such as liver, and fatty cuts of meat.

Use unsaturated fats and oils instead of saturated ones. Corn oil, cottonseed oil, soybean oil, olive oil, and canola oil are good choices. Since the fats in fish and poultry meat are less saturated than those in mammal meat, they are preferable as sources of fat and protein in your diet.

If you are obese, reduce the total intake of fats and calories. In place of fats, use more vegetables, fruits, and grains. Go easy on all types of fat and oil. Most Americans already eat a very high-fat diet, and should reduce their total fat intake to less than 30 percent of total calories.

Become a label-reader.

If necessary, consult a registered dietitian.

EXERCISE AS A TREATMENT FOR HIGH BLOOD CHOLESTEROL

Like diet, exercise has tremendous benefits if it is practiced consistently. Occasional bursts of physical activity, however, carry no more benefit than do intermittent spasms of dieting. Because exercise must be regular and persistent to be of any lasting value, it is important to be realistic about what kind you decide to engage in. The trick is to find something you enjoy enough to do several times a week.

The benefits of exercise include

- Increasing HDL-cholesterol levels
- Lowering triglyceride and LDL-cholesterol levels
- Facilitating weight reduction
- Promoting cardiovascular health through lowering blood pressure and improving heart function, apart from any influence on blood lipids

Picking types of exercise that are safe for you, and that you enjoy enough to keep doing, is much more important than the particular type of exercise you choose. Walking, swimming, bicycling, tennis, gymnastics, aerobics, rowing, racquetball, dancing, skiing, mowing the lawn, digging in the garden, strolling through the mall on your lunch hour, vacuuming, and playing golf without a cart all count. Intending to exercise tomorrow doesn't.

Chapter 11 deals with exercise in detail. Let us simply remind you here that exercise temporarily strains the heart. If you have a history of heart attack or chest pain, or if you are over 40 and not already exercising regularly and successfully, or if you have a high cholesterol level and are therefore at increased risk for heart disease, consult your doctor before embarking on a vigorous exercise program.

MEDICATIONS TO LOWER BLOOD CHOLESTEROL

Drug therapy is usually reserved for those individuals with cholesterol and/or triglyceride levels determined to be in the high-risk range. Even though one of the important medications to treat hyperlipidemia—niacin—is available without prescription, it should be taken only under the direction of a doctor.

Because the measurement of cholesterol can be variable, more than one measurement of your cholesterol level is in order before drug therapy is begun. Remember that drug therapy, like diet and exercise, must take place on a regular basis. Before committing you to ten, twenty, forty, or more years of medications, your doctor will want to assess how well you can do with diet and exercise alone.

The benefits of cholesterol-lowering drugs are *additive* to the benefits of diet and exercise. This means that it is necessary for you to continue a good diet and exercise program while you take these drugs, rather than mistakenly assuming that a medication means you don't have to worry about what you eat or whether you exercise.

The effective medications currently approved for use and available in the U.S. for lowering cholesterol are (1) the bile-acid-binding resins, (2) niacin, (3) drugs derived from fibric acid, (4) probucol, and (5) lovastatin.

Bile-Acid-Binding Resins

The two drugs in this category, *cholestyramine* (sold as Questran) and *colestipol* (sold as Colestid), work in the same manner. They are not absorbed into the body. Taken by mouth, they pass through the intestinal tract and exit in the feces. In so doing, they trap a breakdown product of cholesterol and carry it out of the body. This breakdown product of cholesterol is called bile acid, or bile salt.

Bile acids are natural detergents that are important in digestion. When we eat a meal, the gallbladder contracts and squirts into the intestine a digestive juice known as bile. Bile, which is made in the liver and stored in the gallbladder, contains bile acids that emulsify (disperse finely) the fat in our food so it can be better digested and absorbed. After they have done their work, the bile acids are reabsorbed farther down the intestine and recycled. A small fraction of the bile acid is not reabsorbed and escapes in the feces. The liver makes up for this normal fecal loss of bile acids by manufacturing more bile acids from cholesterol.

Bile-acid-binding resins work by trapping bile acids in the intestine, preventing their reabsorption. Since bile enters the intestine when food arrives there, the resins are best taken with meals, though a bedtime dose also helps. The trapping of bile acids by the resins interrupts the recycling process and carries the bile acids out of the body in the feces. The liver readily compensates for this increased loss of bile acids by breaking down more cholesterol into bile acids. In this manner, bile-acid-binding resins put a drain on body cholesterol stores.

The main side effects of the bile-acid-binding resins are constipation and gassiness. Most people can effectively manage the constipation by adding a natural vegetable laxative made from psyllium seed. These are sold under several brand names. Bile acids bind to them weakly, and they thereby enhance the cholesterol-lowering effect of the bile-acid-binding resins. Like the resins, the psyllium-seed laxative must be taken with water or juice, never dry. You can mix it right in the same glass of juice with the resin, and drink them together. Don't worry—it doesn't taste as bad as it sounds.

The bile-acid-binding resins come in the form of little particles about the size of sand grains. Some people object to their taste and gritty texture, but find them much more palatable if they mix up a day's supply the night before in a jug of orange juice, and let it dissolve overnight in the refrigerator. The next day they simply shake the jug, pour out a glass of juice, and drink it with meals and at bedtime. A few people prefer to take these medications in a newly available "candy bar" form.

Most experts consider these resins the first line in drug therapy for high blood cholesterol. These were the drugs that scientists used to confirm most definitively the lipid hypothesis described earlier. The studies showed that the drugs produced significant drops in total cholesterol, LDL-cholesterol, and heart-attack rates, without serious side effects. Using this treatment, physicians have been able to lower blood cholesterol levels, especially LDL-cholesterol, to prevent heart attacks, and to rid patients of unsightly and unwanted cholesterol deposits in the skin, safely and effectively.

Niacin (Nicotinic Acid)

Niacin, a natural vitamin, effectively lowers cholesterol when taken in huge doses, much larger than those required for its function as a vitamin. When used in such large doses, niacin is considered a drug, even though it is available without prescription. Like other powerful drugs, niacin has side effects as well as benefits.

Like the bile-acid-binding resins, large doses of niacin have been shown to reduce total cholesterol, LDL-cholesterol, and heart attacks. Some practitioners prefer it to bile-acid-binding resins as first-line drug therapy. Most patients, however, find it more difficult to take in adequate dosage than the resins. Like the resins, niacin can usually reduce cholesterol levels by about 15–30 percent.

Niacin appears to work by reducing the production of VLDL particles in the liver. Since VLDL particles become LDL as they give up their triglyceride to body fat stores, taking niacin reduces LDL-cholesterol as well as total cholesterol and triglyceride levels.

Because it slows down production of lipoproteins, niacin works beautifully in combination with bile-acid-binding resins: the resins increase the extraction of cholesterol from the bloodstream while niacin blocks its input. Used together, they can bring cholesterol levels all the way down to normal in many cases of familial hypercholesterolemia.

Large doses of niacin—up to 2,500 milligrams three times a day—

are often required for maximal benefit, though lower doses can offer some benefit. Patients cannot start therapy with such large doses, however, because of side effects, particularly "flushing" (see below) and gastrointestinal upset. Your physician would probably start you with a low dose of niacin in the form of *nicotinic acid* (as little as 50 or 100 milligrams three times daily, if necessary, to minimize side effects), go slowly, and build up gradually. Ulcers of the stomach or duodenum also may reactivate or flare up during niacin treatment. The side effects can be minimized by taking the medication with meals.

"Flushing," the main side effect of niacin therapy, is a feeling of intense warmth and a reddening of the skin, which come on shortly after taking a dose. This is often accompanied by itching. It subsides gradually as you continue to take the same dosage level three times daily. Then you can increase the dosage, patiently go through the flushing and itching again until they subside, and so on up the dosage ladder. If you go off your medication for even a day or two, your symptoms will probably return, and you may have to go back down the ladder to a much smaller dose in order to tolerate the drug, then escalate again. By gradually building up the dose, most patients can tolerate adequate doses of niacin.

If flushing is very bothersome despite gradual escalation of dosage, one can reduce it by taking a single aspirin tablet each morning, or, if necessary, one tablet 30 minutes before each dose of niacin. Aspirin greatly reduces the severity of the flush, and may be needed for only a few days while your body gets used to each new, increased dosage.

To reduce the flushing side effect, many people have tried time-release niacin preparations, which are considerably more expensive than unmodified niacin pills. Published evidence indicates that time-release preparations of niacin are not quite as effective as unmodified niacin, and that while flushing was decreased, other side effects, including nausea, indigestion, diarrhea, fatigue, and liver damage were worse with the time-release niacin as compared to the unmodified pills. For these reasons we seldom prescribe the time-release form of niacin.

Some pharmacists have recommended *nicotinamide* as a substitute for niacin as a way of avoiding the flushing and itching. Although nicotinamide does function as a vitamin, it does not reduce cholesterol levels. It therefore cannot be substituted for niacin in the treatment of blood cholesterol. We repeat: Despite the fact that it is available over the counter, niacin should *not* be used to reduce cholesterol without medical supervision.

Fibric Acids

These are the drugs most widely used throughout the world for lowering cholesterol. In the United States, they are available in two forms, *clofibrate* (sold as Atromid-S), and *gemfibrozil* (sold as Lopid). They usually reduce total cholesterol levels by about 10–20 percent, and have been shown to reduce the risk of heart attack. Their major action is to reduce VLDL (and therefore triglyceride) levels by about 40 percent.

The actions of the fibric acids are complex and not fully understood. They reduce levels of VLDL and raise HDL-cholesterol levels somewhat. Their action on LDL levels is variable and depends on why the LDL is elevated in the first place. Remember that LDL is produced from VLDL. If LDL levels are high because of overproduction, rather than impaired LDL removal, the fibric acids may be effective in reducing them.

Most patients seem to tolerate the fibric acids well, though many side effects have been reported; whether they are suitable for you requires an individualized assessment by a physician of your own specific health risks.

As with any of these drugs, the benefit of the fibric acids should be evaluated by repeated measurements of blood lipids, both before and after starting the drug. Then the degree of improvement must be weighed against the risk of side effects, the expense, and the bother involved in taking the medication.

Probucol

Sold in this country under the trade name Lorelco, probucol is usually about as effective as the fibric acids in lowering cholesterol. It lowers LDL-cholesterol, which should help prevent atherosclerosis, but it also reduces HDL-cholesterol. Many physicians are reluctant to prescribe it because of the possibly deleterious effects of reducing HDL-cholesterol. Convincing proof that probucol prevents heart attacks in humans has not been published, though some animal research looks promising, since the drug has been shown to prevent atherosclerosis in susceptible species.

Lovastatin

Marketed in the United States as Mevacor, lovastatin is the newest drug for treatment of hypercholesterolemia, approved by the Food and Drug Administration in 1987. It is the result of years of research aimed at developing a drug that slows the rate of cholesterol production within the body. Tested widely before its release in this country, lovastatin appears effective and safe when taken with proper medical supervision. It works very well in combination with bile-acid-binding resins, as well as with the resins and niacin combined.

As with any new drug, one must be especially attuned to the possibility of side effects when taking lovastatin. This includes side effects that are unknown at present. Suspicious symptoms must be reported to your physician.

The main side effect of lovastatin, while rare, is a serious condition of muscle pain and muscle breakdown, with resulting kidney damage. This has occurred in patients taking lovastatin in combination with *cyclosporine* (the drug used after heart transplants), niacin, or gemfibrozil. Because of this rare but serious side effect, anyone taking lovastatin who develops widespread muscle pain should stop the drug and contact a doctor immediately.

SURGERY

In some of the most severe cases of familial hypercholesterolemia, in which the patient has inherited a double dose of the abnormal gene, liver transplantation is being tried experimentally, with a high rate of success. For most people with high blood cholesterol, however, surgery plays no role in proper management.

Some people have undergone a surgical bypass of a short segment of the small intestine as treatment for hypercholesterolemia. The operation, which bypasses part of the ileum, causes increased excretion of bile acids in the feces, in a manner similar to the bile-acid-binding resins described earlier. Nevertheless, modern medications can normalize blood lipids in virtually all patients without subjecting them to such surgery and its attendant risks. Consequently, we do not presently recommend ileal-bypass surgery for hypercholesterolemia.

LET THE BUYER BEWARE

Unproven remedies abound for most important health problems, and high cholesterol is no exception. No law prevents an enterprising individual from seizing a shred of scientific information and weaving it into a fabric of false claims. We despair of trying to enumerate and expose these, because they multiply faster than we can subtract. Nevertheless, let us note a couple of the most prominent.

Lecithin

This is an old favorite. Based on the fact that lecithin is an important component of lipoproteins—the tiny particles that dissolve cholesterol in the bloodstream—lecithin has been promoted as a means of dissolving your cholesterol. Unfortunately, scientific studies in which lecithin has been added to humans' diets have not shown any appreciable reduction in their serum cholesterol concentration.

The body makes its own lecithin, and also obtains it as part of a normal diet. It is also an ingredient of many processed foods, such as candy bars, since it is a good emulsifier. When lecithin is administered orally, it is broken down in the intestine prior to being absorbed, then reassembled. *You don't need supplemental lecithin.* It is rich in calories, and can thus contribute to obesity, even though it has been touted as a means of "dissolving" fat as well as cholesterol.

Fish Oils

This is a new favorite. Its entry into health fashion was based on the fact that Eskimos have a low incidence of heart disease despite eating considerable amounts of blubber, which contains fat and cholesterol.

Investigations were launched to discover whether some element of the Eskimo diet might actually protect the heart. Since Eskimos eat fish, and fish oils are highly unsaturated, these oils were nominated as possible explanations for why Eskimos suffer little atherosclerosis. Not only in Eskimos, but in other populations, scientists found evidence of a correlation between eating *fish* and freedom from heart disease. Fish oils are rich in a special type of fatty acid, known as the omega-3 fatty acids. Because seals eat fish, their blubber also contains these special fatty acids.

Fish oil and omega-3 fatty acids, however, have little effect on the total cholesterol level. Sometimes they even reduce levels of HDL-cholesterol—the "good" kind. Fish oils do effectively lower triglyceride levels, and can be used for that purpose. In some individuals with high triglycerides, however, large doses of fish oils taken in capsules can actually increase the level of LDL-cholesterol—the "bad" kind. This may be due in part to the cholesterol content of unpurified fish oils. For example, salmon oil contains about 400 milligrams of cholesterol in every nine grams of oil. Oils from other species of fish, such as menhaden, contain less cholesterol.

Current studies suggest that fish oils may indeed protect the heart, but through mechanisms other than a change in cholesterol levels. For instance, they affect the function of platelets—tiny particles in the blood that promote blood clotting and are thought to participate in atherosclerosis. Aspirin, which interferes with platelet function but has no effect on blood cholesterol levels, indeed has been shown to reduce the risk of heart attacks in certain settings. Aspirin also has definite side effects, which include bleeding. Fish oil, like aspirin, interferes with clotting and causes easy bruising in many people.

Certain species of animals that get atherosclerosis, such as swine fed diets high in cholesterol, show no change in cholesterol levels when they are fed fish oil, but nevertheless do have definite reduction in atherosclerosis. The relevance of these studies to humans, however, is still under investigation, and it is too early to determine the side effects and benefits of taking fish oil supplements, or whether the benefits outweigh the risk.

Until scientific studies clarify the risks and benefits of fish-oil consumption by humans, we suggest you resist the urge to leap on the fish-oil bandwagon. Instead, consider including fish in your diet as a replacement for meat, since fish has been a safe and nourishing part of the human diet for thousands of years, and has been shown to protect against heart attacks when eaten regularly.

6

Obesity: Standards, Degrees, and Patterns

Obesity is a state of having too much body fat. The question of how much fat is too much is not a simple one, since the answer depends partly on individual susceptibility to the effects of obesity, and partly on where in one's body the excess fat is located.

WHO IS OBESE?

To determine whether someone is truly obese, or simply fatter than some statistical, social, or cosmetic standard, one must first define the standards.

Defining Obesity

Social obesity. This is excessive fatness as defined by the standards imposed by cultural and social values, and these values are changing. As we noted earlier, Americans prefer a thinner look today than they did a generation ago. What was considered beautiful by the standards of a century ago could easily be considered obese on the social scale of today.

Whether someone suffers from social obesity depends in part on his or her sensitivity to the opinions of others. If considering this dynamic causes some healthy but heavy persons to contemplate how capricious and arbitrary are the societal norms of today, perhaps they will suffer less from feeling "too fat."

Neurotic (imagined) obesity. This is, of course, a more extreme condition than social obesity, and it is unfortunately all too common. Here the perception of an excess of body fat is based on no objective standard; instead, one perceives one's body as too fat despite the absence of any medical, social, functional, or statistical standard for obesity. Such problems are often classified as "eating disorders," and they usually involve not only abnormal eating patterns, but also distorted perceptions of body image, self-induced vomiting, and sometimes the misuse of drugs and exercise. Apparently psychological in origin, these disorders can have severe medical consequences. (See chapter 3.)

Statistical obesity. A definition of excessive fatness derived from some arbitrary standard based on the average measurements of a given population. Height-and-weight tables used by life-insurance companies employ this approach. On these tables, persons are defined as obese if their weight extends beyond some arbitrary standard such as 20 or 30 percent above average. Besides simply measuring height and weight, such charts also can be employed to measure other body dimensions, such as skin-fold thickness and waist and hip circumference, and use these to define obesity in a statistical way; i.e., that a certain number of pounds above the average for that measurement in your particular group is assigned a value in terms of excess. We have no quarrel with the making of such measurements when they are simple, safe, and inexpensive. The problem comes when these data are used to declare someone obese simply because his or her numbers are above the average of others in a group. Using such a definition, a person could become obese simply by moving to another country or location where the population is slimmer. We think it is more sensible to define obesity in relation to an individual's own particular health-risk profile and intended activities. As we shall see, some statistical measures of obesity do correlate with health risks.

Medical obesity. This is fatness of a degree that causes or worsens one of the medical consequences of obesity reviewed in chapter 2. Whether one's own degree of fatness contributes to premature death or disease depends largely on one's inheritance and predisposition. For example, thirty pounds of adipose tissue might be too much for someone with high blood pressure, elevated cholesterol, and diabetes. Although such a person could be seriously obese from a medical viewpoint, another person with an identical body build might have no such health problems and no genetic predisposition to them, and might therefore not be considered medically obese. Even ten pounds of extra adipose tissue can have considerable medical impact in situations of diabetes mellitus or high blood pressure, yet not be regarded as excessive by social, statistical, or functional criteria.

A person might be medically obese but not socially obese, depending on the society in which that person lives. The societal norm for weight among the Pima Indians of Arizona, for example, is very high when compared to that of the rest of America. Many members of the Pima tribe have diabetes of a type that can benefit dramatically from weight reduction. Most diabetic Pima Indians are obese from a medical viewpoint, but within their society are not heavier than the norm, nor are they made to feel socially uncomfortable on account of their weight. In fact, some Pimas acknowledge a feeling of social pressure to remain heavy.

Functional obesity. As the term implies, this is having too much fat for one's intended activities. Someone too fat to get comfortably in and out of a car would certainly be functionally obese. Functional obesity may not correlate with other definitions of obesity. For example, a Japanese sumo wrestler requires significant amounts of adipose tissue to remain competitive, and might not be considered obese from the point of view of his sport, even though statistically his weight may be in a very high percentile for his height, and medically his fatness might be unhealthy. A person who is underweight for sumo wrestling might be functionally obese in the role of a runner. The same issue applies to ballet dancers, football linemen, and others involved in activities in which the amount of fat is critically important to optimal function.

These are only some ways in which the perception of obesity can vary with the viewpoint of the beholder. And all such factors can determine how much fat is considered too much, including your own perceptions, social and cultural pressures, statistical criteria, your work, your life-style, and your health. It is your health-risk profile, however, largely inherited, that can render you susceptible to the serious medical consequences of having too much fat.

OVERWEIGHT VS. OBESE

Because not only fat, but also bone, muscle, fluid, and other body components all contribute to one's weight, an individual can be overweight without being obese. For example, two men might both be six feet tall and weigh 200 pounds, but one of them might be very muscular and have very little body fat, while the other, at an identical weight, might be fat and flabby. Two women might both be five feet seven inches tall and weigh 160 pounds. But one might be eight months pregnant and very lean, while the other might be decidedly obese. Many athletes are quite heavy when compared to a standard weight for their height, but the extra weight is usually found in muscle, not fat.

UNDERSTANDING BODY COMPOSITION

Using methods we shall describe in this chapter, researchers have found that fat tissue accounts for an average of 28 percent of the body weight in men and 35–40 percent in women. The total content of fat in the body is influenced by a variety of factors, including sex, age, and race. When we are born, our bodies contain about 12 percent fat, a proportion higher than in any mammal except the whale. During infancy, body fat normally reaches a peak of about 25 percent and then decreases to about 18 percent during childhood. At puberty, fat content increases dramatically in females and decreases in males, leading to those differences in body-fat content between the sexes that persist during the rest of adult life.

Fat continues to increase in both sexes after puberty, so that between the ages of 20 and 50 years, the fat content of males approximately doubles, and that of females increases only half as much. Body-fat content increases more than weight because lean body mass (mostly muscle and bone) declines (see Figure 6.1).

Fatness can increase even though weight does not change. The average sedentary American male at age 25 weighs 158 pounds. Researchers have shown that by age 65 he will likely have lost about 26 pounds of lean body mass (mainly muscle). Therefore, even if his weight has not changed over those 40 years, he is 26 pounds fatter, usually around the abdomen. Most individuals do gain weight during their adult lives, however, and therefore accumulate even more fat.

Physical activity influences body composition, and offers a valuable means of lessening the age-associated shift from muscle to fat. With regular physical exercise, the proportion of lean body mass increases while body fat is usually reduced. When this kind of regular training is discontinued, the reverse process occurs. These changes in body composition can occur without any changes whatever in total body weight, and therefore can remain undetected by the scales. Regular

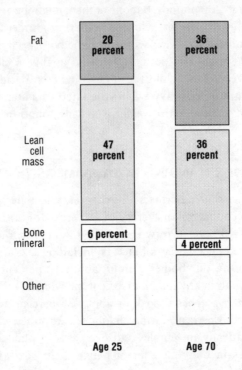

Figure 6.1 Effects of Aging on Body Composition

Body composition changes as we age. The percentage of fat increases, and the percentage of lean cell mass, including muscle, declines.

physical activity maintained throughout life helps minimize the relative decrease in lean body mass and the proportional increase in body fat that accompany aging.

We emphasize this interesting information on body composition because we do not want you to make the common mistake of equating obesity with weight. For example, many people become enthusiastic about a crash diet when they lose five to ten pounds in the first week, not realizing that most of what they have lost is water and lean tissue, not fat. Many dieters try to promote such fluid loss by avoiding salt, not realizing that the water weight will be regained as soon as the diet is interrupted, or as soon as salt intake increases. These shifts in water weight have nothing to do with the logical goal of weight-reduction dieting, which is to eliminate excess body fat. But they are distracting and, at times, needlessly discouraging. Moreover, fluid depletion produces uncomfortable side effects, and should be avoided. Much of the weakness and faintness encountered during dieting is caused by fluid depletion, and it can be avoided by adequate salt and fluid intake.

Unfortunately, many dieters use diuretics to drive down their weight. Diuretics cause loss of salt and water, which will eventually be restored through normal function of the kidneys, pituitary, and hypothalamus, but they do not reduce fat at all. The fluid depletion causes faintness, weakness, and cramps, so diuretics should be avoided unless needed for the treatment of heart failure or high blood pressure. Laxatives, likewise, cause fluid depletion and should not be used for weight control.

Puberty and pregnancy provide us with other examples of how important it is to understand body composition. The regional increases in fat that girls typically experience during puberty are perfectly healthy and normal. Unfortunately, some girls misinterpret them as obesity, and initiate unhealthy attempts to decrease their weight. During pregnancy a woman can actually lose fat despite a gain in weight. Much of the weight gain, of course, occurs in the uterus, with its contents of fluid and fetus. The increase is normal, expected, and healthy, and should not be seen as a reason to starve at a time when the fetus needs nutrition.

As you can see, there are important differences between body weight and body fat. From the viewpoint of health as well as good looks, 20 more pounds of extra fat could be a real problem, while 20 more pounds of lean muscle might be no problem at all.

MEASURING BODY FAT AND ESTIMATING OBESITY

Because the real issue in obesity is not weight but excess fat, in our practice of medicine we seldom make use of height-and-weight charts to decide whether someone is obese, or to determine how much weight our patients should lose. Deciding whether an individual is obese or is simply overweight requires techniques and standards for measuring body fat. Many are available.

Techniques

Visual inspection. A simple and inexpensive but not very quantitative approach is to look in the mirror. This superficial analysis of fatness will reveal increased bulging of the skin or excessive roundness around the midsection, which in most instances suggest increased fatness. Such visual inspection may also be done by another individual.

Belt test. Another simple, inexpensive method for estimating obesity is the "belt test." In this test, you fit a belt snugly around the lower part of your rib cage. Then you try to slip the belt down over the abdomen to the hips without loosening the belt. If you can do so, you pass the test. If you must loosen the belt to get it down over the abdomen, you flunk. An advantage of this test is that it emphasizes abdominal obesity, which is the pattern of excess fatness most associated with health risks.

Clothing sizes. A person who has stopped growing in height can of course follow the progress of her or his weight gain by changes in belt size, dress size, and/or trouser waistline. In doing so, remember that conditions such as pregnancy or severe fluid retention (as in advanced cirrhosis of the liver) can change body size and shape completely apart from any changes in adipose tissue mass.

We mention these simple means of assessing adiposity because for most purposes they are just as useful as the more expensive and complex methods that are now being offered by some health spas, hospitals, and weight clinics.

Somatotyping. Years ago, a popular method for estimating fatness was the assignment of body types based on photographs or renderings of a variety of unclothed human bodies. By matching the subject to these printed visual standards, such as those in the book *Atlas of Men,* by William H. Sheldon, one assigns a degree of roundness (endomorphy), muscularity (mesomorphy), and leanness (ectomorphy). While this method, called somatotyping, is easy and provides crude individual guides, it is not quantitative.

Anthropometric measurements. Measurements of body dimensions offer a good way to analyze indirectly the fat content of the body. These kinds of measurements have been called *anthropometric,* and include height and weight, circumferences of the chest, waist, hips, and extremities, and the thickness of skin-folds in various areas of the body. A description of these methods follows. The most widely used and available are height and weight.

Determining Pounds Over or Under Desirable Weight

Height and weight can be compared to the "desirable weight" in tables provided by the Metropolitan Life Insurance Company. These tables have received wide use. They divide desirable weights into three subgroups based on "frame size." However, they provide no instructions and no data to offer anything more than a crude estimate of whether you are small-, medium-, or large-framed as a guide to which column you should use to evaluate your level of fatness.

These height-and-weight tables are based on data obtained from the pooled experience of the life-insurance industry in the United States. Although they provide data derived from nearly 5 million people, they suffer from the bias introduced by the inclusion of only those individuals who decide to take out life-insurance policies. It turns out that these insured individuals tend to have a longer life expectancy, to be healthier, and in general to be lighter in weight than the general population. The classic 1959 Metropolitan Life Insurance tables are still the most widely used, and are shown here.

Table 6.1   1959 Metropolitan Life Insurance Height and Weight Tables for Adults (corrected for height without shoes and weight without clothes)

Women

Height	Small Frame	Medium Frame	Large Frame
4'8"	89–95 pounds	93–104 pounds	101–116 pounds
4'9"	91–98	95–107	103–119
4'10"	93–101	98–110	106–122
4'11"	96–104	101–113	109–125
5'0"	99–107	104–116	112–128
5'1"	102–110	107–119	115–131
5'2"	105–113	110–123	118–135
5'3"	108–116	113–127	122–139
5'4"	111–120	117–132	126–143
5'5"	115–124	121–136	130–147
5'6"	119–128	125–140	134–151
5'7"	123–132	129–144	138–155
5'8"	127–137	133–148	142–160
5'9"	131–141	137–152	146–165
5'10"	135–145	141–156	153–173

Men

Height	Small Frame	Medium Frame	Large Frame
5'1"	109–117 pounds	115–126 pounds	123–138 pounds
5'2"	112–120	118–130	126–141
5'3"	115–123	121–133	129–145
5'4"	118–126	124–136	132–149
5'5"	121–130	127–140	135–153
5'6"	125–134	131–144	139–158

Men (cont.)

Height	Small Frame	Medium Frame	Large Frame
5'7"	129–138	135–149	144–163
5'8"	133–142	139–153	148–167
5'9"	137–147	143–157	152–171
5'10"	141–151	147–162	156–176
5'11"	145–155	151–167	161–181
6'0"	149–159	155–172	165–186
6'1"	153–164	159–177	170–191
6'2"	157–168	164–182	175–196
6'3"	161–172	169–187	179–201

In 1983 the tables were revised and republished, with somewhat higher weights regarded as ideal. Experience had shown the life-insurance industry that the safe range of weight extended higher than was previously thought. Moreover, mortality rates among very thin people tend to be raised by the inclusion of people who are losing weight because of severe disease, such as lung cancer.

Table 6.2   1983 Metropolitan Life Insurance Height and Weight Tables for Adults (corrected for height without shoes and weight without clothes)

Women

Height	Small Frame	Medium Frame	Large Frame
4'9"	99–108 pounds	106–118 pounds	115–128 pounds
4'10"	100–110	108–120	117–131
4'11"	101–112	110–123	119–134
5'0"	103–115	112–126	122–137
5'1"	105–118	115–129	125–140
5'2"	108–121	118–132	128–144
5'3"	111–124	121–135	131–148
5'4"	114–127	124–138	134–152
5'5"	117–130	127–141	137–156
5'6"	120–133	130–144	140–160
5'7"	123–136	133–147	143–164
5'8"	126–139	136–150	146–167
5'9"	129–142	139–153	149–170
5'10"	132–145	142–156	152–173
5'11"	135–148	145–159	155–176

Men

Height	Small Frame	Medium Frame	Large Frame
5'1"	125–131 pounds	128–138 pounds	135–147 pounds
5'2"	127–133	130–140	137–150
5'3"	129–135	132–142	139–153
5'4"	131–137	134–145	141–157
5'5"	133–139	136–148	143–161
5'6"	135–142	139–151	146–165
5'7"	137–145	142–154	149–169
5'8"	139–148	145–157	152–173
5'9"	141–151	148–160	155–177
5'10"	143–154	151–163	158–181
5'11"	146–157	154–167	161–185
6'0"	149–161	157–171	165–189
6'1"	152–165	161–175	169–194
6'2"	155–169	164–179	173–199
6'3"	159–173	168–184	178–204

A further disadvantage of these life-insurance tables is that they do not take into account the fact that the amount of fat tissue relative to lean body mass normally increases with age, and that some of this increase in body fat is not accompanied by any increased health risks.

Percent Desirable Weight

Weight and height can also be considered by using various ratios. Relative weight is the actual body weight divided by the desirable or standard weight based on height, usually derived from the 1959 Metropolitan Life Insurance tables. Thus a woman who is five feet five inches tall and who weighs 170 pounds would have a desirable weight of about 129 pounds, according to the tables. Her relative weight is calculated by dividing 170 by 129, giving a result of 1.32, or 132 percent of desirable weight.

Body Mass Index

Another widely used and more reliable ratio is the body mass index (BMI), also known as the Quetelet Index. The BMI is the body weight in kilograms divided by the square of the height in meters (weight/height^2). The BMI correlates better with body fat than do other ratios and is not much affected by height. You can use Figure 6.2 or Table 6.3 to derive your own BMI from your height and weight.

A body mass index of 30 or higher is generally agreed to carry increased risks to health and longevity.

Waist-to-Hip Ratio (WHR)

Evidence is mounting that it is worthwhile to assess the relative amount of body fat in the abdomen, as compared to the rest of the body. The ratio of circumference of the waist to that of the buttocks is called the waist-to-hip ratio (WHR), also known by its technical name, abdominal-to-gluteal ratio (AGR). It provides an inexpensive, easily obtainable index of the relative amount of abdominal fat, and it is proving extremely valuable as a guide to health risks. Values of WHR above 1.0 carry a high risk of adverse medical consequences.

You can determine your own WHR by putting a tape measure around your waist, and then around your hips at the area of maximum protrusion of the buttocks. Your waist, for purposes of determining your WHR, is not defined as your girth at the level of your navel. It is your girth at the narrowest part of your torso between the bottom of your rib cage and the top of your pelvis. The lowest part of your rib cage is found on the sides of your body, where your arms hang down. The top of your pelvis is found an inch or two lower, in the same area on the sides of your body. The tape measure should pass between these two landmarks as you measure your waist to determine your WHR. Calculate your WHR by dividing your waist circumference by your hip circumference. Or, if you prefer, simply refer to Figure 6.3 on page 135.

WHRs reflect a characteristic difference between the sexes. Excess abdominal fat is especially common among overweight men, and this condition gives them a high WHR. The distribution of fat more characteristic of women, on the other hand, is mostly on the hips, and gives them a lower WHR. The greater tendency of obesity to cause health problems in men than in women probably relates to the greater tendency of men to store excess fat in their bellies instead of in their lower bodies.

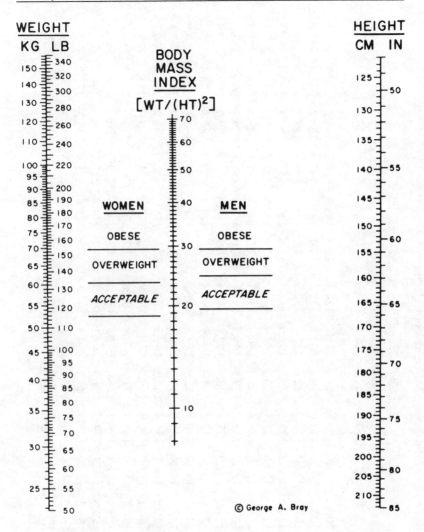

Figure 6.2 Nomograph for Body Mass Index (kG/m²)

Find your body mass index (BMI), or Quetelet Index, by measuring your height and weight, then laying a straight edge across the corresponding points on the two side lines of this nomograph. The straight edge will intersect the BMI line at your body mass index.

Table 6.3 Find Your BMI from Your Height and Weight

Body Weights in Pounds According to Height and Body Mass Index*

Height, Inches	Body Mass Index, kg/m²													
	19.0	20.0	21.0	22.0	23.0	24.0	25.0	26.0	27.0	28.0	29.0	30.0	35.0	40.0
	Body Weight, Pounds													
58.0	90.7	95.5	100.3	105.0	109.8	114.6	119.4	124.1	128.9	133.7	138.5	143.2	167.1	191.0
59.0	93.9	98.8	103.8	108.7	113.6	118.6	123.5	128.5	133.4	138.3	143.3	148.2	172.9	197.6
60.0	97.1	102.2	107.3	112.4	117.5	122.6	127.7	132.9	138.0	143.1	148.2	153.3	178.8	204.4
61.0	100.3	105.6	110.9	116.2	121.5	126.8	132.0	137.3	142.6	147.9	153.2	158.4	184.8	211.3
62.0	103.7	109.1	114.6	120.0	125.5	130.9	136.4	141.9	147.3	152.8	158.2	163.7	191.0	218.2
63.0	107.0	112.7	118.3	123.9	129.6	135.2	140.8	146.5	152.1	157.7	163.4	169.0	197.2	225.3
64.0	110.5	116.3	122.1	127.9	133.7	139.5	145.3	151.2	157.0	162.8	168.6	174.4	203.5	232.5
65.0	113.9	119.9	125.9	131.9	137.9	143.9	149.9	155.9	161.9	167.9	173.9	179.9	209.9	239.9
66.0	117.5	123.7	129.8	136.0	142.2	148.4	154.6	160.8	166.9	173.1	179.3	185.5	216.4	247.3
67.0	121.1	127.4	133.8	140.2	146.5	152.9	159.3	165.7	172.0	178.4	184.8	191.1	223.0	254.9
68.0	124.7	131.3	137.8	144.4	151.0	157.5	164.1	170.6	177.2	183.8	190.3	196.9	229.7	262.5
69.0	128.4	135.2	141.9	148.7	155.4	162.2	168.9	175.7	182.5	189.2	196.0	202.7	236.5	270.3
70.0	132.1	139.1	146.1	153.0	160.0	166.9	173.9	180.8	187.8	194.7	201.7	208.6	243.4	278.2
71.0	135.9	143.1	150.3	157.4	164.6	171.7	178.9	186.0	193.2	200.3	207.5	214.6	250.4	286.2
72.0	139.8	147.2	154.5	161.9	169.2	176.6	183.9	191.3	198.7	206.0	213.4	220.7	257.5	294.3
73.0	143.7	151.3	158.8	166.4	174.0	181.5	189.1	196.7	204.2	211.8	219.3	226.9	264.7	302.5
74.0	147.7	155.4	163.2	171.0	178.8	186.5	194.3	202.1	209.9	217.6	225.4	233.2	272.0	310.9
75.0	151.7	159.7	167.7	175.6	183.6	191.6	199.6	207.6	215.6	223.5	231.5	239.5	279.4	319.4
76.0	155.8	164.0	172.2	180.4	188.6	196.8	205.0	213.2	221.4	229.5	237.7	245.9	286.9	327.9

*Each entry gives the body weight in pounds for a person of a given height and body mass index.

Adapted from G. A. Bray and D. S. Gray, "Obesity: Part I—Pathogenesis," Western Journal of Medicine 149 (1988): 431.

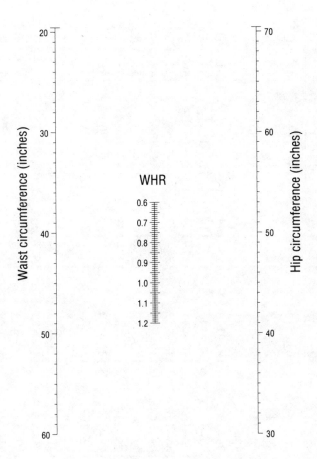

Figure 6.3 Nomograph for Waist-to-Hip Ratio (WHR)

Find your waist-to-hip ratio (WHR) by measuring your waist circumference just above the pelvic bone on the side of your torso, and your hip circumference around the most prominent area of your buttocks and hips. Then lay a straight edge across the corresponding points on the two side lines of this nomograph. The straight edge will intersect the WHR line at your waist-to-hip ratio.

Skin-fold Thickness

Another useful anthropometric measurement is the "pinch test" in its simple and also more sophisticated forms. The amount and, particularly, the distribution of body fat can be assessed fairly accurately

Table 6.4   Age-specific Weight Range for Men and Women as Recommended by the Gerontology Research Center (height without shoes and weight without clothes)

Height	20–29 yr	30–39 yr	40–49 yr	50–59 yr	60–69 yr
4'10"	84–111	92–119	99–127	107–135	115–142
4'11"	87–115	95–123	103–131	111–139	119–147
5'0"	90–119	98–127	106–135	114–143	123–152
5'1"	93–123	101–131	110–140	118–148	127–157
5'2"	96–127	105–136	113–144	122–153	131–163
5'3"	99–131	108–140	117–149	126–158	135–168
5'4"	102–135	112–145	121–154	130–163	140–173
5'5"	106–140	115–149	125–159	134–168	144–179
5'6"	109–144	119–154	129–164	138–174	148–184
5'7"	112–148	122–159	133–169	143–179	153–190
5'8"	116–153	126–163	137–174	147–184	158–196
5'9"	119–157	130–168	141–179	151–190	162–201
5'10"	112–162	134–173	145–184	156–195	167–207
5'11"	126–167	137–178	149–190	160–201	172–213
6'0"	129–171	141–183	153–195	165–207	177–219
6'1"	133–176	145–188	157–200	169–213	182–225
6'2"	137–181	149–194	162–206	174–219	187–232
6'3"	141–186	153–199	166–212	179–225	192–238
6'4"	144–191	157–205	171–218	184–231	197–244

Taken from Reubin Andres, "Mortality and Obesity: The Rationale for Age-specific Height-Weight Tables," in Hazzard, W. R., R. Andres, and E. L. Bierman, *Principles of Geriatric Medicine and Gerontology*, 2nd edition (1990), New York: McGraw Hill, 759–65.

and inexpensively by this approach. We are all familiar with the crude "pinch test" that involves simply gripping a few inches of skin between the thumb and forefinger and squeezing until the two fingers can be squeezed no further. The distance between the two fingers is then an indication of the amount of body fat. If calipers are used, by placing them on either side of this skin fold, the distance between the points of the calipers can be accurately measured. This is called "skin-fold thickness."

Extensive studies in large populations have documented skin-fold thickness at various standard body sites such as over the shoulder blade, over the triceps at the back of the upper arm, and so forth. From these studies, standards have been derived. In some cases, especially in young persons with rather tight skin surrounding lots of fat, the exact measurement can be difficult to reproduce with precision. But the more serious problem with this approach is that it measures only the fat under the skin. As we shall see, some of the more important accumulations of body fat are not necessarily under the skin, but occur, for example, deeper within the abdomen. Sex and ethnic differences also need to be taken into account in interpreting skin-fold measurements. Nevertheless, since half or more of the body fat is located just under the skin, skin-fold measurements are a useful way to estimate body fat and its distribution.

New and More-Expensive Methods

A variety of sophisticated and relatively expensive techniques are now available for measuring the total amount of body fat and its distribution. These include ultrasound, electromagnetic methods, bioelectric impedance, computerized X-ray tomography ("CAT scanning"), neutron activation, and the latest technique, nuclear magnetic resonance imaging (MRI or NMR). As means of measuring fat, they are valuable research tools, but as yet they are of little practical importance. Some health institutions and practitioners offer some of them, perhaps in part as advertising or money-making ploys to capitalize on our societal fixation on fat. Apart from research, however, the availability of such expensive and precise measurement of body fat is of little practical use. One does not need to know whether one's body-fat content is 13 percent versus 18 percent, or how that compares to the fat of a hero in the National Football League. You can decide perfectly well whether you need or want to lose weight without expensive quantitative measurements. You can look in the mirror, do a pinch test, a belt test, a WHR measurement, or simply follow your belt or dress size. Nevertheless, because some of these methods for measuring body fat are becoming so heavily promoted, we will briefly describe each of them.

Ultrasound. This method involves sending sound waves through the body, much like the use of sonar in the ocean. The sound waves are reflected differently by fat, muscle, and other tissues, and they can provide a measure of the thickness of those tissues. From the dimensions of adipose-tissue deposits, the amount of fat in the body can be estimated.

Electromagnetic techniques. These were pioneered by the livestock industry, which has been far ahead of the rest of us in scientific attention to fat. After all, the amount of fat versus lean body mass in livestock sold for meat affects the price to be paid for it. So a pig on the way to the slaughterhouse trots up a ramp into a tunnel surrounded by a big electromagnet. As it moves through the magnet, its lean body tissues, such as meat, which is rich in water, disturb the magnetic field much more than does the fat, which contains very little water. The amount of disturbance of the magnetic field is measured, and is proportional to the pig's lean body mass. The same methods can, of course, be applied to people.

Bioelectric impedance analysis. This is a recently popularized method for measuring the proportion of fat in the body. A relatively inexpensive instrument measures the resistance or impedance to flow of electrical current, which is different for different tissues. The procedure, if done properly, involves applying electrodes to one arm and one leg, and is safe and comfortable. Although this method seems to be accurate in normal individuals, its accuracy in people with varying degrees of obesity and bone density has yet to be established.

Neutron activation. This is a relatively expensive technique in which the body is bombarded by neutrons, and chemical components of the body can be identified by the energy waves they emit.

Nuclear magnetic resonance imaging (NMR or MRI). In this method, the body is subjected to electromagnetic forces and then certain energy waves emitted by various tissues are measured, using a computer to produce an image and analysis of the size of tissues, including fat. The method is safe as long as one's body is free of metallic objects, such as surgical clips or a pacemaker, but it is far too expensive for the routine clinical evaluation of obesity.

CAT-scanning (computerized axial tomography). Multiple X-ray images, analyzed by computer, are used to determine the exact dimensions and shape of various body tissues. The cost and radiation exposure involved make it impractical for the routine measurement of body fat.

Isotope dilution. These techniques involve injecting substances that dissolve in fat or in water, and then measuring their concentration in fat and water to calculate the total quantity of fat in the body.

Underwater weighing. The standard to which all of the above indirect assessments of body fat are compared is the measurement of body fat by underwater weighing. This method is based on the fact that fat is light, or has low density, and that the more fat is in the body, the more readily the body floats. In this procedure, individuals are weighed underwater and again out of water, and the volume of air in the lungs is determined. With this information one can estimate both the fat and the nonfat content of the body. The technique requires specialized facilities and a staff experienced in their use. Consequently, the chief use of underwater weighing is in research.

HOW FAT IS TOO FAT?

Medical scientists generally agree that the following levels of fatness carry significant medical risks: (1) a body mass index (BMI) over 30; (2) a waist-to-hip ratio (WHR) over 1.0; (3) a relative weight (percentage of desirable weight) of 130 percent or more, based on the 1959 Metropolitan Life Insurance tables (adverse health effects are detectable at weights 20 percent over desirable, as defined by the 1959 Metropolitan Life tables, and most experts would agree that at 30 percent or more above desirable weight a person is medically obese); and (4) 50 pounds or more over "ideal" (or "desirable") body weight, based on the same tables.

In a specific individual case, however, a lesser degree of fatness might be definitely detrimental. For example, a five-foot-eight-inch woman with arthritic knees, high blood pressure, and diabetes might be significantly too fat at a weight of 160 pounds, even though her BMI would be only 24, her relative weight 123 percent, and she would be only 30 pounds over her desirable weight as defined by the 1959 Metropolitan Life tables. If her excess fat were mostly on her lower body, she might even have a WHR of less than 0.9. Nevertheless, her degree of fatness could be very unhealthy for her, given her particular illnesses and susceptibility. Another woman of the same age, size, and shape might suffer no ill health effects whatever from the same degree of fatness.

Because of the individual differences in our susceptibility to the medical consequences of fatness, the general guidelines given here are just that—generalities based on population statistics, more applicable to some people than to others.

Age appears to be particularly important in determining what degrees of weight and fatness are healthy. The life-insurance statistics

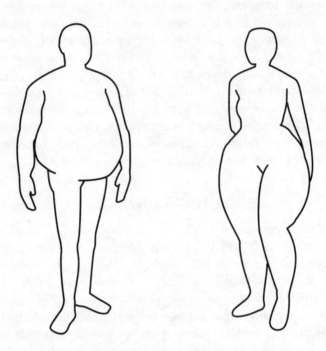

Figure 6.4 Apples vs. Pears

Two important patterns of fat accumulation. The figure on the left shows fat
accumulated in the upper body—a pattern typical of many men as they age and
put on weight. This pattern has been likened to the shape of an apple, and is
referred to as "upper body," "upper segment," "central," or "android" obesity.
It gives a high waist-to-hip ratio (WHR) and is associated with many medical
risks. The figure on the right shows fat accumulated in the lower body—a
pattern typical of many women as they put on weight. This shape has been
likened to that of a pear, and is referred to as "lower body," "lower segment"
"peripheral," or "gynoid" obesity. It gives a low WHR and is associated with
much less medical risk than is upper-body obesity.

presented in Tables 6.1 and 6.2, on pages 129–131, do not take age
into account. When one accounts for age in analyzing such statistics,
the results take on a different aspect, as you can see by comparing
Tables 6.1 and 6.2 with Table 6.4, on page 136.

Table 6.4 takes into account the effects of age on mortality risk in
relation to body size. Ideal weight (the weight associated with greatest life expectancy) increases with age. Evidently, as you age, you

can gain some weight without increasing your risk of premature death. In fact, gaining a little weight as you age appears to protect your life, assuming that you don't have specific medical problems that are made worse by weight gain.

These figures also show that the range of healthy weight for any given height gets broader as people age. As we age, therefore, the range of weight compatible with long survival is not so narrow; it broadens out a bit. On the other hand, particular individuals within these ranges may need to lose weight because of some specific health problems that are worsened by even mild degrees of excess fat.

When the effects of age are analyzed with regard to body mass index (BMI, or the Quetelet Index—see page 131), we see a similar pattern: the degree of fatness associated with lowest mortality increases as one ages, as shown in Table 6.4.

Table 6.5
Body Mass Index (BMI) Associated with Lowest
Overall Mortality in Relation to Age

Age Group (years)	BMI (kg/m^2)
19–24	19–24
25–34	20–25
35–44	21–26
45–54	22–27
55–65	23–28
Over 65	24–29

Adapted from G. A. Bray and D. S. Gray: "Obesity: Part I—Pathogenesis," *Western Journal of Medicine* 149 (1988): 429–41.

These data indicate that unless one has some specific medical condition that should be treated by weight reduction, it is perfectly healthy and normal to put on some weight as one gets older. As shown in Table 6.5 a BMI of 28 would be above the normal range at age 20, but is within the normal range after age 55. These facts should be reassuring to healthy middle-aged people who are finding it difficult to maintain the same weight they had in college.

In addition to one's age, one's particular set of medical problems, and one's individual social and employment situation, an additional factor should also be considered in deciding whether a person is too fat and needs to lose weight: the pattern of distribution of fat within one's body. As we noted earlier, the pattern of fat distribution is a major determinant of whether you are too fat for your own good health. Excess fat deposited in the abdomen carries much more health risk than does excess fat located in the thighs.

PATTERNS OF OBESITY

People differ not only in the total amount of fat they have in their bodies, but also in its pattern of distribution. Gender, age, hormones, and genetic predisposition all affect fat patterns.

Women in general have a larger proportion of their body as fat tissue than do men, and they distribute it quite differently. *"Vive la différence!"* is a common reaction to the characteristic accumulation of adipose tissue about the buttocks and breasts after puberty in women as contrasted to men. This shift in fat distribution is caused by hormones, mainly estrogen. Estrogen-induced regional fat distribution commonly occurs in women who take birth-control pills and in those receiving postmenopausal hormone treatment. It can also be seen in castrated males and estrogen-treated males, in whom the normal relationship between the so-called male and female sex hormones is altered.

Other hormones that influence fat distribution are *cortisol* and its metabolic relatives, such as *cortisone* and *prednisone*. These hormones are known as *glucocorticoids* or *adrenal steroids*. Cortisol itself originates in the adrenal glands. Many of its metabolic relatives, however, are available as pills or shots. Amounts of these hormones taken in excess of daily needs induce accumulation of fat tissue in the central part of the body, the trunk, the neck, and the face. This "steroid-induced" pattern of obesity gives a bloated, puffy appearance above the collarbones, around the abdomen, and behind the nape of the neck (the "buffalo hump" look). Large doses of certain steroid hormones such as prednisone—at times prescribed for severe cases of asthma or arthritis—frequently cause this regional pattern of obesity. Please note that these glucocorticoid steroids are different from the anabolic steroids sometimes abused by athletes. Anabolic steroids do not cause fat accumulation, except around the nipples in some people. This breast enlargement occurs because the liver converts anabolic steroids into estrogen.

Common regional patterns of fat distribution affect the health risks of obesity. These patterns may also influence the likelihood of success in reducing body fat and keeping it off. Historically, physicians and scientists interested in this field have noted two common fundamental patterns of fat distribution in obese individuals. One type has fat distributed throughout the body—just as prominent around the wrists, fingers, legs, and ankles as around the trunk and the chest. This is called peripheral obesity. Because it is more common in women, this form of obesity has also been called "gynoid" obesity. It typically involves the buttocks and legs, and consequently is also called "lower-segment" obesity.

In the other general category of fat distribution, the fat is distributed mainly around the central part of the body—the chest and abdomen—with relatively little extra fat around the extremities. This is called "central," "upper segment," or "truncal" obesity. Because it is more common in men, it is also called "android" obseity. Information from two national health surveys shows that in men the buildup of fat on the arms generally stops after age 35, while abdominal fat continues to accumulate. Women, on the other hand, continue to gain fat both on the limbs and in the central part of the body.

As they put on weight with age, men tend to develop the upper-segment, or abdominal obesity, whereas women tend to develop lower-segment obesity.

Some women, of course, have mainly abdominal obesity, and some men have lower-segment obesity. This has nothing to do with their femininity or masculinity, but often with the age at which they first started to accumulate excess fat. Many people with fat distributed peripherally as well as centrally started becoming obese in early life, and were overweight as far back in childhood as they can remember. Those with more central obesity usually date the onset of their obesity to adult life, and were not overweight as children.

It is now apparent that many of the adverse health consequences of obesity result from excess fat gained in adult life. This seems to be particularly true of Type II diabetes mellitus (the type that usually occurs after age 30), high blood pressure, stroke, high cholesterol, and coronary heart disease. Since adult-onset obesity, especially in males, is usually characterized by fat tissue distributed mainly around the abdomen, simple measurement of this type of obesity becomes important. The belt test and the waist-to-hip-ratio test (WHR) provide these simple measurements. As we noted, abdominal obesity is characterized by a WHR of 1.0 or more, while obesity mainly around the thighs and hips gives lower WHR values.

Racial background is another determinant of regional fat distribution. For example, people of Hispanic and Native American ancestry very commonly accumulate fat in an upper-body, or abdominal, pat-

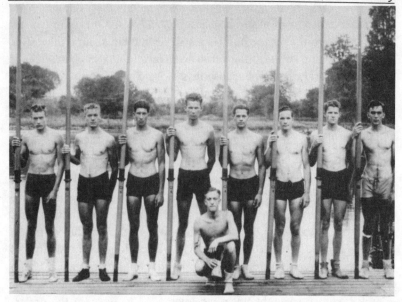

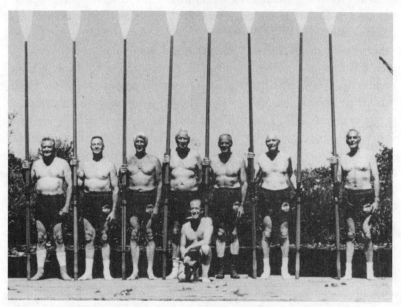

Figure 6.5 Team at Time of Olympic Competition, Then Again in
Same Pose 40 Years Later

The upper photo is of the University of Washington Olympic crew team when
they won the gold medal in the 1936 Berlin Olympic Games. The lower photo
is of the same group 40 years later, at the time of the Montreal Olympics in
1976. Note the typical adult-male pattern of fat accumulation.

tern. This pattern may help explain the very high rates of gallstones and of Type II diabetes mellitus in these groups.

Just as fat usually accumulates around the midsections of adults who were not previously obese, weight reduction in such people tends to subtract fat from the same area. Adipose tissue around the thighs and hips is relatively resistant to change, as calorically restricted diets usually reduce fat tissue around the abdomen. It appears as though the body prefers the LIFO ("last in, first out") method of accounting to the FIFO ("first in, first out") method often used by accountants. Because the abdomen is usually where fat accumulates last and recedes first, adults often realize significant health benefits from relatively minor amounts of weight reduction. As abdominal fat is lost, the WHR returns toward safe levels, and "apple" shapes start to normalize. "Pear" shapes, on the other hand, may be accentuated as abdominal fat shrinks, while lower-segment fat acquired in childhood resists reduction.

Since excess abdominal fat is often the first to go during weight reduction, health risks may decrease dramatically with the first 20 or 30 pounds of weight loss. Many obese people do not need to get all the way down to ideal body weight to improve their health dramatically. Blood cholesterol, blood pressure, and their tendency to diabetes often vanish with the first 20 or 30 pounds lost, typically with a disproportionate reduction in abdominal fat.

ABDOMINAL OBESITY: A WARNING

A potentially very important new development has been the discovery by CAT-scanning techniques that abdominal obesity can be further subdivided into two types, with only one of these types being associated with some of the medical risks. In some people the abdominal fat tissue lies mainly just under the skin of the abdomen (*subcutaneous abdominal obesity*), while in others the fat resides predominantly *inside* the abdominal cavity, around the internal organs (*visceral abdominal obesity*), as shown in Figure 6.6.

It is visceral abdominal obesity that appears to correlate most closely with high blood pressure, diabetes mellitus, heart disease, high blood cholesterol, and premature death. This observation calls into serious question the wisdom of trying to treat obesity by surgically removing subcutaneous fat, as by liposuction. If weight is later regained, the fat is more likely to grow back in the deeper sites within the abdomen, because subcutaneous fat deposits have been partly destroyed. These

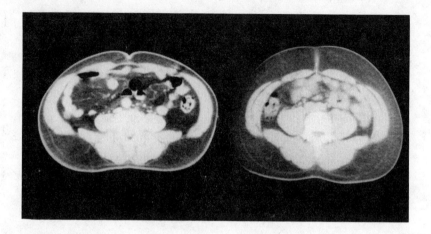

Figure 6.6 Visceral vs. Subcutaneous Distribution of Abdominal
Fat

Patterns of fat distribution within the abdomen. These cross-sectional views of
the abdomen were obtained by computerized axial tomographic X-ray scanning
("CT scanning"). In these photos, fat appears dark, while skin, muscles,
vertebral bone, and contrast material within the intestines looks white. The
individual on the right has lots of fat lying just beneath the skin. We call this
subcutaneous or *superficial* fat. The person on the left has much less
subcutaneous fat, but has more fat deep within the abdomen, surrounding the
intestines inside the wall of abdominal muscles. This deep pattern of fat
deposition appears to carry greater health risk than the more superficial pattern
illustrated by the person on the right.

deeper and apparently more dangerous visceral fat depots are not
accessible to liposuction.

FAT CELLS: TOO MANY VS. TOO LARGE

More than 20 years ago, investigators at Rockefeller University in
New York City devised a technique for estimating the total number
of fat cells in the body. The technique involves removing a tiny piece
of fat tissue from under the skin with a syringe and needle, much like
obtaining blood from a vein. The size of the fat cells in the tissue can
be measured under a microscope, and from body measurements and
the weight of the sample of fat tissue, the total number of fat cells

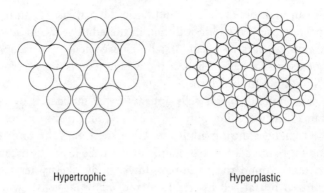

Hypertrophic   Hyperplastic

Figure 6.7 Hypertrophic vs. Hyperplastic Fat Tissue

When someone accumulates fat, the mass of adipose tissue enlarges, either by becoming hypertrophic (made up of large fat cells) or hyperplastic (made up of many smaller fat cells).

in the body can be calculated. These investigators showed that while all obesity was characterized by fat cells swollen with triglyceride, some obese individuals had an excessive number of fat cells in the body. They called this *hyperplastic* obesity, as distinguished from *hypertrophic* obesity, in which the fat cells were enlarged but not exceptionally numerous. Hyperplastic obesity generally corresponds to juvenile-onset obesity, with distribution of fat in the legs in addition to centrally, and with relative body weights more than 60 percent above desirable. Hypertrophic obesity is more characteristic of adult-onset obesity, with a preponderance of fat distributed in the abdomen.

While hypertrophic (swollen) fat cells can shrink during weight reduction, the total number of cells does not decrease. There is some evidence that these greatly distended fat cells give up trigylceride more readily than do smaller, more numerous fat cells. This may account for the fact that regions of more-recent weight gain, such as the abdomen, tend to surrender their fat more readily during weight reduction than do areas with adiposity of juvenile onset, such as the thighs.

While scientists once believed that the total number of fat cells was fixed very early in life and couldn't be changed, we now know that fat cells can multiply even into adulthood. Hyperplasia is more likely to occur, however, in childhood than in the adult years. In adult life, weight gain appears to occur first by enlargement (hypertrophy) of already-existing fat cells. Then, if the weight gain is not reversed, the fat cells multiply (hyperplasia).

The total number of fat cells appears to be influenced by genetic inheritance, early feeding patterns, puberty, and perhaps pregnancy and other changes during adult life. Consistent with the difficulty in reducing fat tissue distributed mainly around the lower body, in contrast to that around the abdomen, lower-body obesity tends to be characterized by fat-cell hyperplasia (too many fat cells), while abdominal-type obesity is mainly hypertrophic.

7

The Causes of Obesity

Understanding of the factors that cause obesity is finally emerging from the realm of mythology into that of science. The scientific evidence firmly discredits the popular misconception that all obese individuals are gluttons who constantly overeat. We now realize that obesity can have several different causes, and the known causes do not include either deficient willpower or personal wickedness.

One informative way to look at the causes of obesity is to take a "macro-economic" view that considers an entire society and the influences that contribute to the prevalence of obesity. A second, equally informative approach is "micro-economic," looking within the individual at the processes governing the intake, storage, and expenditure of calories.

OUR ECONOMIC AND SOCIAL ENVIRONMENT

It is estimated that the prevalence of obesity has increased 500 to 800 percent in the United States since the turn of the century. Unquestionably, much of this rapid rise is due to the fact that Americans are expending approximately 75 percent fewer calories in physical activity than they did 90 years ago. With fewer calories expended, more calories will be stored as fat. In addition, Americans have increased the proportion of calories they consume as fat by 31 percent over the same period. And more fat intake means more calories (see chapter 4). Americans, on the average, consume more than 35 percent of their total calories as fat, while the worldwide average is under 25 percent.

Immigrants entering the United States from underdeveloped countries are often astounded by the tremendous availability of food in this country. A woman who immigrated from Central America reported that one well-stocked American refrigerator contains more food than an entire grocery store in her native city. During her first year in America, she gained more than 30 pounds. Many other immigrants report similar experiences. Japanese who move to the United States tend to acquire many American customs, and as a group they also acquire a dramatic increase in the prevalence of obesity and obesity-related health problems, such as heart disease.

The island of Nauru provides an accelerated and dramatic example of parallel environmental changes. Nauru is a tropical island in the Pacific that, for many years, had a subsistence economy. Nauruans had to work hard for a limited income and enjoyed limited supplies of high-calorie food. Then someone discovered that large portions of their island were made up of bird droppings. Indirectly, this discovery led to a rapid increase in obesity among the islanders.

For centuries, countless seabirds have perched on the hills of Nauru, leaving behind high-phosphate excrement that makes wonderful fertilizer. Enterprising islanders began mining these hills, and developed a very profitable fertilizer industry. Island leaders saw to it that the entire population shared in the revenues derived from this industry. Per-capita income shot up dramatically. The islanders spent a good deal of this income on food, which they could now easily afford to import. With their rapidly rising caloric intake, and the decline in their physical activity as a result of the automation of the fertilizer-mining operations, more calories were being consumed, and fewer expended. The stage was set for weight gain. As the average weight of the islanders rose sharply, there was an onslaught of the medical complications of obesity. Within a generation, Nauru islanders developed very high rates of diabetes. Their economy had become "modernized," with obesity and its medical consequences as by-products of successful industrialization. Similar changes in America have taken place more gradually, but with much the same result.

Obesity runs in socioeconomic classes. An important study conducted in midtown Manhattan showed that obesity was five times more prevalent among the poor than among the rich. Starting life in a low socioeconomic class more than tripled a girl's chances of eventually becoming obese; 26 percent of adult women who had been raised in poor families became obese, as compared with only 7 percent of women born into the highest socioeconomic class.

One's environment, of course, includes television, the eating habits of one's parents, the availability of high-calorie, prepackaged foods, and means of transportation and employment that do not require much physical exertion. One's social and economic environment also includes social pressures to eat or to drink, or to be slender. Many such environmental factors appear to play a role in causing excess weight gain.

From a "macro" viewpoint, there is no question that our American life-style, with lots of high-calorie foods and little necessity for exercise, contributes to the great increase in obesity. On the other hand, these societal changes do not explain why some Americans, or some Nauruans, *become* obese, while others do not. A "micro" look into the factors governing weight gain in individuals is necessary to understand why one person gets fat while his sibling or neighbor does not. To comprehend what can go wrong to make someone gain too much weight, one must first understand the processes that normally govern the accumulation and storage of fat.

THE PSYCHOLOGY AND PHYSIOLOGY OF FAT ACCUMULATION

Fat storage occurs when someone takes in more calories than he or she expends. (Because the calorie is a unit of energy, we use the terms *calories* and *energy* interchangeably in what follows.) Obesity—excessive fat storage—occurs when this energy imbalance is severe, or when it persists for a long time. Figure 7.1 diagrams this simplified overview of the causes of obesity.

Just like the amount of money in one's bank account, or the amount of water in a reservoir, the amount of fat in one's body is determined by the balance between intake and output. This explanation raises further questions:

- What determines how much one eats?
- How is energy expended?
- How does the body regulate the balance between energy intake and expenditure?

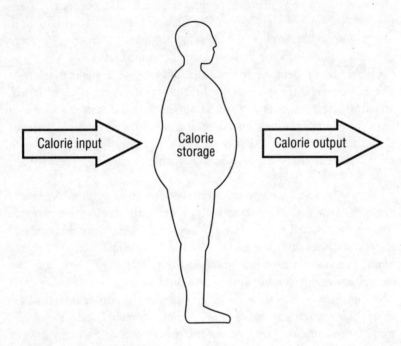

Figure 7.1 Causes of Obesity

Taking in much more energy (calories) than one expends leads to obesity—the accumulation of excess fat.

Questions like these have led investigators to study many interesting details of the processes that control calorie intake and output. Their studies have opened new levels of understanding of the causes of obesity. In greatly simplified form, the next level of understanding might be diagrammed as in Figure 7.2.

A scientist could spend an entire career investigating the details of any one of the listed components, such as the impact of emotion, or of aroma, on calorie intake.

A CASE HISTORY

Sharon was a shy young woman whose parents divorced when she was 11 years old. During junior high and high school, she lived with her mother. Always apart from the crowd, Sharon was never involved

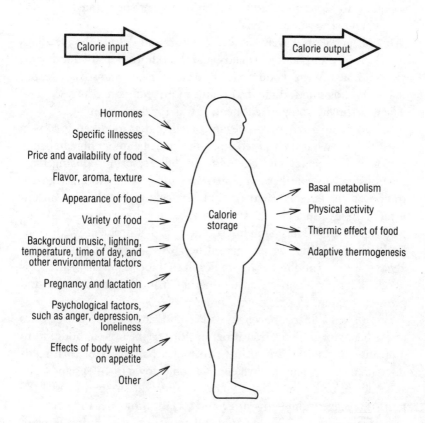

Figure 7.2 Causes of Obesity

Calorie intake, storage, and expenditure are complex matters, each involving several components. Derangement of any of these components could alter the balance between energy intake and expenditure and lead to obesity.

in school sports, student government, or more than an occasional school activity. She was always on the sidelines, watching, and felt hurt and left out of the school's social life. In her loneliness, she consoled herself with food. As the years went by, she continued to use food as a way of compensating for her sense of emptiness, isolation, and frustration. By age 19, at five feet four inches tall, she weighed 173 pounds. She frequently craved sweets, but any quick food would suffice. Sharon tried many diets, but none were successful. Although she had heard of bulimia, and even tried to vomit a few times, it didn't feel good to her, and it didn't accomplish what she wanted. She was lonely, and she wanted food.

In college, Sharon weighed 220 pounds, and despite the pleadings of her mother and her few friends, and the exhortations of her doctor, she continued to eat. Food was her "drug." She had no social life, but only her studies and food. She became more and more depressed, and when she finally sought treatment, it was for depression.

In psychotherapy, Sharon began to realize that food had become a substitute for what she wanted most: the love of another human being. Her fear of intimacy and closeness, in the face of her longing for a relationship, quickly became apparent to her. In addition, her frustration at her parents' divorce, and her feeling that she was an unwanted child—an unloved and unlovable inconvenience—gradually surfaced as well. Her "simple" solution to this problem was to eat. Food never said no, never rejected her, was never too busy. It was always there. In addition, Sharon began to understand that the excess weight kept people away, insulating her from her greatest fear and greatest longing: closeness with other people.

Sharon was able to lose weight with a moderate diet of 1,200 calories and a behavior-modification program for weight loss, in addition to individual psychotherapy. After two and a half years of this multidisciplinary treatment, her weight had come down to 140 pounds. She still had difficulty in social situations; after all, she had missed the normal teenage training in dating and socialization. Her therapist had to help her with the simple social skills that others took for granted. Initially she was afraid of the new "thin" person that emerged from her protective corpulency. She feared being attractive to men. She was tempted to start eating, and regained 20 pounds before realizing that she really wanted to progress, not escape back to obesity. Eventually, Sharon worked through all these problems, and found herself fully capable of giving and receiving love. She maintained her weight loss and went on to have a successful marriage and a satisfying career.

Sharon's case illustrates the complexity and individuality of each person's weight problem. A complete appreciation of all the causes of her compulsive eating is beyond our current understanding; no doubt psychological and societal influences played a role, and biologic mechanisms of food intake and metabolism were involved. Keep in mind, however, that our understanding of these matters is incomplete and still evolving.

WHAT REGULATES OUR APPETITES?

Energy Intake and Storage

We take in energy in the form of food. We eat when we are hungry, when food is available, and when it is tasty and appetizing. As illustrated by Sharon's case, other influences also play a role. Current evidence points to two ways in which the body regulates food intake through appetite and hunger. One takes place over a short period of time (usually minutes to hours). This short-term response is linked to the feeling of an empty stomach. The other occurs over a longer time period, usually several days. In this type of long-term response, feeding drives appear to be modulated by the amount of fat one has stored in the body.

In theoretical engineering terms, we can visualize feedback loops that control appetite. (See Figure 7.3.) The "short loop" of appetite regulation involves both the appeal of the food—whether it be the social setting or the tempting smells and tastes—and the empty stomach. Good smells and tastes signal the brain to begin the reflexes and motions that impel us to sit down at the table, pick up the fork, and begin to put food into the mouth. The empty stomach and intestines operate at a far less conscious level, sending out hormonal signals (chemical messages in the bloodstream) and nervous-system signals (electrical messages transmitted through our network of nerves) to an important part of the brain called the *hypothalamus*. These messages that the stomach is empty and that good food is available converge in the hypothalamus and trigger feeding behavior. Likewise, unpleasant tastes and smells inhibit eating behavior. Food entering the body generates other immediate signals, some of which stimulate more eating—as described in the French proverb, *"L'appétit vient en mangeant"* ("Appetite comes with eating")—and some of which inhibit food intake (such as a feeling of fullness). These mechanisms and signals operate fairly immediately, and provide short-term regulation of food intake.

In the hypothalamus are so-called regulatory centers—groups of nerve cells that turn on and turn off when the stomach is full or empty. All animals have this basic hypothalamic mechanism in the brain controlling appetite and satiety (the feeling of fullness). If all we had was this short-feedback loop, we could continue to eat in excess of our energy needs so long as food was available and appetizing. This

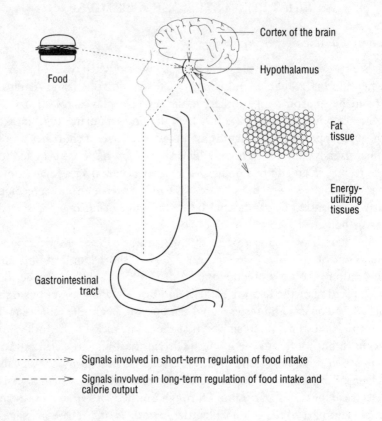

Food

Cortex of the brain

Hypothalamus

Fat tissue

Energy-utilizing tissues

Gastrointestinal tract

- - - - - - - - -> Signals involved in short-term regulation of food intake

- - - - - -> Signals involved in long-term regulation of food intake and calorie output

Figure 7.3 Theoretical Diagram of Signals Involved in Energy Intake and Storage

The intake of food appears to be under both short-term and long-term regulation. Both types of regulation operate through the portion of the brain called the hypothalamus.

could lead to an immense accumulation of fat. Fortunately, as Figure 7.3 shows, we seem to have built-in systems for long-term monitoring of how much fat tissue is in the body. In other words, the brain somehow senses the mass or the size of fat cells present in the body, in a way that influences our feeding behavior. According to this idea, when fat accumulates beyond a certain point, signals are sent to the brain, and the drive to eat is reduced. The precise nature of these signals is unknown, but as we shall see shortly, they certainly appear to exist.

By the same token, when fat tissue shrinks beyond a certain point, the lack of adequate fat stores is thought to stimulate the hypothalamus to increase feeding behavior, and also to reduce the rate of metabolism so that energy is expended more slowly and fat tissue is thus preserved. This long-feedback mechanism occurs over a period of days, and its existence probably accounts for why most people don't vary their weight and fat mass very much, despite wide variations in day-to-day food intake. Superimposed on all these mechanisms, and capable of controlling food intake at least briefly, is the *cerebral cortex*, where conscious thought processes and decisions also influence food intake.

While these short- and long-feedback loops for appetite regulation remain theoretical for humans, there is considerable evidence for their existence in animals. In studies where animals have been purposely overfed through a tube inserted through the abdominal wall into the stomach, they voluntarily decrease their food intake, even though nothing has passed through their mouths for 24 hours, demonstrating the likely presence of this kind of short-feedback loop. Blood serum extracted from such overfed animals will decrease food intake even when injected into hungry recipient animals. The blood evidently carries a chemical message, produced in response to food intake, which inhibits eating.

In other studies, rats have been surgically joined like Siamese twins so that their blood circulation is completely mixed but they have otherwise totally separate bodies, including separate brains and intestinal tracts. Scientists have then put electrodes into the hypothalamus of one of the rats to stimulate electrically those nerve cells that promote eating behavior. Stimulating one of the rats to eat in this way soon causes the other rat to stop eating. The feeding rat evidently releases a chemical message into its bloodstream that signals satiety, or fullness. One rat has eaten and become full, and the other rat, which should still be hungry, nevertheless stops eating.

Other cross-circulation experiments have involved strains of genetically obese rodents that spontaneously overeat and become fat. One of these strains seems to lack the chemical message that signals satiety, and for this reason keeps eating and gets fat. Another strain seems to produce the satiety signal, but its own hypothalamus does not respond to it.

Such experiments indicate that there is a short-term satiety factor that is fairly potent and is probably released from the gastrointestinal tract. You may have heard of one prominent candidate, a hormone (blood-borne chemical messenger) called *cholecystokinin,* or CCK. When injected into animals, CCK causes them to stop eating.

We do not know whether an inability to produce or to detect such a chemical "satiety factor" causes humans to be obese. Theoretically, such a deficiency could represent an inherited biochemical cause of obesity. Moreover, if one could identify satiety factors and then produce them in pill form, one might have a wonderful treatment for certain forms of obesity. Drug companies are keenly aware of such possibilities, and actively sponsor scientific research to find natural or artificial satiety factors that they might then sell as appetite suppressants to cure obesity.

With regard to the long-feedback loop for appetite regulation, involving detection of body-fat content, scientists have studied animals that hibernate, such as squirrels. Just before hibernation, squirrels eat enough to produce large deposits of body fat. Researchers have removed as much as half of the squirrels' fat surgically. As a result, one might expect the squirrels to go on to develop only half as much fat, because they have only half as much adipose tissue. Instead, however, they put back on the total amount of fat needed. Somehow the squirrel's brain knows how much fat is present in its body, and how much is needed. Once the needed amount is stored, feeding slows down.

Such observations have led to the "set point" theory of obesity. The idea is that the hypothalamus promotes food intake until a certain amount of body fat has been accumulated. Once enough body fat has been accumulated, feeding slows down because the feedback signal derived from all that fat is now strong enough to inhibit eating behavior. It is the sensitivity of the hypothalamus to the feedback signal that determines the "set point," or the amount of fat that will be stored. A decrease in the sensitivity of the hypothalamus to these long-term feedback signals, such as might occur in autumn prior to hibernation, would cause increased calorie intake and fat accumulation. An increase in hypothalamic sensitivity would cause weight reduction. The implications of such studies for human obesity are enormous. For example, if your hypothalamus has a "set point" for food intake that is governed by your body-fat content, reducing body-fat content through dieting or surgery may simply stimulate more food intake.

In other studies, when poodle dogs are allowed unlimited access to food, they will generally eat only enough to maintain normal weight. They behave as though they have a rather sensitive hypothalamic mechanism that suppresses food intake readily in response to fat buildup. One might say they have a low "set point," because something turns off their eating before very much body fat has accumulated. For this reason, you will seldom see a very fat poodle. Hounds, on the other hand, keep on eating when allowed unlimited access to food, and become obese. In this regard, some people seem to behave like poodles, maintaining fairly constant weight despite unlimited access to food. Other people's behavior more closely resembles the nonregulating conduct of hounds.

There is evidence for the existence in humans of a mechanism by which the hypothalamus monitors body fat content. For example, the menstrual cycle is controlled by the hypothalamus, and women do not menstruate when their body-fat content is below a certain critical amount. Excessive thinness stops women from menstruating, whether it is due to famine, athletic training, dieting, or anorexia. Moreover, women do not resume menstruation until they gain back to that critical level of body fat. In this way, the human hypothalamus appears to possess means of detecting how much fat is present in the body.

In addition to the short-term and long-term signals that regulate food intake, higher brain centers appear to play a role in how much we eat. The "gray matter" on the surface of the brain is known as the cerebral cortex. It is involved in functions such as thinking, and is highly developed only in higher mammals, including humans. The human cerebral cortex can, at least temporarily, function to overrule eating impulses from the hypothalamus, which appears to operate as a computer center integrating the short- and long-term signals described above. A person can consciously decide to eat, even though he or she feels full already. A person also can decide not to eat, even though he or she may feel hungry. These conscious decisions involve the function of the cerebral cortex.

The compulsive overeating illustrated earlier in the case of Sharon exemplifies the influence of the cerebral cortex over food intake. Sharon's psychotherapy was directed at influencing the thought processes of her cerebral cortex, and she eventually succeeded in reducing her calorie consumption.

Most present-day treatments of obesity focus on the cerebral cortex and on the conscious decisions we make about food intake and exercise. Future treatments—such as, perhaps, a pill to curb appetite—may succeed better by influencing the short- or long-term signals integrated by the hypothalamus. In particular, current research hotly pursues the nature of signals from adipose tissue regulating the long-term control of food intake in response to body-fat content. The dis-

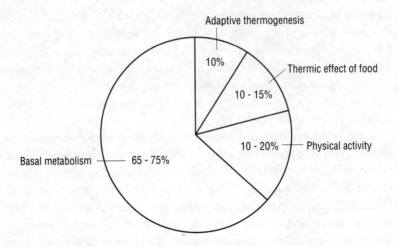

Figure 7.4 24-Hour Energy Expenditure

Most of the energy we expend is devoted to keeping our tissues alive, warm, and healthy; this is called *basal metabolism*. A variable amount of energy is expended through *adaptive thermogenesis*—heat production and calorie expenditure that adjust to influences such as illness, injury, weight gain, weight reduction, and starvation. In addition, we expend energy in digesting food, processing and biochemically transforming it for storage or use as fuel. This metabolic expense of food intake and processing is called the *thermic effect of food*. The other, and most flexible, component of energy expenditure is exercise, or physical activity.

covery of such factors could have important implications for our ability to prevent and treat obesity.

Energy Expenditure

We burn calories simply by staying alive. In fact, the largest component of energy expenditure is *resting energy expenditure,* or REE. (See Figure 7.4.) The rate at which we burn calories in this way is also called the *resting metabolic rate,* or sometimes the *basal metabolic rate,* or BMR.

More than two-thirds of the calories we expend are devoted to basal metabolism—the work of breathing, pumping blood through the heart and blood vessels, and running our vital organs, such as the brain, liver, and kidneys. Even when we are asleep, we are burning calories at this basal rate.

Another component of energy expenditure is the one related to eating and digesting food. It includes the work of propelling foods through the gut for digestion and absorption, and the energy expended in processing and storing food once it has been absorbed into the body. This component of energy expenditure is called the *thermic effect of food.*

A small fraction of the calories we burn is "adaptive." *Adaptive thermogenesis* is part of the body's means for controlling the amount of calories stored as fat. It explains the changes in how efficiently we use fuels when we are under- or overfed. For example, if individuals overeat for an extended period of time, their metabolism will adapt, and fuel is, in essence, wasted. On the other hand, during prolonged undernutrition, calories may be more effectively utilized. Body temperature falls, because fewer calories are being burned. In some species, brown fat (see chapter 3) plays an important role in adaptive thermogenesis. In these animals, brown fat acts like a furnace, consuming calories and producing heat. The importance of brown fat in human energy expenditure is not well understood.

An astonishingly small fraction of our 24-hour energy expenditure occurs in nonresting activities including walking, running, and moving our arms and legs in any way. This third component of energy expenditure, *physical activity,* or exercise, is the part that is obviously modifiable. Although it is a small fraction of the total, it is nevertheless the most significant way we have at the present time for influencing energy expenditure.

While we store a little energy as carbohydrate in the form of glycogen, or animal starch, in our livers and muscles, most of our energy stores are in the form of fat. In order to dip into our energy stores, and reduce them, we must either start expending more calories or eating fewer, or both.

If we cut our calorie intake to a level below calorie expenditure, our body will call on its stored calorie reserves. Enzymes within these tissues break them down and release their constituents into the bloodstream. One such enzyme, located within fat cells, is called *hormone-sensitive lipase.*

This enzyme breaks triglyceride down and releases it from the fat cell into the bloodstream as glycerol and free fatty acids. The glycerol is taken up by the liver and converted to glucose, a simple sugar that is needed by the brain. The free fatty acids can be taken up directly by muscle, and used for fuel. In fact, fatty acids mobilized from adipose tissue are the primary fuel for all tissues of the body except the brain and some blood cells. They are also taken up by the liver, which chemically chops them into small fragments known as *ketone bodies* or *ketone acids,* or simply as *ketones.*

Think of ketones as little, bite-sized pieces of fat, ready for use as a fuel. Ketones can be used by muscles and by the brain for energy. When one fasts for a long time, lots of ketones build up in the blood-stream in response to the breakdown of fat. This condition is called *starvation ketosis.* The ketones also appear in the urine, and can be detected easily by routine tests. Because ketones are acids, too many of them in the bloodstream can cause serious chemical disturbances. Certain dangerous diets cause the body to produce excessive amounts of ketones (see chapter 9).

As calorie expenditure continues to exceed intake, fat tissue and muscles start to shrink. They are "cannibalized" so that other vital organs, such as the brain and heart, which need a constant supply of energy and nutrients, can continue to function. In this way the body protects the functioning of its vital organs, sacrificing its stores of nutrition and energy. It gives up these stores grudgingly, however, as you know if you have ever tried to consistently curtail caloric intake below the level of expenditure. Rather than run a deficit, the body signals the brain to start eating, so that energy stores can be main-tained. It is difficult—seemingly impossible for many people—to keep caloric intake curtailed enough to lose a lot of weight and keep it off.

To summarize: The body regulates energy balance and fat storage by altering both energy intake and energy expenditure. Energy intake involves appetite, hunger, and food-seeking behavior. Energy storage involves metabolic processes providing for the more or less efficient formation or breakdown of fat. Energy expenditure involves metabolic adaptations that lead to the more or less efficient burning of calories. It includes resting energy expenditure, adaptive thermogenesis and the thermic effect of food, and physical activity. The human organism is a finely regulated machine, and it is very difficult to modify severely any of the aspects of this regulation over a long period of time.

Energy expenditure does decline with age, and caloric requirements normally decline with it. Unless one reduces the intake of calories, one will therefore gain weight as one ages. While we cannot at present safely reverse the decline in resting energy expenditure that occurs with aging, we may safely restrict caloric intake and maintain our level of physical activity. Because exercise is one of the few aspects of energy regulation over which we have easy and conscious control, it is a particularly valuable way to avoid the tendency to put on weight with age.

OBESITY: A COMPLEX SYMPTOM WITH MULTIPLE CAUSES

As you contemplate the mechanisms governing obesity and weight control, you will realize that they are diverse and complex, and not simply a matter of willpower. Obesity has many different causes. With so many steps involved in the control of fatness, the reasons for excessive fatness are likely to differ from one person to another. In general, however, the different causes of obesity result in too much calorie intake, or not enough calorie expenditure, as diagrammed in Figure 7.1.

OBESITY AS A RESULT OF VARIATIONS
FROM NORMAL PHYSIOLOGY

Increased Calorie Intake

Several lines of scientific evidence support the conclusion that some obese people get that way through increased caloric intake. Scientists have observed that some obese people eat more calories, and eat them faster, than thin people. For example, when researchers watched adolescents select and consume food in a school cafeteria, obese subjects ate more calories than their lean schoolmates. Moreover, when the caloric density (calories per volume) of food was increased, obese subjects did not cut down on the amount of food consumed as much as lean subjects did. Some obese people increase their eating in response to external environmental cues, such as noise level, lighting, time of day, and attractiveness of the food, more than slender people do. In ways like this, increased caloric intake contributes to some cases of obesity.

When diet histories are used as the means of determining how much someone eats, however, obese people report caloric intake lower than normal-weight people. This finding suggests that as an underlying cause of their excessive eating, some obese people may lack normal awareness or monitoring of their caloric intake.

Increased food intake probably also accounts for obesity resulting from brain damage, hypothalamic disorders, and the intake of certain drugs (see page 169). Our societal abundance of high-fat foods undoubtedly contributes as well to increased caloric intake, as do the psychological dynamics of compulsive overeating illustrated by Sharon's experience. Many obese persons, however, do not eat any more than normal-weight persons do. In these individuals, the obesity must result from decreased energy expenditure.

Decreased Calorie Expenditure

As shown in Figure 7.4, decreased energy expenditure could be caused by a decrease in physical activity, a decrease in resting metabolic rate, or a decrease in thermogenesis.

Researchers have explored the possibility that obese individuals may utilize fuels more efficiently than do slender people, and thus have more calories left over for storage. However, neither diet-induced thermogenesis (the thermic effect of food, described earlier in this chapter) nor adaptive thermogenesis appears to be abnormal in obese people.

Slow Metabolism

Recent evidence shows that some obese people have a slower rate of resting energy expenditure, or basal metabolism, than do normal-weight people. This causes a tendency to gain weight. Since resting energy expenditure accounts for about two-thirds of our calorie usage, it is easy to see how very small, almost immeasurable changes in the efficiency of energy expenditure could cause obesity. Two recent studies support this idea. In one, some Pima Indians in Arizona, who as a group are unusually obese, were carefully tested to determine their resting metabolic rates. Over the next several years, those who had the lowest resting metabolic rates were found to gain the most weight. In another study, scientists measured the resting metabolic rate of certain infants and followed their rate of weight gain. Those with the lowest rate of resting energy expenditure gained the most weight. Especially interesting was the fact that a low resting metabolic rate appeared to be inherited—it ran in families. Although the resting metabolic rate varied widely among families, it tended to be quite similar among members of the same family.

Not all obesity is caused by an abnormally slow rate of resting energy expenditure. Many people, especially in our society, are obese largely because of lack of physical activity.

Lack of Physical Activity

Observations on playgrounds and at summer youth camps have shown that some obese children and teenagers are less physically active than their thinner companions. Other observations have shown that obese people are more likely than thin people to take an escalator instead of the stairs. It is difficult to conclude, however, that their decreased physical activity is the cause, rather than the effect, of their obesity. Physical activity requires greater energy expenditure when one is obese, so an obese person can burn up more calories than a slim person doing the same task. Studies of the efficiency of muscle contraction have shown no differences between thin and fat people.

Lack of physical activity undoubtedly contributes to the considerable increase in obesity in this country since 1900. Although calorie consumption by Americans has *decreased* by an average of 10 percent during this century, Americans have become an average of 14 percent fatter. The increasing weight of Americans, therefore, cannot be blamed on increased eating. It is due instead to the decrease in energy expenditure, which outweighs the drop in caloric consumption.

At the turn of the century, the average person ate more but also expended a great deal of energy in the workplace—whether farming, manufacturing, or homemaking—and was leaner as a result. As forms of employment have become more sedentary, the prevalence of obesity has risen rapidly.

The Bell Telephone Company conducted an informal experiment and found that when their linemen were switched to desk jobs, they gained an average of ten pounds in six months. The company has estimated that having a standard extension phone causes the loss of energy expenditure equivalent to fifteen pounds of fat every ten years, simply because people have less far to walk to answer the phone.

The modernization of transportation is another element in our declining level of activity. While pioneers walked across the continent, for example, we fly in a few hours, with a meal served in flight. And one of the earliest studies of the effects of automobile driving on weight, done in 1951, was prophetic. Test drivers in an automobile factory were asked to drive 400 miles a day for six days a week as part of their jobs. They were encouraged to eat whenever they were hungry. One driver gained six pounds in the first week, the second driver ten pounds over eight weeks, and the third driver 26 pounds over eight weeks.

Perhaps the most common example of a reduction in physical activity leading to weight gain is the athlete who stops practicing his or her sport, or who sustains an injury and is thus forced to exercise less. Many such people gain weight. Consider the former college football players or retired professional football players you may have seen. Many have not cut back their calorie intake concomitantly with their drop in physical exertion. Not all people who stop exercising, however, gain weight. The ones who cut back their calorie intake to match their reduced energy expenditure remain slim. Those who keep on eating as though they were still more active, and become obese, appear to have a weak or deficient coupling between their level of physical activity and their level of food intake.

Studies clearly show that we Americans, on the average, eat fewer calories as we age. Our tendency to gain weight with age, therefore, is not due to increased caloric consumption, but to decreased caloric expenditure. As we noted earlier, part of the decrease in caloric consumption is due to a loss of lean body mass. Even though our weight is going up, our muscle mass is going down. Since muscle has a higher rate of basal metabolism per pound than does adipose tissue, therefore, resting energy expenditure slows. Continuing to exercise as one ages thus offers a double benefit: the increased lean body mass stimulated by exercise keeps resting energy expenditure high, and the exercise itself expends calories.

Some evidence in animals and humans suggests that a lack of exercise may actually increase appetite. The effect is most apparent in the cattle feedlot or the modern chicken farm, where animals are kept confined without exercise in the presence of ample food, and gain weight rapidly with an apparently enhanced hunger. In some ways the modern, white-collar life-style is similar to the feedlot, with ample food and little physical activity.

Genetics

Obesity tends to run in families. We have already noted the inherited tendency to gain weight because of slow metabolism. Some of the family tendency toward obesity, however, could be due to environment rather than to genetic inheritance. Studies of infants adopted out of their biologic parents' home have helped sort out how much of the familial tendency to obesity is due to genetic inheritance, and how much is environmental.

In a study of 800 adopted Danish children, scientists found no relationship between the degree of obesity in the children and their adoptive parents, but a definite correlation between the biologic parents and their children who had been adopted and raised by others. This study suggests that genetic inheritance is more important than family environment in causing obesity.

Another way to sort out the relative roles of genes versus environment is to observe twins. Identical twins share identical genetic inheritance, while fraternal twins do not. If genetic inheritance were very important in determining obesity, one would expect identical twins to be much closer in degree of fatness than fraternal twins. Dr. Albert Stunkard, the same scientist who conducted the study of Danish adopted children, studied 1,983 pairs of twins. He found that the identical twins had higher correlations in degree of fatness than did the fraternal twins, and was able to calculate that almost two-thirds of their variation in weight could be attributed to genetic inheritance. In another study, Dr. Stunkard and his colleagues compared 673 pairs of twins in Sweden. A group of 93 pairs were identical twins who had been reared apart, in separate homes; they shared identical genes but different home environments. A separate group of 154 pairs were identical twins but had been reared together, sharing both the same genes and the same environment. A third group of 218 pairs were fraternal twins reared apart, sharing neither identical genes nor identical environments. The last group consisted of 208 pairs of fraternal twins reared together. The study showed that about 80 percent of the variation in obesity among all these individuals was due to genetic inheritance rather than to any specific home environment.

Similar studies by Dr. Claude Bouchard in Canada also have shown that genetic inheritance plays a strong role in determining who gets fat and who does not. One of Dr. Bouchard's recent landmark studies involved 12 pairs of identical twins who were housed in a locked dormitory at Laval University in Quebec City. All of the twins were kept under 24-hour supervision for 17 weeks. Throughout the study, calorie intake was carefully measured and physical activity was kept constant. For the first two weeks, the subjects were kept at the same weight, and the number of calories per day required to maintain weight was determined for each subject. For the next 14 weeks, each subject was fed exactly 6,000 calories per week more than the amount required to maintain his or her weight. When the resulting changes in body composition were measured, it was found that identical twins gained nearly identical amounts of weight and had very similar gains in fat versus lean tissue. Moreover, the pattern of fat accumulation—subcutaneous versus visceral—was very similar for each pair of identical twins. Considerable differences were noted, however, in the amount of weight gained, the percentage of that gain going into fat, and in the overall pattern of fat accumulation. The study showed that heredity plays a significant role in determining how much weight one gains from overeating, how much of that weight gain becomes fat, and how the fat is distributed throughout the body.

Not only obesity, but also the pattern of obesity, can be inherited. This appears to be especially true for the abdominal, or upper body, obesity which predisposes one to medical problems such as diabetes. Mexican-American children, for example, have a pronounced upper-body pattern of fat distribution whether or not they are obese.

Genetic factors undoubtedly account for some of the tendency for certain ethnic groups, such as Pima Indians and Polynesians, to become obese. Father Eusebio Francisco Kino was an early explorer in the American Southwest. He lived among the ancestors of the present-day Pima and Papago Indians, who as a group are among the most obese people in the world. His writings record experiences with those indigenous farmers eking out a living in the desert regions now represented by Arizona and Mexico. They tell of his life among these people for a season, and then of his departure and later return, after an abundant harvest. In his absence, the people had become so obese that he could hardly recognize his friends among them. They had a remarkable ability to put on weight.

Anthropologists have surmised that these desert farmers were able to survive in the harsh conditions of the Southwest American desert in part because of "thrifty genes." This theory holds that genetically inherited traits, such as a slow metabolism, enabled them to accumulate lots of fat, and consequently to survive periods of famine and starvation.

A similar theory applies to some Polynesian peoples, such as Nauru Islanders, who also tend to become obese when food supply is unlimited and continuous. The ancestors of the Polynesians are thought to have migrated across the Pacific, and those who were able to gain abundant weight before the long ocean voyage were more capable of surviving the trip. They therefore passed "thrifty genes" on to their descendants. Now, when food supply is more reliable and predictable, these same genes may predispose them to obesity.

Genetic inheritance is definitely the cause of certain very rare congenital syndromes (disorders present from birth) of obesity. These include Bardet-Biedl syndrome, Carpenter syndrome, Cohen syndrome, and Alstrom syndrome. Some of these disorders also involve mental retardation, deformities such as extra fingers or toes, and deficient function of the testicles or ovaries. More common is Prader-Willi syndrome, in which varying degrees of mental retardation and mild deformities occur. Although not clearly inherited, Prader-Willi syndrome sometimes involves a damaged chromosome. In these syndromes, brain centers that regulate eating behavior appear to malfunction. The unfortunate individuals who suffer from Prader-Willi syndrome are not only prone to obesity, but show other evidence of malfunction of the hypothalamus, such as delayed or absent sexual maturation. At times, they feel an insatiable demand for food, and are subject to fits of rage when food is not available. It has been suggested that in this disorder, the hypothalamus does not recognize that sufficient fat has already been stored in adipose tissue.*

Brain Damage

Some unusual cases of obesity are caused by brain damage. For example, individuals who have suffered skull fractures have been known to gain as much as 100 to 200 pounds within a year or two after the accident. In other situations, tumors have developed in and around the hypothalamus, with the same result. Thus, in these rare circumstances, damage to the brain—by trauma or tumor—causes obesity.

Injury to the "computer center" of the brain, the hypothalamus, can cause this rapid weight gain. Because the normal circuitry is damaged, the body no longer regulates energy intake, storage, and expenditure normally. Rare diseases of the hypothalamus that are present from birth can also cause marked obesity. The most notable of these is Prader-Willi syndrome, noted earlier as sometimes involving a damaged chromosome.

The Effects of Drugs

Certain drugs prescribed for psychiatric conditions may cause hypothalamic disturbance resulting in rapid weight gain. Among their

*If you have a child with Prader-Willi syndrome, contact the Prader-Willi Syndrome Association, a national association of parents and professionals working together to help families provide optimal care to the victims of this disease. The national headquarters is at 6490 Excelsior Boulevard, Suite 102, St. Louis Park, Minnesota 55426, telephone (612) 926-1947. In addition, you may want to read *Management of Prader-Willi Syndrome,* edited by Louise R. Greenswag and Randell C. Alexander (New York: Springer-Verlag, 1988).

other effects on the brain, some of these drugs appear to stimulate appetite. For instance, the treatment of depression with tricyclic antidepressants, such as *amitriptyline* (usually sold under the brand name Elavil), is often accompanied by the gain of 20 or more pounds of excess weight. Another widely used group of drugs with similar side effects are the *phenothiazines*. These are known as "major tranquilizers" or "antipsychotics," and are widely used in the treatment of psychiatric disorders. Common brand names include Thorazine (chlorpromazine), Prolixin (fluphenazine), Mellaril (thioridazine), Stelazine (trifluoperazine), and Trilafon (perphenazine).

Another class of medications that promote weight gain are those used to treat diabetes—insulin and the so-called oral hypoglycemic drugs. As we noted in chapter 2, people with diabetes have high blood levels of sugar, fat, and amino acids because they lack insulin, or are resistant to it. The hormone insulin promotes the transfer of sugar, fat, and amino acid out of the bloodstream and into body tissues. In other words, it promotes the storage of calories. A deficiency of insulin prevents the storage of calories in body tissues, while the administration of insulin promotes calorie storage and weight gain. So do oral hypoglycemic medications, because they stimulate the production of insulin within the body. The tendency to gain weight with these medications is not a problem for diabetic patients who are underweight, but many diabetics are overweight. In fact, obesity is an important cause of diabetes, since it renders tissues resistant to the calorie-storage effects of insulin.

Because insulin and oral hypoglycemic medications produce weight gain, doctors prefer to treat obese diabetics with exercise and calorie restriction. Those diabetics who cannot control their blood sugar through diet and exercise, however, require either insulin or oral hypoglycemic medications. Obese individuals with diabetes who must take these medications should redouble their efforts to diet and exercise, lest they experience a worsening of their obesity.

Fat-Regulating Enzymes

The enzymes involved in adipose tissue metabolism play a central role in the efficiency with which the body stores and mobilizes fat. We have already noted two key enzymes involved in energy storage in adipose tissue. One is lipoprotein lipase (LPL), which facilitates the transfer of fat from the bloodstream into fat cells for storage. The higher the activity of this LPL enzyme, the more fat is stored. On the other side of the coin, hormone-sensitive lipase liberates triglyceride from the fat cells during weight reduction. While LPL ushers fat into our adipose tissue for storage, hormone-sensitive lipase ushers it out, back into the bloodstream for consumption as fuel.

Obese individuals have high levels of LPL activity in their adipose tissue. This may explain some of their tendency to store lots of fat. When obese individuals lose weight, their LPL activity becomes even higher. This suggests that adapting the activity of this key enzyme is one of the body's protective devices to prevent permanent weight loss. Someone with very active LPL enzymes may thus find it particularly difficult to avoid obesity, as opposed to another person with normal LPL activity. In fact, individuals with Prader-Willi syndrome have the highest activity of LPL ever measured.

With regard to the enzymes governing fat mobilization, evidence for regional differences within the body is now emerging. In some people, certain regions of fat deposits are resistant to the hormones, such as adrenaline, that produce fat breakdown. For example, the hormone-sensitive lipase in the gluteal fat of some people with lower-body obesity responds poorly to the fat-mobilizing hormone adrenaline.

Another hormone, insulin, stimulates LPL and suppresses hormone-sensitive lipase. Both of these actions promote calorie storage. Too much insulin is thus an example of a hormone imbalance that can cause obesity.

Hormone Imbalances

Imbalances in the signals and hormones that govern food intake and utilization are responsible for some cases of obesity. These hormones include cortisol, thyroid hormone, insulin, and probably also estrogen.

Cortisol is a hormone that is known to affect appetite, and is closely related to the common medication cortisone. An overproduction of cortisol in the adrenal glands, or receiving excessive amounts of cortisone or similar medications, produces a rare disease known as Cushing's syndrome. In this condition, fat tends to accumulate especially around the abdomen, chest, and neck. Excessive cortisol also causes thin, bruised skin with very prominent stretch marks, a tendency to high blood pressure, and fragile, easily broken bones. Cushing's syndrome represents one of the few specifically treatable causes of obesity, for the underlying cause can be eliminated. Depending on the exact circumstances, the treatment of Cushing's syndrome might consist of simply reducing the patient's dosage of cortisone, biochemically blocking the production of cortisol within the body, or of surgically removing a tumor that is producing too much of the hormone.

Another biochemical messenger important in human energy balance is thyroid hormone. Made in the thyroid gland and secreted into the bloodstream, thyroid hormone influences the resting metabolic rate of tissues throughout the body. Deficiency of thyroid hormone, known as hypothyroidism, thus results in a reduced rate of resting energy expenditure. It also causes fatigue, so that energy expenditure through physical activity is also diminished. With a reduced resting metabolic rate and reduced activity level, fat tends to accumulate. Other than weight gain and fatigue, typical symptoms of hypothyroidism include constipation, feeling colder than other people, dry skin, muscle cramps, and fluid retention. The symptoms themselves are not necessarily conclusive, since other conditions can cause the same feelings. Fortunately, however, modern blood tests provide definitive diagnosis. Treatment is with thyroid hormone, taken orally. In proper dosage, this treatment reverses all the manifestations of hypothyroidism. By normalizing the slow metabolic rate, thyroid hormone treatment makes it easier for the hypothyroid patient to correct obesity through exercise and calorie restriction.

A third hormone that promotes weight gain is insulin. Released by the pancreas, insulin signals body tissues to take calories out of the bloodstream and store them away. For example, insulin stimulates the LPL enzyme that promotes fat storage and blocks the enzyme (hormone-sensitive lipase) that promotes fat breakdown. It also activates the enzymes that promote the storage of carbohydrate and protein in body tissues. Excessive amounts of insulin, resulting either from a tumor of the pancreas or from overtreatment of diabetes, produce excessive weight gain. While instances of weight gain due to too much insulin definitely occur, they are usually mild. The treatment of this rare cause of obesity is to surgically remove the tumor that is overproducing the insulin, or, in the case of an overtreated diabetic, to reduce the dosage of insulin being administered.

The so-called female sex hormones, especially estrogen, are produced by the ovary and the placenta, and are found in oral contraceptives. Some susceptible women gain as much as 20 or more pounds when they start taking oral contraceptives or when they become pregnant. We do not know why some women are more susceptible than others to weight gain during pregnancy or during oral contraceptive usage, but these female hormones appear to contribute to the weight gain. Estrogens do have tissue-building properties; they promote fat deposits in the typically female distribution, predominantly about the hips and in the breasts. Some girls become alarmed when they start to gain weight at puberty. They mistakenly believe that they are getting fat, and need to be reassured that their fuller shape is the result of normal development rather than of obesity.

Another situation in which high estrogen levels and obesity are linked is the rather common condition known as *polycystic ovary syndrome,* or *Stein-Leventhal syndrome.* Women who suffer from this disorder tend to have irregular menstruation, excess facial and body hair, high levels of estrogens, and often obesity. It is not known whether the high estrogen levels help cause the obesity in this syndrome, but the condition is another example of how people with high estrogen levels tend to gain weight.

Now that you know obesity can arise from abnormalities in the genes, in the environment, in the brain, in adipose tissue metabolism, in any of the signals between the brain and fat tissue, or from still other causes, you know it involves far more than a lack of willpower. Much research is currently in progress to uncover the chemical signals that flow between fat cells and the brain, in the hope of discovering more about the causes of human obesity. We suspect that these mechanisms are keys to the delicate balancing of energy intake and expenditure that normally prevents excess weight gain. Understanding them may lead to new and better ways to prevent and treat obesity.

8

Maintaining a Reduced Weight: Why It's So Difficult

About 95 percent of people who intentionally lose weight regain it. Among the Pima Indians of Arizona, for example, volunteers whom researchers considered medically obese were paid to enter a metabolic research ward and lose large amounts of weight through diet and exercise. Two such men lost 220 pounds each, and were still medically overweight. They then returned to their homes on the reservation, and to their previous life-style. Both reported that they felt better at their reduced weight, and both expressed a desire to keep from regaining weight. When they were followed up fifteen months later, however, each had regained virtually all his lost weight, and was within five pounds of his initial, pre-reduction weight. This striking example is actually typical of most of us as we lose, then regain, smaller amounts of weight.

Many people have the following idea about maintaining a reduced weight: "Although I'm fat now, I'm not gaining. Since my weight is stable, I'm probably not overeating. If I could just drop 20 pounds on a diet, then I could go back to the way I eat now, and maintain my new, lower weight." This thought process is mistaken. The error in the logic derives from the fact that at our reduced weight, we will no longer have those particular 20 pounds of flesh to burn up calories from the diet. Either we will have to exercise more to burn up those calories that the 20 pounds of flesh used to expend, or we will have to eat proportionally that much less.

No matter what method of weight loss you use, it is extremely difficult to maintain a reduced weight. The vast majority of successful weight reductions are followed by a disappointing regain. Many factors combine to facilitate this weight regain, not the least of which are the causes—environmental, hereditary, metabolic, and psychological—that produced the excess weight gain in the first place. In the future, researchers may develop safe methods to prevent hunger or to waste calories. For the present, however, rational attempts to maintain weight reduction must focus on our consuming fewer calories, getting more physical activity, and controlling our environment.

A person who has lost weight no longer has as many pounds of flesh to consume calories through basal metabolism. In a man, each pound of flesh consumes about 12 calories every day simply in staying alive; in a woman the figure is about 11 calories per pound of body weight. A man who has lost 100 pounds therefore has a resting energy expenditure about 1,200 calories lower than he did prior to losing the weight. Those 100 pounds of flesh are no longer there to consume calories. Consequently, if he eats and exercises as he did before losing weight, he will have a calorie excess of about 1,200 calories each day, and gain back about a third of a pound per day. The examples of two men, both of whom lost weight, will serve to illustrate this important principle.

Larry is a 49-year-old engineer who has just lost 84 pounds in a commercial weight-loss program. For about 20 years prior to losing this weight, he averaged 284 pounds. It took Larry more than a year to lose the weight, and he now weighs an even 200 pounds. He's very pleased with his weight reduction, and he's determined to maintain it. Let's contemplate what it will take for him to maintain his new weight.

Larry works long hours at a desk job, and he is also a busy father with three children. His wife also works, and he shares responsibility for dishwashing and other light housework and yardwork. He doesn't have much free time to devote to new physical activities, such as fitness programs.

Most men like Larry, with the same kind of sedentary life-style, expend about 12 calories a day maintaining each pound of body weight. At 12 calories per pound, and 284 pounds, he expended an average of 3,408 calories each day (12 times 284) to maintain his weight. Since Larry has lost 84 pounds, he now expends 12 times 84, or 1,008, fewer calories each day to maintain his weight than he did prior to the reduction. Therefore, if he is to maintain his new weight, he must make a 1,000-calorie-per-day change in his life-style to compensate for the 1,000-calorie-per-day decrease in spontaneous energy expenditure that has taken place.

The task of weight maintenance for Larry boils down to these 1,000 calories. Just keeping those 84 pounds alive and moving used to utilize 1,000 calories a day. Now those 84 pounds are gone. If he eats as much as he used to without exercising more, Larry will have a daily excess of 1,000 calories that his body will store as fat. And since each pound of fat contains about 3,500 calories, he would gain about one pound every 3.5 days, or two pounds per week.

How can Larry eliminate those 1,000 extra calories from his day, every day, so the weight doesn't reaccumulate? He has only two options: increased physical activity and decreased calorie intake. One thousand calories of exercise every day, or eating 1,000 less each day, would get the job done. Or he could achieve some combination of exercise and decreased eating totaling the 1,000 calories. But he must find all 1,000 *every day* on average, or he will inevitably regain the weight he has lost.

It is these 1,000 calories per day, or 7,000 per week, that account to a great extent for why Larry will have a hard time maintaining his new weight. Changing your eating habits and life-style by so much isn't easy, and the challenge isn't made any easier by the fact that, like everyone who loses weight, Larry now expends *fewer* calories than he used to in doing the same everyday activities.

Now that he weighs 200 pounds, it takes less energy (i.e., fewer calories) for Larry to take out the trash or to climb the stairs to his bedroom than it did when he weighed 284 pounds. In fact, it takes about 30 percent fewer calories, because he has lost about 30 percent of his body weight. After all, energy expenditure with most forms of physical activity is proportional to your weight. Consequently, if Larry wants to burn off calories by walking, he must now walk 1.3 miles to burn the same number of calories that he used to burn by walking one mile.

Fortunately, Larry does have some important assets to support him in maintaining his new weight. First, he feels better since losing weight, less fatigued and more inclined to go out and exercise. Second, his wife is genuinely pleased with his weight reduction, and is not subtly trying to sabotage his success, a sad dynamic that takes place in many households where the weight loss of one member strains established relationships between couples or with other family members. She will help with environment control by bringing home fewer doughnuts and other pastries, choosing fruit instead of ice cream for dessert, and serving lower-fat foods. She doesn't mind substituting swordfish or turkey breast for red meat at dinner. She likes baked potatoes, which are low in calories, as much as she likes french fries, which have so many more calories because of the oil they contain, and is happy to eliminate french fries from their diet. Third, Larry likes to walk, and he lives only two and a half miles from work. If he walks to and from work, he will burn about 670 calories for each round trip at his new, reduced weight. Since he works five days a week, this walking alone will expend 5 times 670, or 3,350, calories out of the 7,000 calories he must eliminate each week.

Even walking off those 3,350 calories going to and from work each week, however, Larry still has to eliminate 3,650 more calories each week to reach the weekly 7,000-calorie deficit (1,000 calories per day) needed to keep those 84 pounds off. Unless he makes further changes, he will gain back about one pound per week, since 3,500 excess calories make one pound of fat. Because he doesn't have time for any more exercise, those other 3,650 calories will have to come from Larry's caloric intake. By eliminating the alcohol he used to drink before dinner every night, and making the dietary substitutions sketched above, he can save another 550 calories a day—3,850 calories per week—and thereby balance his calories and maintain his new weight.

How easy will it be for Larry to give up his beer, steaks, and french fries? And when the weather turns bad, the pressure increases at work, and the kids are sick, will he be able to continue his daily five-mile round-trip walking? These are major life-style changes—feasible, but not easy. Of course, Larry doesn't have to give up steaks completely. He can simply cut down on the number he eats. He can also substitute mustard for mayonnaise on his sandwiches, which can save him 80 calories a day. And we haven't even broached the questions of his afternoon snacks of peanut-butter bars, or his riding the elevator to his fifth-floor office instead of taking the stairs. Larry can decide for himself which changes are most practical for him. But the point is that unless such substantial changes take place—and *stay* in place—the fat will reaccumulate.

In addition to these life-style issues that make it difficult for Larry to keep his weight off, powerful biologic forces may also be at work. If the "set point" theory (see chapter 7) is correct, Larry may experience more severe hunger at his reduced weight than he did prior to his weight loss, and his expenditure of calories through adaptive thermogenesis may decrease. The severity of hunger is difficult to measure scientifically. The usual way of evaluating it is simply to measure the number of calories eaten. While we know that calorie intake usually increases after one goes off a diet, and that weight is usually regained, the degree to which a "set point" plays a role in this tendency is not known. Nevertheless, people's weight generally behaves as though some set-point mechanism were driving it back to the previous level.

Consider now the case of Chris, who owned a liquor store, and whose idea of exercise was to walk to the door of his store from his Cadillac parked in front of it. Chris is alcoholic, but he worked full-time and had an apparently stable family life. For lunch he drank something from the shelf at work, and before driving home for dinner he braced himself with another drink. He also drank after dinner at night in front of the TV. His alcohol intake contributed an average of 900 calories to his daily energy input. This, and his sedentary lifestyle, helped keep him fat.

During the years he lived in this way, Chris's stable weight was 320 pounds. Now, however, he maintains his weight successfully at 195 pounds, a resounding 125 pounds less than he used to weigh. Multiply those 125 pounds by 12 calories per pound, and you'll see that Chris now requires 1,500 calories per day less to maintain his weight than he used to. How does he do it?

First, Chris no longer drinks alcohol. With his wife's encouragement, he sold his liquor store, and he and his family moved to a new home in the suburbs. This is a particularly dramatic example of the approach to reduced-weight maintenance known as "environment control." Chris changed his environment in order to make it easier for him to behave in a way that would allow losing weight and keeping it off.

In addition, Chris became a bicyclist. Except during bad weather, he pedals through the rolling hills near his suburban home at least 15 miles a day. When the weather is bad, he uses his exercise bicycle indoors. He hasn't really changed his diet much except for the alcohol, which used to contribute about 900 calories per day to his fat stores. He feels very gratified about the changes he has made, and is confident that he will continue to maintain his current weight, as he has already for several years.

Chris made a couple of very significant and dramatic changes in his life-style, and these changes enabled him to eliminate the 1,500 calories he needed to maintain a 125-pound weight loss. But not everyone can afford a new home in the suburbs, or even an exercise bicycle, nor is it true that everyone has to make such dramatic changes. Learning to enjoy lower-calorie snacks can be vital to weight maintenance, and walking provides a very effective and inexpensive means of expending calories. Again, the point is that one way or another, the adjustments in calorie intake and calorie expenditure must be made, or the lost weight will be regained.

KEEPING IT OFF: A REPRISE

What are the biologic mechanisms that make it so difficult to undertake and enforce a major change in eating and expending calories? How does the body defend its adipose mass so effectively?

Several factors combine to make weight maintenance difficult:

1. The environment that helped you become obese doesn't necessarily change because you have lost weight. The delicious, easily available, high-calorie foods, and the motorized, mechanized society in which we live, contribute to weight regain just as they contributed to weight gain in the first place.

2. Eating habits, which helped you get fat in the first place, are hard to change, as are habits of physical activity.

3. Resting energy expenditure falls with weight loss because there is less tissue around to consume those calories required simply to stay alive.

4. Calorie restriction itself triggers a reduction in adaptive thermogenesis as the body "defends its territory." This slowing of energy expenditure may persist for many months.

5. Energy requirements for physical activity are lessened because the weight-reduced person has less bulk to lug around.

6. Fat storage becomes more efficient, as reflected in heightened activity of the lipoprotein lipase (LPL) enzymes that promote fat accumulation.

7. Unconscious mechanisms involved in regulating fat storage may stimulate food-seeking behavior.

8. Other matters, such as social pressures or psychological barriers in adjusting to a new body shape, add to the difficulty of weight maintenance in certain instances.

Many individuals appear to be "programmed" to a certain range of weight, with a relatively constant adipose-tissue mass and fat-cell size. This hypothetical "set point" or "set range," around which an individual maintains his or her own weight, may help explain the ease with which we are disposed to return to our former weight after weight loss.

Evidence for a body-fat set point includes the fact that when individuals deviate from their usual weight, mechanisms to maintain fat storage come into action. When we examine an individual who was once obese and now has lost weight and is trying to maintain this reduced weight, we can observe (1) increased food-seeking behavior; (2) increased efficiency in the utilization of calories; (3) increased efficiency of fat formation and storage by adipose-tissue cells; (4) decreased calorie output through thermogenesis.

We do not know how the brain detects the amount of fat in our bodies, or whether there is a specific anatomical structure in the brain or elsewhere that controls our weight. Neither do we know why some people appear to have a higher set point than others, nor why the set point appears to shift upward in Americans between the ages of 20 and 50, nor why Americans in the twentieth century behave as though their set points were higher than those of their ancestors in the nineteenth century. Some researchers contend that a balance of environmental and internal forces maintain our weight in a constant range without any central regulatory mechanism, as demonstrated by the following analogy to water level in a lake.

Lake Superior maintains a fairly constant water level, not because of a set point affecting the rates of rainfall, runoff, and evaporation that determine water level, but simply because these processes tend to balance each other out. When water levels in Lake Superior fall, seepage of water into the ground, evaporation, and runoff into the Mississippi River are automatically reduced because there is less water around to escape. When water levels rise, runoff and ground seepage increase because there is more water in the lake to seep into the ground and run into the Mississippi River. So the lake maintains a fairly stable water level, year in and year out. To someone unaware of the climatic and geological determinants of the amount of water in Lake Superior, its tendency to return to a normal, average level might give the appearance of a set-point mechanism.

Likewise, when an obese person loses weight, the particular forces that we have described tend to return the weight to its previous level. As illustrated in the story of Larry, fewer calories are burned during daily chores because there are fewer pounds to carry around. Moreover, with fewer pounds of tissue to consume energy, resting energy expenditure falls, thus favoring regain of the weight which has been lost.

As we have noted, we do not really know to what extent an internal set point regulates our weight, or whether a discrete anatomical location serves that function. We do know that weight is relatively easy to maintain within a certain range, and that environmental influences affect that range. We also know that achieving a lasting reduction in weight below that range is both difficult and unusual unless the kinds of changes we have described are sustained.

There are two theories about the location of the apparent set-point mechanism in humans. One theory holds that the hypothalamus, where signals governing food intake appear to converge, monitors and regulates the amount of fat stored. (See pages 155–160.)

A second version of the set-point theory locates the regulatory mechanism for fatness in the number and size of fat cells within a person's body. The idea is that small fat cells make us hungry, and large ones, full of fat, do not. In other words, fat cells depleted of triglyceride somehow trigger feeding behavior. Once refilled, they calm down and stop screaming for food. In support of this theory are observations that (1) fat cells resist the accumulation of additional fat when they are already stuffed full of fat; and (2) people with lifelong obesity—whose adipose tissue is hyperplastic, with many fat cells (see chapter 6)—have a harder time losing weight and keeping it off than do people with adult-onset obesity, whose adipose tissues contain fewer but larger fat cells.

This theory implies that surgical removal of fat should effectively reduce the drive to eat and thus provide a permanent cure for obesity. Unfortunately, however, we see the same tendency to regain weight after the surgical removal of fat as after the removal of fat by diet and exercise.

As this discussion shows, we do not know all the reasons why it is so difficult to maintain weight at a reduced level. While we can observe that there are natural compensatory mechanisms that tend to restore weight to its previous levels, it is uncertain whether these mechanisms involve some central set point or, like the level of water in a lake, may simply give the appearance of a coordinated scheme to maintain a constant level. In either case, however, we do know that whatever caused a person to become obese in the first place tends to cause the obesity to recur. And because the causes of obesity are multiple and range so widely (see chapter 7), there must be multiple causes for regain. When the underlying causes of obesity can be pinpointed and reversed, as occurs when hypothyroidism is diagnosed and treated, the remission of obesity is likely to last. When those causes include life-style habits, genetics, and other biologic mechanisms, they are more difficult to correct.

No matter what the causes for obesity and its tendency to recur, the task faced by the person who has lost weight remains the same. She or he must eliminate 11 or 12 calories each day for every pound that has been lost, or the excess fat will reaccumulate.

Theoretically, there are many points at which effective intervention might be applied to achieve weight maintenance in the future. For example, safe and effective drugs that interfere with hunger and food-seeking behavior might be developed, or surgery might be devised that can safely and selectively interfere with the absorption of fat. From a practical standpoint at present, however, the key to success still depends on making conscious changes in habits and life-style to increase physical activity and reduce calorie intake.

If you are to maintain your weight loss, the change in calorie intake and calorie output must be sustained. If you continue to eat and exercise as you did prior to your weight loss, the lost weight will return. Making those lasting changes in eating and physical activity is the task faced by anyone who would maintain a reduced level of body fat.

PART III

The Treatment of Obesity

9

The Benefits (and Risks) of Weight Reduction

"If I could only lose weight . . ." How would you finish this sentence? If you could lose weight, would you be happy? Would your high blood pressure go away? Would your diabetes disappear? How about your heartburn? Would your marriage or other current relationship improve, or would it deteriorate? Would you get that job or promotion? Would your wardrobe fit? Would your self-esteem improve? Would you regain the weight, and lose self-esteem?

Questions like these are worth considering. When we long for something—money, status, a new car, accomplishment, a mate, a particular friend, or a new body shape—we may develop unrealistic expectations of the happiness that attaining it may bring. But what can you realistically expect—in benefits and in difficulties—if you lose weight?

PHYSICAL BENEFITS AND RISKS

Weight reduction brings definite health benefits to obese persons, but it also entails risks. Certain health risks, for example, such as gallstones and gout, are increased in the short run during weight reduction, but they are lessened in the long run, once weight reduction is achieved and maintained. Let's survey the possibilities.

Blood Pressure

When a person starts to lose weight by going on a low-calorie diet, an initial loss of body fluids takes place. This accounts for the rapid, easy loss of several pounds experienced during the first week or two on any low-calorie diet. Loss of body fluids reduces the volume of blood, and this in turn reduces blood pressure.

If you have normal blood pressure and go on a diet, you may soon experience low blood pressure, especially when standing. You may notice a sensation of dizziness or faintness when you stand up. This faint feeling occurs because your blood pressure is no longer sufficient to pump enough blood upward, against gravity, to the brain. When blood flow to the brain is compromised, we feel faint or dizzy. Fainting is the brain's way to make us lie down, so that the heart no longer has to pump the blood upward against gravity, and so that blood flow to the brain can improve.

Much of the faintness and dizziness experienced by people who are losing weight on a low-calorie diet is due to this reduced fluid volume, a problem that can be alleviated by taking in more salt. Salt intake boosts fluid retention, thereby raising the volume of blood and, consequently, raising one's blood pressure.

On the other hand, people with high blood pressure, or hypertension, may benefit from the drop in blood pressure caused by calorie restriction: their blood pressure may come down to normal. And if medications have been required to control their blood pressure, they may be able to discontinue taking the drugs, or at least to reduce the dosage. Since all blood-pressure medications involve expense, nuisance, and potential side effects, the correction of hypertension can be a very valuable benefit of weight reduction.

It is not only in the initial week or two of calorie restriction that blood pressure is lowered. Once an obese person has completed weight reduction and is at a stable, reduced weight, the blood pressure is usually significantly lower than it was prior to weight loss. Weight reduction is thus an important part of treatment for high blood pressure.

Blood Lipids

Cholesterol and triglycerides are the main fats, or lipids, carried in our bloodstream (see chapter 5). Calorie restriction promptly reduces blood lipid levels. As with blood pressure, this effect may begin promptly after calorie intake is restricted—even before appreciable amounts of weight have been lost. Moreover, after weight loss has been completed, and weight is being maintained at a reduced level, the cholesterol and triglyceride levels remain lower than they were before the loss of weight. High blood lipid levels are a very good reason to try to lose excess weight.

People whose obesity is predominantly abdominal in distribution are particularly liable to have elevated blood lipid levels. Weight reduction in these cases is especially likely to improve blood levels of cholesterol and triglycerides.

In most people, triglyceride levels respond to weight reduction more dramatically than do cholesterol levels. But don't be discouraged if your own cholesterol doesn't drop very much with weight loss; you may well have done yourself more good than is reflected simply by your total cholesterol count. Even though *total* cholesterol levels may not come down very far, the *type* of cholesterol improves.

Cholesterol comes in several types, as described in chapter 5. To recapitulate briefly, one of these types, known as HDL-cholesterol, helps prevent heart attacks. HDL-cholesterol levels *increase* with weight reduction, even as total cholesterol levels decrease. Following weight reduction, therefore, most people have a more favorable pattern of blood lipids, and a diminished risk of heart attack.

Considering that heart attacks are the leading cause of death in this country, the reduction of elevated cholesterol levels provides a very sensible reason for many obese persons to lose weight.

Congestive Heart Failure

The correction of cholesterol levels is, of course, not the only cardiac benefit of weight reduction in the obese. Obesity causes congestive heart failure by loading the heart with more work than it can handle—more fluid to pump and more miles of blood vessels to pump it through. Weight reduction relieves the heart of these excessive work demands, enabling it to cope more easily with what remains.

To treat congestive heart failure, doctors often prescribe medications that drain fluid from the body, dilate blood vessels, and strengthen the heartbeat. Losing weight can reduce or eliminate the need for such drug therapy, with its high costs and unpleasant side effects. The treatment or prevention of congestive heart failure is thus another good reason to lose excess weight.

Type II Diabetes Mellitus

Obesity plays an important causative role in the most common form of diabetes. It does so by making body tissues resistant to insulin—the hormone that normally keeps blood sugar levels normal. Weight reduction makes tissues more responsive to insulin and thereby allows the metabolism to return toward normal.

Early in the course of Type II diabetes, reducing one's weight through diet and exercise may bring about a remission of the disease, and a return to normal metabolism. It is important to point out, however, that to be beneficial, the weight loss must occur by calorie restriction and exercise, not merely by leaving the diabetes out of control.

Uncontrolled diabetes itself causes weight loss, but not in a beneficial way. In uncontrolled diabetes, blood sugar and fat levels increase hazardously because insulin-resistant tissues cannot assimilate these nutrients. Calories are wasted in the form of sugar and ketones in the urine. Weight loss occurring in this manner does not improve the diabetes, and is detrimental to one's health. On the other hand, when the obese diabetic loses weight through exercise and calorie restriction, blood sugar and fat levels come down toward normal. The pancreas may recover part of its ability to secrete insulin, and tissues respond better to insulin by clearing calories out of the bloodstream.

This remission of diabetes, with normalization of body metabolism through weight reduction, occurs quite frequently in obese persons who have become diabetic shortly before initiating exercise and calorie restriction. After several years, however, weight reduction becomes much less effective in inducing a full remission of the diabetes. Therefore, if you have developed Type II diabetes within the past few years, and are obese, it is imperative that you promptly start losing weight through calorie control and exercise. As a result, you may enjoy years free of diabetes.

If you are an obese person who has had diabetes for years, you will still benefit from weight reduction, but probably not with a complete remission of the disease. Your diabetes may become much easier to control, however, with less need for medication to control the blood glucose. It is not uncommon for someone who required large doses of insulin to control diabetes while obese to enjoy normal blood sugar levels without any insulin injections once excess weight has been lost. Improved control of Type II diabetes mellitus is thus a very valuable benefit of weight reduction.

Type II diabetes mellitus runs strongly in families. Evidence suggests that persons with a family history of diabetes may be able to forestall, or perhaps prevent entirely, the onset of diabetes by avoiding weight gain. Consequently, if you have a strong family history of diabetes, and if you are starting to become obese, you should work on normalizing your body weight. One of the benefits of so doing may be to avoid, or at least postpone, developing diabetes yourself.

Gallstones

Obesity is a major contributing cause of gallstones (see chapter 2). But while avoiding obesity may enable you to avoid developing gallstones, and although losing weight ultimately results in a lower likelihood of forming gallstones, the process of weight reduction temporarily *increases* the chance of forming gallstones.

Gallstones form in bile—a digestive juice formed in the liver and stored in a little sac known as the gallbladder. They range in size from tinier than a grain of sand to over an inch in diameter. Gallstones come in two main types, cholesterol and pigment. Pigment stones are composed of breakdown products of hemoglobin, the substance that carries oxygen in our bloodstream, and they are common in persons with blood diseases such as sickle-cell anemia. The risk of pigment gallstones is not related to obesity or to weight reduction. Cholesterol stones, on the other hand, are the more common type of gallstone in this country, and are definitely found more often in obese persons. Obesity causes excessive secretion of cholesterol into bile, with resultant formation of cholesterol crystals and stones. Weight reduction slows the secretion of cholesterol into bile. Therefore, *after* an obese person has lost weight and is maintaining the reduced weight, his or her bile is less saturated with cholesterol and is less likely to form gallstones. *During* weight loss, however, the risk of gallstone formation temporarily increases.

As one loses weight, the body develops a partial deficiency of bile acids, the substance in bile that keeps cholesterol dissolved. This deficiency permits cholesterol crystals to form, thus increasing the risk of gallstones and painful gallbladder attacks. Taking a certain type of bile acid (ursodiol) by mouth has recently been shown to reduce the risk of gallstone formation during weight reduction. However, details of the risks, benefits, and appropriate dosages of this treatment have not yet been fully established. Current research is actively addressing these important issues because this treatment promises to prevent cholesterol gallstones, one of the most significant medical risks of weight reduction.

Many people lose weight and regain it, then lose and regain it again, in a familiar yo-yo pattern. These people probably increase their chances of getting gallstones. The unusual person who loses weight and keeps it off, on the other hand, remains less likely to form gallstones than if he or she had remained obese.

Heartburn and Esophagitis

Abdominal obesity tends to push stomach acid up into the esophagus, or "food pipe" (see chapter 2), and this helps cause heartburn. When stomach acid enters the esophagus repeatedly, it causes esophagitis—inflammation, tissue damage, and scarring of the esophagus. Weight reduction often ameliorates the problem.

Back Pain

Obesity imposes severe stress on the back, and stretches out the abdominal muscles that stabilize and protect the lower spine. Losing weight alleviates these abnormal stresses. It also allows the abdominal muscles to firm up and provide needed support to the spine.

Low-back problems usually respond to conservative measures, including weight reduction and exercises to strengthen the abdominal muscles, without the need for surgery.

Arthritis

Arthritis, or inflammation of the joints, has several causes. The type of arthritis caused by mechanical trauma is called *osteoarthritis*. Obesity traumatizes weight-bearing joints such as the knees and ankles by increasing the load they carry. In this way, obesity helps cause osteoarthritis at those sites. Weight reduction lessens the load on these weight-bearing joints, decreasing the trauma with its consequent damage and pain. Osteoarthritis of the knees, ankles, and hips can be somewhat eased by lightening one's load through losing weight.

Gout, another form of arthritis, results from tiny, needlelike crystals of uric acid that form within joints. Obesity raises uric-acid levels, and thus contributes to gout. After an obese person has reduced weight, his or her uric-acid levels tend to become lower. As a result, attacks of gout become less frequent once weight reduction has been completed and maintained. However, the risk of gout, like that of gallstones, increases temporarily during weight reduction.

Uric-acid levels usually rise during weight loss because a chemical product of fat breakdown inhibits the excretion of uric acid through the kidneys. As explained in chapter 7, when fat is broken down during weight reduction, weak acids known as *ketones* are formed. Like uric acid, ketones are acids and are excreted through the kidneys. In fact, both of these types of acid utilize the same pathway through the kidneys into the urine. When lots of ketones are present, not as much uric acid can get through into the urine, and so uric acid builds up in the bloodstream during weight loss. The heightened blood levels of uric acid may lead to formation of uric-acid crystals in joints, with a resulting gout attack.

Gout attacks are usually experienced as severe pain, redness, and swelling in a single joint. Most often the joint at the base of the big toe is involved, though gout may attack other joints as well.

The risk of gout attacks during weight loss may be reduced by drinking lots of water, but sometimes medications are required to prevent uric-acid buildup.

Certain diet plans are deliberately designed to produce ketones. These are the high-fat diets. Through high-fat, low-carbohydrate intake, such diets encourage the processing of lots of fats and the consequent production of lots of ketones. The underlying theory of these diets is that ketones kill the appetite, and that their excretion in the urine accelerates calorie wastage and weight loss, but those who are considering such a diet should think again. They increase the risk of gout, can raise blood cholesterol, and can deplete the body of potassium, leaving one weak and susceptible to irregular heartbeat.

Electrolyte Problems and Sudden Death

Our bodies contain certain essential salts that dissolve in body fluids. In their dissolved state, they exist as individual particles, or ions, that carry an electrical charge and are thus called *electrolytes*. Among the important electrolytes in our bodies are sodium, potassium, chloride, magnesium, bicarbonate, hydrogen, calcium, phosphate, and sulfate. Their presence in normal concentration is essential for the normal functioning of most of our organs and tissues, including the intestines, the heart, and the brain.

Obesity does not disturb the healthy balance of electrolytes, but weight reduction can cause life-threatening electrolyte disturbances.

Some of the deaths that have occurred during severe dieting, such as when liquid-protein diets were first introduced, are attributed to electrolyte problems. The detection and correction of electrolyte abnormalities is an important reason why medical supervision is mandatory during rapid weight loss.

As we noted earlier, severe calorie restriction causes an initial loss of body fluids, and these fluids contain sodium and chloride. The resulting deficiency of sodium and chloride can cause feelings of weakness and faintness while standing. Muscle cramps also result from the deficiency of sodium and chloride. These side effects of rapid weight reduction can usually be avoided simply by increasing one's intake of sodium chloride—common table salt.

As the body loses sodium and chloride, the kidneys and adrenal glands secrete hormones to conserve these electrolytes and maintain blood pressure. In conserving sodium, however, these hormones increase the urinary excretion of potassium and hydrogen. A deficiency of potassium can thus develop, with resulting weakness, fatigue, and interruption of the normal rhythm of the heart's beating. Heart-rhythm disturbances due to severe potassium depletion can be fatal, which is why doctors supervising intensive weight-reduction programs regularly measure their patients' potassium levels.

A normal intake of electrolytes is important to balance the excretion that normally occurs through urine, sweat, and stool. Diets that are too low in any of the essential electrolytes can eventually lead to depletion, with potentially dangerous biochemical imbalances. This caution applies equally well to the vitamins and trace minerals that are also required for the normal functioning of our body organs and tissues. A diet deficient in any of the necessary electrolytes, vitamins, or minerals can thus eventually lead to malnutrition and disease. This is why we need a "balanced" diet—one that contains all necessary nutrients—and why fad diets that overemphasize one or a few nutrients can be dangerous.

Calcium and Osteoporosis

Calcium functions in the body both as an electrolyte (dissolved ions in body fluids) and as a salt (crystallized into solids that give bone and teeth their structural strength). Calcium deficiency in a diet usually goes undetected in blood tests, because the bones readily release calcium into the blood to maintain normal concentrations of this important electrolyte. This allows tissues that require calcium, such as the nerves and muscles, including the heart, to function normally despite a diet deficient in calcium—at the expense of the bones.

To maintain healthy bones, an adult should average *at least* one gram of calcium intake daily. This is approximately the amount of calcium found in a quart of milk. Many Americans do not take in this much calcium even when they are not dieting, and many diets do not provide sufficient calcium intake. This can contribute to osteoporosis: bones that are brittle because they do not contain enough calcium to maintain their structural strength. Osteoporosis is a major cause of death, disability, and disease in the elderly, who suffer fractures of the hip and other bones as a result. People predispose themselves to this preventable problem by following diets insufficient in calcium. If you do not or cannot consume a quart of milk per day, you should discuss with your physician the use of calcium supplements.

Women are more prone to osteoporosis than men are. They build a less rugged skeleton during childhood and young adulthood than men do, and menopause deprives women of estrogenic hormones that help maintain strong bones. Women are also more likely than men to go on diets. Consequently, women need to be particularly conscious of adequate calcium intake, and to consider with their physicians the pros and cons of hormone replacement therapy after menopause. For most women, the benefits of estrogen therapy, including the prevention of osteoporosis, appear to exceed any potential drawbacks, such as fat deposits in the usual female pattern (see chapter 6).

Obesity protects against osteoporosis. The added mechanical stress imposed on bones by excess weight causes them to retain calcium. Estrogens formed in fat tissue may also contribute to the prevention of osteoporosis. In losing weight, therefore, a person increases the likelihood of developing osteoporosis unless the following steps are taken to maintain bone strength: (1) assure adequate calcium intake; (2) exercise, to provide the mechanical stresses necessary to keep bones strong; and (3) avoid tobacco and alcohol, both of which predispose one to osteoporosis. These measures should more than suffice to make up for the loss of protection against osteoporosis occasioned by a loss of obesity.

Breathing Problems

The lungs have a twofold task: to obtain oxygen for the rest of the body, and to rid the body of carbon dioxide. Both tasks are accomplished through breathing, with which extreme obesity interferes.

Excess weight not only increases the body's demand for oxygen, but also impairs the lungs' ability to obtain it. Each breath involves expanding the chest cavity. A heavy chest wall, laden with fat, increases the work of breathing. Breathing also involves the contraction of the diaphragm—the sheet of muscle that separates the chest cavity from the abdomen. An abdomen that is distended with fat pushes up on the diaphragm, making it more difficult for this muscle to contract. Eventually, obesity makes the work of breathing so great that the lungs start to fail in their task of obtaining oxygen and getting rid of carbon dioxide. The patient may become drowsy and lethargic, unable to engage in physical activity or even to concentrate mentally. This potentially lethal problem is reversible by weight loss. Lesser problems, such as breathlessness with exercise, also improve as body mass decreases.

Surgical Risks

Obesity increases the risks of surgery (see chapter 2). Blood-clot problems, wound infections, hernia formation at the site of an incision, and postoperative pneumonia are among the surgical complications that are more likely to occur in obese persons than in those of normal weight. Weight reduction reverses these added risks, and makes surgery safer. The absence of a thick layer of fat in the abdomen also makes operating in the belly technically easier for the surgeon.

Physical Mobility and Ease of Function

Many simple acts commonly taken for granted are difficult or impossible for the very obese. Like a release from prison, weight reduction restores these daily functions that the rest of us take for granted: being able to lace and tie your own shoes; getting through the turnstile at a grocery store or ballpark; going for a walk without breathless exhaustion; carrying your own groceries up the stairs to your apartment; fitting into normal-sized chairs, so that you can go confidently to a restaurant or movie theater; functioning normally in sex; climbing a ladder safely; mowing the lawn, or just bending over to pull weeds. Even swimming is impractical for the extremely obese; although fat is lighter than water and improves buoyancy, very obese persons report that they cannot enjoy swimming until they have lost weight.

Regaining these functions is even more gratifying to many people than knowing that their blood cholesterol and blood pressure have improved to the point that their life may be prolonged. The ability to perform such simple functions makes a longer life seem worthwhile.

Cosmetic Appearance

Whether you look better or worse when you have lost weight is a matter of individual taste and preference. Some people prefer robust roundness, while others love a lean, hungry look.

If you are young, weight reduction may not leave you with sagging skin. Many people, however, even those in their twenties or thirties, develop definite sagging of skin with major weight loss. Vigorous exercise may help to keep one's skin elastic and taut, but with weight loss many people develop loose skin folds under the chin or on the neck, arms, abdomen, buttocks, and legs, even though they exercise abundantly. Although these can be eliminated with plastic surgery, such surgery is often expensive, and is seldom covered by health insurance. In good hands, plastic surgery usually goes well. Any such surgery, however, entails risks such as infection, bleeding, scarring, and adverse reactions to anesthesia.

Wrinkles in skin are often accentuated by weight reduction, which makes some people look older after they have lost weight. Since our society prizes youthfulness, some people feel that they look worse rather than better after losing weight.

SOCIAL AND PSYCHOLOGICAL BENEFITS AND RISKS

For many people, obesity is even more detrimental mentally than it is physically. Painful feelings of depression, worthlessness, and helplessness are typical. A sense of disgust about the inability to control one's own body and appetites is demoralizing indeed.

Losing weight successfully brings a great sense of accomplishment. Many of those who do it perceive themselves as overcoming a major obstacle to their personal development, and feel substantially more empowered and worthwhile. Their shyness and sense of shame become replaced by self-confidence and a sense of self-mastery, and the change sets the stage for progress in other areas as well.

While many obese and overweight people are obviously well adjusted, with healthy attitudes and good self-esteem, many others do not have such a healthy outlook, nor is their experience after weight loss necessarily a happy one. Some people feel threatened by the increased attention and sexual attractiveness engendered by their slimmed shape. They may not feel ready to cope with the demands and pressures of dating, and they may even sabotage their own success by intentional overeating in order to avoid the discomfort of having to deal with new social opportunities and challenges.

Others become so enthralled with the new feelings of control and self-mastery that, for them, weight control becomes an unhealthy obsession. In going from overweight to a weight loss so extreme that it verges on anorexia and/or bulimia, a person may become psychologically worse off than he or she was before losing weight. Many such people report that their dieting and exercising just seem to "take over." Rather than being a means to an end, weight control becomes the dominant focus of their existence. They become obsessed with being "in control" of their bodies, and feel desperate panic if they eat a big meal or gain a few pounds. This danger of developing an unhealthy obsession with weight control and becoming bulimic or anorexic is one of the most serious risks of weight reduction (see chapter 3). The results can be devastating physically as well as psychologically.

Another psychological risk of weight reduction is disappointment. Many people feel that losing weight in itself will make them happy, and they are terribly disappointed to find that they have the same hang-ups and problems when they are slim as they had when they were many pounds heavier. It is important to realize that weight loss will not remake your personality. Being thinner does not turn a pessimist into an optimist or make a nervous person calm, a shy person gregarious, a dour grump cheerful, or a socially awkward person easy and gracious. Just as remodeling a house doesn't fundamentally change the family life of the people living inside, changing your physical shape won't fundamentally transform your character. You will still have to live with yourself, with your personality strengths and weaknesses, even though your physical shape has changed. Happiness is not found simply in a new body shape, or in the ability to say no to one's appetite for food.

Disappointment may occur not only when weight loss fails to magically remake our own personalities, but also when it fails to alter the behavior of others toward us. Losing weight may not produce the invitations, promotions, compliments, or whatever else one fantasized that it would elicit. In fact, from some people it may evoke jealousy or even rejection.

Personal change can destabilize interpersonal relations, and the loss of 60 pounds, for example, is a huge personal change. The social consequences of such a change are difficult to predict, and sometimes unpleasant. Consider the story of Jenny.

A CASE HISTORY

Harold and I had a reasonably happy marriage until I started to lose weight. We were both about ninety to a hundred pounds overweight and wished we weren't so fat. We teased each other in good humor, but we accepted each other and felt secure together. We enjoyed eating out, going to movies, watching TV together, and socializing with friends.

Then, unexpectedly, one night I went to the hospital with chest pain. The doctor informed me I had suffered a heart attack, and also that my blood pressure was too high and that I had diabetes. I had not previously been aware of having any of these problems, though diabetes runs in my family. I had thought I was just fat, not sick.

The nurses taught me about the complications that diabetes can cause, and then I really got scared about my health. I figured I might not survive to see my grandchildren unless I changed my ways. So, after recuperating from the heart attack, I got going on a serious diet-and-exercise program.

By the time sixty pounds had come off, people were very complimentary about how much better I looked. I felt better too, both physically and emotionally. I felt I was really doing myself good. Harold, however, just seemed to get jealous. He kept saying how I wouldn't be satisfied with him anymore, now that I was getting my figure back. He became suspicious and started accusing me of being interested in other men, which was not true. His beer-drinking increased, and his weight crept upward as mine was coming down. My progress in weight reduction seemed to trigger a downhill guilt trip for him. He wasn't interested in taking me out anymore. We got into serious arguments, which we had never done before. Finally, Harold and I decided to get some marital counseling. It has helped some, but I'm still not sure that our marriage is going to survive.

Jenny's experience is far from unique. The social consequences of weight change are frequently not as positive as anticipated. Some people who lose weight do so with the expectation that their social lives will greatly improve once they are slimmer, only to find out that they still can't attract the attention of the person they long for. This kind of disappointment often sets the stage for regain of weight.

When the motive for weight loss is based on such unrealistic hopes and expectations, it is difficult to remain motivated enough to continue the exercise and eating behaviors that permit weight maintenance. This can start cycles of weight gain and loss and regain.

The "yo-yo syndrome" of repeated weight loss and regain is especially demoralizing. Most people know about it, but assume that they will so enjoy their reduced weight that they will never regain. Yet the statistics show that lost weight is usually regained, and after losing and regaining several times, people tend to become either discouraged or desperate. These feelings very often lead to depression and/or to fanatical, dangerous methods of weight reduction.

Depression also occurs *during* weight loss in many people, especially when their method for losing weight is severe caloric restriction. People who are starving themselves often feel deprived, depressed, and uncomfortably restrained, not to mention just plain hungry. Exercise, on the other hand, seems to cause less depression than severe dieting. Gastrointestinal surgery as a means to weight reduction also seems to cause less depression than dieting does, though it should be undertaken only with the greatest of caution (see chapter 13).

Although weight reduction brings definite social and psychological risks, most people find that the benefits outweigh the risks—that is, if a reduced weight can be maintained. Enhanced self-esteem and reduced social isolation and exclusion are rich rewards for losing weight. For many people, they are even more meaningful than the benefits that accrue to physical health.

ECONOMIC AND EDUCATIONAL BENEFITS AND RISKS

It is expensive to be obese. Large-sized clothing carries a premium price tag and seldom goes on sale. Moreover, when obesity is progressive, one grows out of clothing before one wears it out. Weight loss, of course, brings the same problem in reverse, unless one has saved the clothing one grew out of. Even then, the clothing outgrown ten years ago may be hopelessly out of style by the time one shrinks back into it. So whether you are going up or down the scale, changing size can temporarily but substantially boost your clothing bills.

Life insurance costs more for obese people than for those of normal weight. Weight reduction can reduce your premiums, if you have maintained your weight loss for a year or more.

Health-insurance premiums are also rated higher for the obese, since disease and injury occur more frequently among people who are seriously overweight. Since employers bear the brunt of paying for health care, they may be reluctant to offer employment to obese persons. This financial consideration simply reinforces the prejudice against obesity that many employers share. Weight reduction may thus make it much easier for a person to find employment as well as to acquire affordable health and life insurance.

In certain jobs, such as in sports, in ballet, in the military, and in police and fire departments, physical mobility is legitimately integral to job performance, and weight reduction may open employment opportunities in these fields to otherwise qualified individuals. There are very few lines of work in which obesity is an advantage and in which one's employability may be impaired by weight reduction.

Many other career opportunities depend on slimness. Fashion modeling is probably the most obvious example, but the immense physical-fitness industry, including health spas, weight-reduction programs, athletic equipment stores, and so forth, tends to offer employment only to those slender enough to serve as role models for the slimness they are trying to market. Weight reduction can thus open the door to many job opportunities denied to obese but otherwise qualified persons.

The prejudice against obesity that characterizes our society extends into the academic realm as well. As we noted earlier, research shows that obese applicants are less likely to be accepted to college than equally qualified slimmer applicants.

In short, if you lose weight, your opportunities for economic and academic advancement might well improve. You might also realize significant psychological and social benefits, such as enhanced self-esteem and an expanded circle of friends. Your health might improve, especially if you have diabetes, high blood pressure, high cholesterol levels, back pain, heart failure, or another physical problem that is worsened by obesity. Your physical mobility and your ability to enjoy many simple, daily activities could greatly improve.

On the other hand, if you lose weight, some of your friendships and even your marriage or other primary relationship might be destabilized. You might become depressed during dieting, or discouraged if you begin to regain some weight. The person you thought would like you better might still ignore you. You might even become obsessed with weight loss and become anorexic or bulimic. This, or some dangerous unsupervised diet program, could even cost you your life. Even on a sensible weight program, you could become dizzy or develop muscle cramps, gallstones, gout, fatigue, or weakness. And, having gone to all the bother of losing weight, you might gain it back again.

With your doctor's help, you should carefully consider the risks and benefits of weight reduction in your own particular case, and decide whether it is worth the effort for you.

10

Diet

The English word *diet* dates back to Chaucer's *Canterbury Tales*. Dieting—restricting one's caloric intake in order to lose weight—is an ancient activity, deeply ingrained in our Western culture. Between 1806 and 1811, for example, we know that Lord Byron was upset about his weight of over 13 stone (182 pounds) and went on a vinegar diet to reduce his weight to nine stone (117 pounds).

Throughout Western history, the restriction of food intake has served four main purposes: as punishment in a penal institution, as mortification of the flesh for religious purposes, as a means of improving body shape for purposes of vanity, or as a means of promoting health. All of these elements persist in our current preoccupation with diet, shape, and fitness.

For many people, diets are a source of guilt and anxiety. "Cheating" is how we describe eating food that is not included in our particular program, as though adherence to such a program were a moral issue. Some of the moral, judgmental overtones that surround dieting come from our culture's view of obesity as a sin. When obesity is experienced as sinful, and dieting as penance, then to deviate from one's diet shows a moral defect and reflects upon one's individual worth. Thomas Jefferson wrote, "One rarely experiences guilt or remorse as a result of food not eaten."

With its deeply ingrained overtones of guilt and morality, is it any wonder that dieting depresses us? Is it any wonder that diets fail as a means of controlling weight in the long run?

If by dieting one means following the latest miracle food fad, the practice is to be condemned. Temporary, "crash" diets always end in crash landings. Overweight people do not need a difficult, deprived, unrealistic food prescription to which no normal person could stick for long. If, on the other hand, by dieting one means the long-term cultivation of eating habits that provide good nutrition and calorie levels low enough to avoid obesity, then it is something to be encouraged.

Because dieting carries such negative connotations of deprivation, guilt, and failure, we suggest that you think in terms of "eating a healthy diet" rather than "being on a diet." Eating a healthy diet is not a temporary adventure in masochism, but a practice to be cultivated and continued permanently.

To renounce the idea of a "crash" diet might not be so easy. We are a nation of dieters, and dieting is an activity and a concept with which we are preoccupied. As we noted earlier, studies have shown that as many as 80 percent of high school girls are on a diet at any given time. Up to 50 percent of our population starts a new diet each year. Americans have an insatiable appetite for fad diets. Publishers know that all you need to sell a magazine is to advertise a new diet on its cover. If you need an idea for a best-seller, create a title that promises to take off pounds magically, quickly, and with no effort.

Reliable statistics are hard to come by, but it is estimated that on the average, diets produce about 10 to 12 pounds of weight reduction. Yet within a year, more than 95 percent of people who have lost weight by dieting have gained it all back. Many gain even more than they lost. This rebound, of course, provides an incentive to diet once again, usually with a "new" and, it is hoped, better diet.

Diets also provide far more than weight reduction. Since dieting is often a group activity, it also provides sociability, though perhaps not on a conscious level. To read a diet book that your friend is reading, and to share focused discussion and dietary activity, can be a pleasant social experience. Discussing how good your friend looks this week, or what he or she thought of the shredded-cabbage soufflé, may provide a certain bond that creates more intimacy than talking about the weather. Many commercial diet programs bring you into contact with concerned counselors and with those who share your struggle. Such common concerns and enterprises can become the basis for real friendship. For many people, this social involvement is as rewarding as any weight they may—or may not—lose.

On the other hand, diets also provide people with feelings of failure, frustration, and discouragement. Indeed, unrealistic, impractical diet plans are prescriptions for failure. The "yo-yo syndrome" that we have referred to describes the familiar pattern of losing weight on a diet, then regaining it, then losing it again, only to regain it yet once more. Closely related is the "failure syndrome"—the familiar cycle of unrealistic vows to restrict food intake, eventual failure to adhere to the restrictions, and then giving up and overeating, feeling guilty and hopeless about ever achieving weight control. Such feelings are themselves obstacles to successful weight control. No one achieves major positive personal changes without morale and enthusiasm, and the failure syndrome demoralizes the dieter, destroying enthusiasm for the challenge of lasting weight control. By setting people up for a full-blown case of failure syndrome, fad diets contribute to the problem of persistent obesity.

The effectiveness of dieting as a means of achieving long-term weight control has not been documented much better than the other approaches described in this book. Investigators in Israel, however, tracked down 27 patients 14 years after they had lost weight on a 550-calorie diet. The 27 patients had lost an average of 30 pounds each on the diet. Fourteen years later, 19 of the patients were within a few pounds of their original, pre-diet weight. Five patients, on the other hand, had succeeded in maintaining a great deal of their weight loss. These five had lost an average of 25 pounds each, and 14 years later they had lost an average of four pounds more, making them an average of 29 pounds lighter than they were before the diet. The other three of the 27 patients had regained all the lost weight, plus an average of 62 pounds more by the end of the 14-year period.

We don't know what any of these patients would have weighed if they had never gone on the diet. But we do know that for two-thirds of them, dieting did not produce any lasting weight change. Did it prevent them from winding up even fatter? We have no way of knowing what might have been. We do know that for five of the 27 patients (19 percent), the diet appeared to be a first step toward lasting weight reduction.

One factor that affects the likelihood of success in dietary therapy relates to the age at which a person first became obese. Those who become obese in adulthood tend to lose weight and keep it off better than do people whose obesity dates back to childhood. This distinction probably applies to all forms of obesity treatment, including exercise.

A GENERAL PERSPECTIVE
ON EATING AND WEIGHT CONTROL

There is no "quick fix" for obesity. The only route to long-term weight control is a lasting decrease in caloric intake and/or a lasting increase in caloric expenditure. If a weight-loss diet were the first step to a lifetime of improved eating habits, it would be a great benefit to the obese person who undertook it. But few diets have any lasting impact on eating habits. In fact, the more fanciful a diet is in terms of content and timing of food intake, the less likely it is to have lasting impact.

Implicit in the concept of successful dieting is the notion of gaining a measure of lasting control over one's behavior. Dieting thus goes far beyond lists of foods that are recommended or forbidden. A successful diet must

- capture the attention of the dieter
- motivate the dieter to adhere to the program
- teach new eating skills, including the ability to change the environment so that lasting reductions in food intake are maintained
- develop personal characteristics such as persistence and the ability to forgive oneself for straying from one's diet
- cultivate the capacity to cope with the normal variations in weight that all human beings experience

Overweight people need not only to lose weight, but to modify permanently their tastes and food choices toward lower-calorie foods. In practical terms, this means learning to enjoy foods with a lower content of fat, since it is fat that carries the most calories. If you enjoy Chinese food, healthy dieting may mean learning to enjoy it cooked in a dry wok, instead of with the usual generous amounts of oil. It could include learning to substitute mustard for mayonnaise in your sandwiches, thereby saving about 85 calories with each tablespoon. It doesn't mean *never* having pizza, but it may mean *usually* choosing something less fattening. It may mean learning to substitute skim milk for whole milk. In this sense of changing one's food selections toward lower calorie intake, dieting is indispensable to the successful treatment of obesity. It is possible to make these changes, however, without ever embarking on a rigid, temporary "diet" that specifies precisely what can and cannot be eaten.

Think of successful weight control as a talent, or as a series of skills—like playing the piano. These skills can be practiced and acquired. Many of them involve choosing foods that are low in calories. Just as a person who is broke can learn to balance a budget, a person who is fat can learn to balance calories. Someone with high blood pressure can learn to eat—and like—low-sodium foods, and someone with obesity can learn to choose—and enjoy—low-calorie foods. The skill of consuming calories at a level below one's calorie expenditure can be successfully cultivated. So can the skills of manipulating one's environment to make it easier to choose low-calorie foods. For example, you can learn to keep high-calorie snack foods out of sight, or even out of the house. Acquiring and applying such skills are indispensable parts of sensible eating for weight control.

As a concept and an endeavor, "going on a diet" is not a sufficient response to the challenge of obesity (see chapter 7). For this reason, dietary therapy for obesity should not be employed without additional measures. It is one essential part of a comprehensive approach to weight management, and should be combined with regular exercise, modification of one's habits of eating and thinking, and, in many cases, group support and individual counseling. In certain extreme cases, even surgery may be needed as part of the overall plan.

If there were a special diet that would make it easy to maintain a reduced weight, you would already have read about it in headlines, and its inventors would have received the Nobel Prize. Unfortunately, no such diet exists. What the world needs now is not one more delicious recipe for tofu casserole à la bean sprouts, but a means of maintaining weight reduction that is practical for ordinary people. At present, the only safe and practical means available is a generous and sustained level of physical activity, and a curtailing of calorie consumption through better habits of eating and food selection.

There is no secret or new information about foods that will "melt away" or dissolve fat, despite claims to the contrary. The basic nutritional facts have been known for some time, and it is important for you to understand them. A calorie is a calorie, whether it comes in burgers or bean sprouts. Neither lecithin nor grapefruit "burns" calories. In fact, since both contain calories, you could get fat by eating too much of either of them.

It has been claimed that the "thermic effect of food"—also known as "specific dynamic action"—plays an important role in successful dieting. These phrases refer to the calories expended by the body in processing various types of food. The idea is that the body processes fat more efficiently than protein or carbohydrate, and consequently that excess carbohydrate and protein calories don't count as much as fat calories do. Technically, this is true. The body does expend a few more calories to process dietary protein and carbohydrate (such as beans and bread) into fat for storage, than it does to process dietary fat (such as butter). The differences, however, are small. Besides, there are plenty of other good reasons to reduce dietary fat.

The overall principle of dieting, of course, is that there must be a *calorie deficit;* more energy must be expended than is taken in. The difference is made up from body fat stores. The greater the deficit, the faster the weight loss. A calorie deficit can be created either by decreasing calorie intake (diet) or by increasing physical activity (exercise), or both.

NOTHING TO EAT

The diet that creates the greatest calorie deficit is to eat nothing at all. This is the epitome of a dangerous and unrealistic diet that cannot be continued for long. It does, however, have the advantage of simplicity, as it entirely eliminates choices and decisions about portion size and food selection. In general, diets in which the food is very simple and repetitive are easier to follow than ones in which one must choose among tasty alternatives and decide how much to eat. And what could be simpler than consuming nothing but water? The other advantage of total starvation is that it enables a person to lose fat rapidly—the exact rate of weight loss depending upon one's level of physical activity, metabolic rate, and size. (The bigger one is, the more calories are consumed by basal metabolism and by any given activity.)

Total starvation is dangerous unless it is used only for brief periods, and then *only under close medical supervision.* The degree of medical supervision required for safety with this "diet" can be quite expensive. Physician visits, blood-chemistry tests, and, if required, hospitalization make bills mount quickly.

Physicians have used this diet successfully for brief periods in overweight patients with diabetes of the type that does not require insulin. By completely eliminating caloric intake for 24 to 96 hours, some diabetic patients can restore their blood-sugar levels promptly to normal. As with all very-low-calorie diets, liberal fluid intake and vitamin and mineral supplementation are necessary.

Metabolic disturbances on a zero-calorie diet can endanger health and life. These disturbances include the depletion of various body salts, the buildup of uric acid (which can damage the kidneys and cause the painful arthritis known as gout), and dangerous heart-rhythm problems. Moreover, total fasting results in breakdown of muscle—including the heart—and depletion of body protein stores. It is preferable, of course, to conserve muscle and protein while losing fat, and this can be accomplished by adding some protein and carbohydrate back into the diet (see below).

Those who successfully employ the brief total fast do so under strict supervision, and as a brief prelude to less severe, continuing restriction of caloric intake. Used properly, it is a way of getting off to a fast start; it is not a long-term dietary strategy. Some people believe that starting with this brief total fast makes subsequent dieting less painful. Do not undertake it without a doctor's supervision.

VERY-LOW-CALORIE DIETS (VLCD, OR "PROTEIN-SPARING MODIFIED FASTING")

Since total fasting is not safe or practical as a method for losing much weight, let's look at what needs to be added back into the diet to reduce risk, yet still permit a negative calorie balance. Two items, besides vitamins, minerals, and liberal fluid intake, are essential for any reducing diet to be safe and healthy: sufficient high-quality protein, and enough carbohydrate to minimize loss of muscle and fluid. The early versions of such very-low-calorie diets did not have these characteristics, and were not safe.

The "liquid protein" diets of the 1970s were implicated in almost 60 deaths. Weight loss was rapid—about one-half pound per day—but medical supervision was often inadequate or altogether absent. In many instances, the nutritional quality of the protein used was poor. And not enough carbohydrate or total calories were present to permit the partial maintenance or sparing of body protein stores. Autopsies of patients who died during or after such diets showed shrinkage and weakening of heart muscle attributed to protein malnutrition, of the kind that can be seen in victims of concentration camps or starvation by famine.

After these tragic experiences, researchers at the Case Western Reserve University Hospital in Cleveland found that by adding carbohydrate to the diet formula, and improving the quality of the protein, many of the negative physical consequences of starvation could be lessened while the rate of weight loss was maintained. In the original studies, patients were hospitalized for the initial seven days to establish the supplemented fast. They received five equal portions of formula food between 8:00 A.M. and 11:00 P.M. Group meetings were held for the purposes of nutrition education, exercise training, and family support. Routine blood chemistries, including potassium and uric acid, were obtained every two weeks, and an electrocardiogram and a blood count were done every four weeks. Weight loss was rapid, and many patients' medical conditions, such as diabetes and high blood pressure, improved remarkably on this program, which came to be known as a "protein-sparing modified fasting diet."

In the past few years, these physician-supervised, very-low-calorie diets (VLCDs) have become very popular in the United States. Many commercial companies have entered the market in response to the rising demand. They sell their liquid diet formulas to physicians and hospitals, which in turn make them available to patients, usually with some accompanying educational program. This approach is proving to be an effective way to achieve major weight loss.

Because of the risks, time, and expense involved, VLCD therapy is not recommended as the initial method of weight loss. It is appropriately reserved for people who require major weight reduction, such as 50 pounds or more, for significant health reasons, and who have failed to control their weight with less drastic measures.

The VLCD diets generally supply from 400 to 800 calories per day. Most of them come in powdered form, in individual-serving-size packets. The powder formula is usually mixed in a blender with water and ice, or simply stirred into either hot or cold water. Calorie-free flavorings may be added. In some programs the dieter is encouraged to consume nothing except the formula, with the exception of copious quantities of calorie-free liquids. In other programs the formula is intended to be used in addition to such items as fruits and vegetables. In some cases the formulas contain all necessary vitamins and minerals, while in others these are taken separately as a supplement. The nutritional content of these formula diet programs tends to be quite similar, and is generally adequate if one takes the full number of packets prescribed each day.

In an attempt to achieve lasting weight maintenance, VLCD programs also typically include a weekly one-to-two-hour group session aimed at behavior modification, nutrition education, promotion of physical activity, and, in some programs, psychotherapy. This makes the programs time-consuming as well as expensive.

Although most people are able to lose between two and four pounds per week on these programs, many do not stick with the programs until they achieve their goal weight. Some drop out because of the expense—as much as $750 per month during the fasting phase. Others do not adhere strictly to the fast, become discouraged, and drop out. In most programs, less than half of the patients who sign up to start a VLCD fast actually get all the way down to their goal weight. Joining such a program, therefore, is not a sure-fire way of eliminating excess weight. Unfortunately, no good method yet exists to predict in advance which patients will succeed in sticking with the fast and getting down to their goal weight, and which ones will not.

Once people have lost weight in a VLCD program, weight regain is often rapid and considerable. The programs have not yet proven that they can achieve long-term cure (such as five years or more) or control of obesity in a substantial percentage of their patients. This issue—the ability to maintain reduced weight—will be the crucial test that determines the future of the VLCD programs.

Because these programs are still so new, not enough follow-up data yet exist to assess their long-term benefits. Early data on their long-term success, however, are quite discouraging. For example, a group of patients treated by VLCD in Denmark lost an average of 22 kilograms (48 pounds) each. Five years later, only 3 percent of the patients had managed to keep off at least 10 kilograms (22 pounds) of the weight.

A study at the University of Pennsylvania looked at patients three years after the completion of a program combining VLCD and behavior-modification therapy. The patients had lost an average of 19 kilograms (42 pounds) in the program. Three years later, the average amount of weight loss maintained was 6.5 kilograms (14.3 pounds). And even to maintain that fraction of the original reduction, most of the patients had participated in other weight-loss efforts.

In another study, 56 percent of the patients had regained more than half their original weight at a 22-month follow-up. Although all of the patients were unhappy with their weight regain, all wanted to go back on the modified fasting program.

The above statistics, preliminary as they are, show clearly that VLCD therapy for severe obesity is still unproven as an effective means of achieving long-term weight control. They also point to the importance of combining dietary therapy with additional means of inducing lasting changes, including exercise and behavior modification. There is, of course, a great financial incentive for companies to develop effective means of weight maintenance, and this may occur. In addition, as techniques of behavior modification, group support, and exercise motivation improve, long-term results should improve. At present, however, patients who choose this form of therapy should realize that while short-term weight reduction is often gratifying, long-term weight maintenance has yet to be shown for the majority of patients.

The important differences among the various VLCD programs do not lie in the flavor or the nutritional content of the liquid formulas. The taste varies from one brand to the next, and is a matter of individual preference. The practical differences are found in the quality and effectiveness of their respective behavior-modification programs as regards their ability to sustain the long-term maintenance of the weight reduction achieved. Unfortunately, adequate statistics that would allow us to compare these programs are not yet available. Moreover, it is highly likely that within any of these programs, the effectiveness of the group therapy is dependent in part on the quality of the individual group leader. Someone with the skills and personality to effectively help people change is likely to have better long-term results than a group leader without these attributes, even within the same VLCD program.

With modern, nutritionally complete formulas, good patient compliance, and competent medical supervision, these programs are proving to be relatively safe. It must be emphasized again, however, that medical supervision is mandatory. The potential risks of such programs include heart problems due to inadequate intake of high-quality protein and upsets in the chemical balance of salts such as potassium and magnesium. To avoid these problems, it is essential that patients *maintain* close medical follow-up, including frequent blood tests and doctor visits. They should report symptoms promptly to the supervising physician, and take the full amount of formula prescribed (instead of skipping packets to speed up weight loss). Other potential problems include weakness and fatigue, muscle cramps, and faintness while standing up. Diarrhea and/or constipation are frequent but easily managed. Dry skin and temporary hair loss are also frequent complaints. The most serious frequent complication of very-low-calorie dieting is gallstones, with painful gallbladder attacks—sometimes serious enough to require surgery. These risks and problems are shared by all weight-reduction diets, but they are more likely to occur with the kind of severe calorie restriction we are describing. The prevention and management of these problems are outlined at the end of this chapter.

The high cost of VLCD programs—as much as $750 per month during fasting—make them inaccessible to many patients. Health-insurance companies are reluctant to pay for this treatment, especially since long-term cure or control of obesity has not yet been demonstrated. Moreover, insurance companies tend to regard the powdered formula (which constitutes a portion of the expense) as food—as opposed to drugs—and therefore not reimbursable. To cut down the expense for their patients, some physicians have prescribed homemade substitutes for the formula in these diets. For example, an approximate substitute for the formula can be achieved by consuming four glasses of skim milk per day, plus a serving of chicken breast or water-packed tuna, some fruits and vegetables, vitamin and mineral supplementation, and lots of water. Such a substitute program, however, still requires medical supervision and behavior-modification therapy, and a registered dietitian should assess the nutritional adequacy of the food eaten. As a result, effective, inexpensive alternatives to the current commercial VLCD programs are yet to be developed.

One serious drawback to very-low-calorie modified fasts is that their participants do not learn new and better eating behaviors. The consumption of normal food is suspended during the period of rapid weight reduction. It is crucial that the issue of weight maintenance be addressed before one starts such a program, and especially when one goes off the diet. Once they have resumed intake of normal food, patients need a prolonged period of training, encouragement, and problem-solving as they practice improved behaviors of eating and exercise. This behavior-modification component of VLCD programs is critical for long-term success. If you decide to try a VLCD program, look for the one with the best follow-up and maintenance provisions. While impartial publications have not yet compared these various programs with one another, there are a number of steps you can take on your own to evaluate a behavior-modification program. And since the behavior-modification components of VLCD programs are the elements most essential for long-term success, you will want to study them (see chapter 14) before selecting such a program. In any event, medical supervision is indispensable.

RESIDENTIAL PROGRAMS

As expensive as the VLCD programs are, they pale in comparison to the cost of residential, or inpatient, weight-loss programs. For thousands of dollars per week, you can check into one of these facilities and enjoy intensive nutrition instruction, exercise classes, recreational facilities, close medical supervision, and room and board. The "board," of course, consists of the facility's diet presented in its most delectable form. With a great deal of support, weight loss in these programs gets off to a fast start. Patients typically come home two to six weeks later, feeling rested, refreshed, and enthusiastic about managing their weight through controlled eating and exercise. In that time they may have lightened their bodies by ten to twenty pounds, and their bank accounts by $6,000 to $16,000.

Employers and insurance companies sometimes cover a portion of the expense. For example, the Pritikin Longevity Center in Santa Monica, California, charges approximately $5,500 for a 13-day stay, and about $9,400 for a 26-day stay. About 20 percent of the charges are attributed to the medical services provided, and, depending on your policy, may be covered by medical insurance. The remaining charges cover the room, maid service, classes, meals, and so forth, and are generally not covered by health insurance.

Most residential programs provide more than just weight loss. Some have a spiritual focus, others a psychiatric approach. Certain facilities provide a broad-based medical approach to better health and living habits. Others emphasize relaxation, with amenities such as massage, recreation, and socializing prominent in the program. Some centers offer cosmetics and fashion advice.

Statistics on rates of success in sustaining weight reduction through such programs are not available. We know of no reliable evidence that these residential centers are any more effective than other, less costly, programs at producing permanent weight loss. Because of the dearth of statistics demonstrating long-term efficacy, advertising generally takes the form of testimonials by individuals who *have* achieved successful weight reduction in these programs—at least for the time being.

It would be valuable to have unbiased statistics as to which of these residential treatment programs have the highest rate of success, but such comparative data are not available. It would be extremely helpful to have a means of predicting what kinds of people will succeed in this type of program, or to preselect which program will work best for a given individual. Unfortunately, no reliable answers are available to these fundamental questions. The business aspects of these programs remain far more advanced than their scientific medical components, and, as with other therapies for obesity, what works for one person may not work for another.

Three People—Three Responses

Jeff was an overworked, overweight executive who took several medications to control diabetes mellitus, high blood pressure, and high blood cholesterol. His company sent him and his wife, all expenses paid, to a well-known California health center for a one-month "tune-up." They both loved it. It was a refreshing vacation, and a chance to focus on long-neglected health issues. Jeff came back from the program having stopped, with the supervision of the facility's medical department, the four medications he had been taking; his tests now showed better levels of blood pressure, blood sugar, and blood cholesterol than the ones he had had before he entered. His weight had decreased by 14 pounds, and he was enjoying daily exercise in the form of walking with his wife. Jeff felt very good about himself and the program. He warmly recommended it to friends and to his doctor.

A year later, however, Jeff has regained his weight and is back on most of the same medications. He reports that while his eating habits are better than they were before he entered the program, he has not kept up the exercise. He is hoping to persuade his employer to send him back for another month at the center.

Not everyone regains all the weight he or she has lost at such inpatient programs. Consider Mary and Phyllis, television writers who enrolled together in a six-week residential program that specialized in treating food, alcohol, and drug addiction.

Mary and Phyllis had been obese for many years, and had each tried many diets without success. Mary's insurance company agreed to pay all but $1,600 of the over-$20,000 fee. Phyllis had to pay her own bill. Both were excited and optimistic as they traveled from California to Florida to enter a residential program.

The facility they entered employed the "twelve step" program of Alcoholics Anonymous and Overeaters Anonymous. After a thorough initial evaluation, the treatment consisted of a 1,400-calorie "eating program," individual and group psychotherapy, lectures, recreation such as tennis and boat rides, and educational activities such as going out to restaurants to practice controlled eating and selection of healthful foods.

Phyllis lost weight rapidly during her stay, but has since regained it all and feels she has received no lasting benefit from her participation. She says she has no interest in ever trying such a program again.

Mary, on the other hand, states that the experience "saved my life."

Having completed the six-week residential program, she continues to lose weight at home, and is almost down to normal weight—approximately 100 pounds less than what she had weighed prior to entering the program. She attends several Overeaters Anonymous meetings each week, and finds the approach very well suited to her personality and her needs.

The experiences of Jeff, Mary, and Phyllis demonstrate a point that applies as well to other modes of treatment for obesity: Individuals differ, sometimes substantially, in their responses to the same basic therapy.

In summary, if you can afford a vacation at a residential facility that focuses on weight control, you will probably lose a few pounds. You may even manage to keep some of the weight off in the long run. These programs usually get weight reduction off to a fast, enjoyable, and enthusiastic start. Most of them provide at least some written take-home material intended to encourage continuation as an outpatient. Some programs provide follow-up groups and/or a telephone "hot line" for support as needed. The likelihood of maintaining your weight reduction as an outpatient after attending one of these programs, however, is unknown. It is probably no better than after undertaking traditional, stay-at-home, crash diets.

OUTPATIENT SUPERVISED DIETING: A SAMPLING

Closely supervised dieting on regular food while living at home is becoming very popular as a way to lose weight. Several commercial programs are available. What follow are descriptions of some of the older, nationally known programs, but many local competitors are entering this fast-growing market as well.

Diet Center. This is a chain that has been in the market since 1971, and it operates more than 2,000 franchises throughout the United States and Canada. Despite the program's having treated almost 5 million patients, carefully tabulated results of Diet Center treatment never have been published in any independently reviewed scientific journal. This lack of data on the long-term results of treatment is typical of other, competing commercial programs as well, as is the fact that statistics are not available to answer such important questions as what percentage of people who start the program actually achieve their goal weight, and what percentage of people who do achieve goal weight are still maintaining that weight one, two, and five years later.

The distinguishing feature of the Diet Center approach is a daily

(Monday through Saturday) weigh-in and one-on-one meeting with a counselor. The client meets with whichever counselor is available at the time. Most of the counselors are people who have completed the program as clients themselves, and have been trained by the company, but have no formal training or accreditation as dietitians, teachers, or psychologists. Although the diet is nutritionally adequate, some of the guidance given—such as that all patients curtail salt intake and avoid certain vegetables—is not scientifically sound.

The prescribed diet uses food bought at the grocery store, including fruit, vegetables, meat, and eggs. Diet Center itself sells a variety of crackers, salad dressings, seasonings, and protein preparations, but these are not required as part of the diet. Diet Center does insist, however, that clients buy from it about $30 per week of its own vitamin, mineral, and food supplements. These food supplements contain sugar and are taken between meals "to stabilize the blood sugar," a concept of dubious validity.

Weekly group meetings, with video presentations and discussions led by a company counselor, cover a core curriculum in ten weeks. The ten weekly classes each last 60 minutes, with about 30 minutes devoted to nutrition and 30 minutes to behavior modification. The same counselor usually leads all ten group sessions.

Although discounts are often available, typical charges are as follows: $100 for lifetime membership; $240 for the ten weeks of classes, including written handouts; $30 per week for daily visits with the counselors and for supplements during weight loss; and $100 for a year of brief weekly visits after completion of weight loss, for "stabilization and maintenance." Assuming that one lost an average of two pounds per week on the diet, and purchased no Diet Center foods except the required supplements, total charges for a 50-pound weight loss would come to $1,190.

While Diet Center is one of the major providers of diet therapy, and has many customers, no reliable estimate of the efficacy of this treatment approach is available. Anecdotal evidence suggests that many people lose weight in the program, but that weight regain is very common. Similar conclusions apply to its major competitors.

Nutri/System. Like Diet Center, this company operates an extensive network of storefront franchises. Unlike Diet Center, however, Nutri/System sells nearly complete diets of already-prepared foods. These include entrees (there are about 30 different ones from which to choose), vitamin and mineral supplements, snacks, and desserts. In addition, clients purchase fruits, vegetables, and nonfat milk from the grocery store to make up a daily diet totaling from 1,000 to 1,500 calories. The diets are generally low in sodium and nutritionally adequate. Some of the food is freeze-dried (dehydrated), and some is retort-packaged (heat-sterilized but not dehydrated).

Clients come into Nutri/System stores once a week to buy a week's worth of prepared meals, to be weighed, to talk privately with a counselor, and to attend a class centered on nutrition and behavior modification. Many of the personnel in Nutri/System are licensed and university-trained as nutritionists, nurses, and counselors. While other programs employ video presentations, at Nutri/System the counselors themselves present the educational material.

Nutri/System promotes itself as a convenient and good-tasting way to lose weight. It is growing fast and enjoying tremendous commercial success. For example, it claims to have served 750,000 clients in 1988. More than 1,300 Nutri/System franchises are in operation, and approximately two new ones open each week. Despite this substantial commercial success, Nutri/System cannot provide detailed information on success rates in either achieving or maintaining weight loss. Neither does it disclose the rate of drop-out of its clients from either the weight-loss or weight-maintenance phase of its program.

The costs of losing weight at Nutri/System vary from time to time with the competition, but in 1990 an up-front fee of $348 covered the initial evaluation, the counseling and education services and written materials, the vitamin supplements, and a one-year maintenance program. In addition, the food costs an average of $70 per week. Assuming, as we did with Diet Center, that one might lose two pounds every week, 50 pounds of weight reduction would cost approximately $2,100. Some of this expense is partially offset by the reduced level of expenditures on groceries, restaurants, and alcohol, since 21 meals per week are included in these costs.

Can you assume that you would indeed lose an average of two pounds per week for 25 weeks with Nutri/System? Unfortunately, the company does not provide data as to the percentage of customers who enjoy such success, or to the success rate of their customers in keeping their weight off.

Jenny Craig Weight Loss Centres. This is another large and rapidly growing franchise chain, competing directly with Nutri/System. In many ways, Jenny Craig appears to be patterned after Nutri/System, but there are certain differences.

Like Nutri/System, Jenny Craig Weight Loss Centres has its clients come in weekly for weigh-in, individual and group counseling, and purchase of vitamin and mineral supplements and already-prepared food, to be supplemented with fruit, vegetables, and nonfat milk from the grocery store. Unlike Nutri/System, however, some of the Jenny Craig foods are frozen; others are retort-packaged.

Group education at Jenny Craig consists of a video presentation, followed by discussion led by a staff counselor. The staff has been trained by the company, but its members often lack university training in nutrition, nursing, or counseling.

Clients at Jenny Craig pay an initial $185 fee, plus $99 for the one-year maintenance program. If not subscribed to at the outset, the maintenance program doubles in price to $199. The food costs around $65 per week. A series of optional educational, motivational tapes sells for $75–$95, depending on whether a special promotion is in progress. Assuming a consistent two-pounds-per-week rate of weight loss, one would thus pay Jenny Craig approximately $1,900 for 50 pounds of weight reduction. As with Nutri/System, some of these costs are offset by savings on groceries, alcohol, and restaurants.

Like its competitors, the company does not compile comprehensive data on the percentage of customers who attain their goal weight, the percentage who drop out, or the rate of success in maintaining a reduced weight.

Weight Watchers International. Now more than 25 years old, this is the oldest and largest of the major weight-reduction chains. Weight Watchers combines dietary instruction with encouragement of exercise and behavior modification, all at weekly group meetings. Although the parent company, H.J. Heinz, markets food under the Weight Watchers label, the program utilizes regular supermarket groceries. Clients are taught to weigh foods and follow a low-fat, low-calorie diet plan. Since there is no individual counseling, and there are no prepared meals to buy, the costs are considerably lower than those of the other programs described here.

The Weight Watchers registration fee is $26, and the weekly group sessions cost $8 to $12 each. After reaching goal weight and paying for six weeks of maintenance at $8 per week, one then can attend meetings free of charge so long as one remains within two pounds of goal weight and attends monthly. A 50-pound weight reduction, accomplished in 25 weeks, would therefore cost only $226.

As with the other companies, Weight Watchers International does not say, and claims not to know, how many of its clients achieve goal weight, how many maintain their reduced weight, or what percentage of people drop out en route.

In deploring the lack of long-term statistics for all of the above programs, we do not necessarily condemn the treatments they offer. Plenty of individuals have benefited from them. The programs generally take a sensible approach of encouraging people to eat nutritious foods restricted in fat content, to exercise regularly, and to work on improving their eating habits. No one company has yet proven that it accomplishes these worthwhile objectives more regularly or effectively than other, competing programs. There is, however, tremendous financial incentive to do just that. We expect that such commercial programs will increase their effectiveness in response to market demand. And when they do, we hope they will document that effectiveness in a reliable, scientific manner, so that consumers in the future will have a solid basis for choice.

FINDING THE WEIGHT-REDUCTION DIET THAT'S BEST FOR YOU

Should You Consult a Dietitian?

The standard medical approach to weight-reduction dieting is for a physician to refer a patient to meet individually with a registered dietitian. When the reason for the referral is a disease, such as diabetes or high blood pressure, the expense may be covered by medical insurance. Depending on your area of the country, the services of a registered dietitian might cost anywhere from $45 to $85 per hour. An initial visit would typically take one to one and a half hours, and follow-up visits 15 to 30 minutes.

Registered dietitians have a college degree in nutrition, plus practical experience and training, and have passed a competency examination in order to be registered by the American Dietetic Association. As with other medical professionals, dietitians' education must continue in order to maintain their credentials. Their training includes nutrition, biochemistry, and physiology, as well as principles and methods of teaching. They assist people in modifying their diets according to individual needs and preferences.

A visit to a dietitian typically starts with a dietary and life-style history, analyzing the adequacy of one's current diet and its impact on whatever disease or other complaint might be present. The dietitian takes into account individual dietary preferences, the presence of current drug therapy, and such practical issues as the availability and affordability of various foods, and works out an individually tailored diet plan. In assuring that the diet is nutritionally adequate, the dietitian calculates the caloric content to achieve a satisfactory but safe rate of weight loss. Follow-up visits are encouraged, during which the patient is assisted in complying with the diet. If necessary, the dietitian will revise the diet to suit changing preferences or needs. Recipes, shopping tips, ideas for dining out, and basic behavioral modification techniques might all be conveyed, as needed. Some dietitians organize patients into groups for the added efficiencies and benefits of group support.

Many group nutrition programs taught by dietitians are available at hospitals and medical clinics. For a reasonable cost, such as $100 for a ten-week program, these classes offer training in diet, exercise, and behavior modification.

Why do some patients succeed in losing weight with dietitians, while others fail or drop out? As with other programs for weight control, an important element is one's own willingness to make necessary changes. To succeed, one needs to be ready to modify one's diet and life-style. In addition, certain patients seem to relate more effectively to one dietitian or another, just as they may relate better to one doctor than another. There is no practical way to predetermine which patients will actually change their diets and life-styles for the better by consulting a dietitian, and which will not. At present, doctors tend to refer to dietitians any patient who needs to lose weight for medical reasons and who will accept this kind of help. The expense of consulting a dietitian is minimal when one considers the long-term benefits of a properly established eating pattern. Because of their backgrounds, dietitians can provide a well-rounded approach to weight loss, encompassing behavior modification as well as the medical implications of a change in diet.

Evaluating Diets on Your Own

Many patients prefer to forgo the cost of an individually tailored diet and to find a published diet that offers some of the same assurances. If a published diet looks appealing to you, a dietitian can help you evaluate it and make the adjustments that will incorporate it into your particular life-style. If you want to evaluate a new diet on your own, you may be able to find a review of it in a reliable nutrition newsletter, such as the *Tufts University Diet and Nutrition Letter, The Mayo Clinic Nutrition Letter,* or *Nutrition Forum.* You can subscribe to these by writing to *Tufts University Diet and Nutrition Letter,*

P.O. Box 57857, Boulder CO 80322-7857; *The Mayo Clinic Nutrition Letter,* Rochester MN 55902-9915; or *Nutrition Forum,* Journal Fulfillment Dept., J.B. Lippincott Co., Downsville Pike, Route 3, Box 20-B, Hagerstown MD 21740, phone 800-638-3030.

EATING WELL

A weight-reduction diet should restrict your total calories to a level that allows a safe rate of reducing your weight while it provides all essential nutrients. In other words, even with a shortage of calories, your diet should supply complete nutrition. By not eating as many calories as are required to maintain our weight—a shortage we call a *calorie deficit*—we force our bodies to expend their fat stores. This process should take place at a rate that is slow enough to avoid complications, while providing all nutrients necessary to avoid malnutrition.

A calorie deficit is the number of calories expended in excess of those consumed. To achieve a calorie deficit, you need to increase physical activity (calories expended) and restrict calorie intake. When a person consumes 3,500 calories less than he or she expends, that person has achieved a 3,500-calorie deficit. And since one pound of adipose tissue contains 3,500 calories, a deficit of 3,500 calories produces a one-pound weight loss.

To be safe, medically unsupervised weight loss should not exceed two pounds per week, even for a very large person. Since one pound contains 3,500 calories, this means a calorie deficit of not more than 7,000 calories per week, or 1,000 calories per day. Reducing your weight any faster than this requires medical supervision.

As mentioned previously, women expend approximately 11 calories each day in maintaining each pound of their weight, and men expend about 12 calories per day per pound (see chapter 8). Thus, a 300-pound man with a sedentary life-style requires about 3,600 calories per day to maintain his weight. To lose weight, he must consume fewer than 3,600 calories, or else he must significantly increase his energy expenditure. If he ate no calories at all, he would initially have a daily calorie deficit of 3,600 calories and lose about one pound of fat per day, plus some fluid and muscle protein. Total fasting, however, is dangerous, as we have noted. To achieve a more reasonable and safe calorie deficit, this man might instead modestly restrict his daily calorie intake—let's say to 3,000 calories. This would give him a deficit of 600 calories, and if he would then also increase his daily calorie expenditure by walking an extra two miles each day, he would add another 400 calories to his deficit. The combination of increased activity and decreased calorie intake would thus generate a calorie deficit of 1,000 per day. In a week, this equals 7,000 calories, or two pounds. A lighter person would need a lower calorie intake, or more exercise, to lose weight at this rate.

The point here is that despite the calorie deficit, a weight-reduction diet should provide all needed nutrients. An adult should consume about 60 grams of protein daily. The actual recommended daily allowances are 44 grams of protein for adult women and 56 grams for adult men. Most Americans eat far more protein than this recommended minimum; to be sure of adequate protein intake, it's best to plan on about 60 grams per day.

Here are some good sources for protein:

- Nonfat milk contains 8–9 grams of protein per cup, or 32–36 grams per quart. It is the skim part of the milk, not the cream, that contains the protein, so nonfat milk is far preferable to whole milk when it comes to getting your protein while curtailing fat and calories. Low-fat buttermilk and low-fat yogurt have similar nutritional values.
- Cottage cheese contains 27 grams of protein per cup. Cottage cheese comes in low-fat varieties, which are obviously preferable for anyone trying to cut down on calories. It also contains quite a bit of sodium, but this is a problem only for people with high blood pressure or problems with heart failure. Other low-fat, soft cheeses (pot cheese or farmer cheese) are similar in protein content.
- Lean meat, poultry, fish, and shellfish contain about seven grams of protein per cooked ounce. Meat is also a major source of minerals, including iron and zinc. To minimize calories, choose the low-fat varieties, such as white poultry meat, water-packed tuna, and the leanest of the red meat cuts. Avoid frying or adding back fats or oils as you prepare the meat.
- Legumes, such as peas, beans, and lentils, are excellent sources of protein. They also make great soups. If ham must be used in preparing split-pea soup, it should be very lean, though leaving the ham out altogether is preferable in order to minimize fat and calories. Likewise, in preparing the beans, leave out the bacon, lard, and other sources of fat, though small amounts of lean ham may be added for flavor. Seasoning with thyme, parsley, bay leaf, and onion lends flavor, without fat, to beans and lentils. (Although

peanuts are also technically legumes, they contain too much oil—
and therefore too many calories—to be a good source of lean
protein.)

In addition to protein, a healthy diet should contain about 1,000
milligrams of calcium to keep the bones strong. This is the amount
of calcium in four glasses of milk. Again, nonfat is just as good as
low-fat or whole milk, since the calcium is in the skim part of the
milk, not the cream. Calcium supplements can also be taken to help
supply this requirement, although calcium in general is better absorbed
when it is contained in food as part of the diet.

At calorie intakes of less than 1,200 per day for an extended period,
it is wise to take vitamin and mineral supplements, since decreased
food intake affects the total amount of nutrients available. However,
most of the required B vitamins are present in grains, and vitamin C
is present in many fruits and vegetables. Vitamin A, which is also
needed, is available as beta-carotene in deep orange vegetables such
as carrots, and in leafy green vegetables such as spinach. A well-
balanced diet includes all these components: grains, fruits, and a variety of vegetables.

In obtaining all these nutrients, you should consume at least 1,200
calories per day, even if your weight loss is less than a pound per
week. The rest of the calorie deficit can be contributed by exercise.
Diets that are calorically restricted more severely than this should be
medically supervised.

Adequate fluid intake is another component of a healthy diet. When
you are losing weight rapidly, certain waste products tend to build up
in the bloodstream as body fat is being broken down. A generous
intake of fluid helps keep these by-products safely diluted in the blood
and urine, and also helps maintain normal bowel function.

In addition to adequate supplies of nutrients and water, a weight-
control diet should contain bulk in the form of fiber, not only because it provides satisfying bulk to meals, but so that bowel function
can continue uninterrupted. In practical terms, fiber means vegetables, whole grains, and fruits. These foods tend to have low caloric
density—that is, to contain relatively few calories in terms of the
amount of food they supply. They provide bulk without adding a lot
of calories.

Of course, foods of high caloric density, especially oils and fats,
should be restricted; after all, the point of producing the calorie deficit
is to allow your body to consume the animal fat that is already draped

around your own waistline. Since most Americans already eat more fat than is healthy, and since fats contain more calories (nine per gram) than the other food constituents (four calories per gram for carbohydrate and protein), it makes sense to limit fat intake. The American Heart Association, the Surgeon General's Report, and the National Academy of Sciences all recommend that we reduce our fat intake to 30 percent or less of our total caloric consumption. The U.S. Senate Select Committee on Nutrition has recommended that we eat only 28 percent of our calories as fat, instead of the 42 percent now being consumed. A reduction in fat intake will help control cholesterol as well as obesity (see chapter 5).

What about alcohol? To maintain a healthy and successful weight-reduction diet, your intake of alcohol should be reduced to one "light" beer or four ounces of wine or one ounce of liquor per day maximum; better yet, it should be eliminated completely. Since alcohol is nutritionally worthless, its calories have been aptly termed "empty." Alcohol contains seven calories per gram—almost as much as fat. As you look for calories to cut out of your diet, alcohol is a good place to start.

These two changes—reducing the intake of fat and of alcohol—will provide a healthy and sufficient calorie deficit for most overweight Americans if they are also combined with increased physical activity. No other special diet would be necessary.

Where are the overabundant fats that might be trimmed from a typical American diet? They are found mainly in the following seven types of foods:

1. Red meats, such as beef, pork, and lamb. Red meat should be prepared by trimming visible fat, and it should be cooked by low-fat methods, such as broiling. Not all cuts of red meat are very fat. Lean cuts of beef include eye of round, top round, top loin, tenderloin, and round tip. Lean cuts of pork include loin, center loin, and loin chops. It is possible to find boneless ham with only 5 percent fat by weight, which is about 20 percent of calories from fat. Many other cuts of meat from these animals, however, contain over 50 percent of calories as fat, even though the fat is almost invisibly "marbled" throughout the meat.

2. Animal-based processed foods such as sausage, hot dogs, salami, and other "lunch meats."

3. Fatty fowl. Much of the poultry currently available in this country is heavily laden with visible fat. Skin the bird and trim off the fat.

4. Certain dairy products such as butter, cream, whole milk, and cheese, or anything made from these, such as sauces or pizza. Cheeses high in fat include the hard cheeses (such as Swiss, American, cheddar, muenster, and feta), Brie, Neufchatel, and cream cheese. Butter is of course generously incorporated into many sauces, candies, and pastries.

5. Animal fats, such as lard, bacon fat, and gravy made from the drippings from roasted or fried meat or fowl.

6. Vegetable oils and shortening, such as are found in breaded meats and fried foods, in many sauces, dressings, margarine, and mayonnaise, in some baked goods, including pastry, candies, cookies, crackers, and pie crusts, and in many snacks and "granola" products. Although vegetable oils such as olive and safflower are not saturated and therefore reduce cholesterol, they are high in calories and therefore help you gain weight. Whether liquid (unsaturated) or hardened (saturated), they are fats containing nine calories per gram. Fats and oils are fattening, whether they are unsaturated or saturated, animal or vegetable in origin.

7. Nuts and seeds, including their products, such as peanut butter and oils.

As you educate yourself to read the labels in supermarkets, be especially aware that many commercial foods promoted as health-enhancing—even some "health food" cereals—contain hydrogenated oils and other such fats.

Many people confuse calories with the effect of foods on blood cholesterol levels. They mistakenly assume that if something is good for their cholesterol level, it can't be fattening. They have heard, for example, that olive oil is "good for you." Insofar as its effects on blood cholesterol are concerned, olive oil *is* good for you. But it is still just as fattening as any other oil or fat. Just because vegetable oils are unsaturated, and consequently help lower blood cholesterol levels, doesn't mean they are not fattening. Despite their beneficial impact on cholesterol, vegetable oils are just as fattening as animal fat. Since most Americans eat too much fat, correcting obesity means that we should reduce our intake of *all* fats, including vegetable oils.

The seven types of high-fat foods listed above include so many American favorites that you may wonder if there is anything left to eat that is healthy. Be assured that there are many delicious foods left for you to choose from, and we note some of these beginning on p. 228. A number of cookbooks containing good, low-fat recipes are available. And a dietitian can help you revise your own favorite recipes to reduce the fat content.

Many Americans believe they are already eating a healthy, low-fat diet. Let's examine the typical day's menu of such a person. For purposes of illustration, let's say that you are a man who weighs 220 pounds, and that on a particular work day you consume the following food:

For breakfast, three and a half ounces of granola cereal with six ounces of whole milk, and two cups of coffee with dried nondairy creamer.

During your 10:00 A.M. break, a big (unbuttered) bran muffin.

For lunch, a large tuna-salad sandwich on a croissant, with a wine cooler.

For dinner, a broiled 12-ounce porterhouse steak with visible fat trimmed off, served with stir-fried Chinese vegetables, a light beer, and no dessert.

Let's analyze the fat and calorie content of this day's diet. First, granola, which seems so virtuous a choice, contains vegetable oil, seeds, and nuts, all of which are high in calories. The nondairy creamer in the coffee and the cream in the cereal milk are both fats, containing nine calories per gram. All together, this breakfast totals about 600 calories, mostly from fat (including oils). Even the bran muffin of your midmorning snack isn't blameless; commercial muffins contain a lot of oil, and modern-day muffins are bigger than their ancestors. An average commercial muffin contains 350 or more calories. The tuna in your sandwich at lunch provided high-quality protein, but in becoming tuna salad, it was mixed with lots of mayonnaise, each tablespoon of which contains about 100 calories. The croissant was nice and flaky precisely because it had been made with butter, so the sandwich added up to 750 calories. The wine cooler contributed another 150, making this a 900-calorie lunch. At dinner, the steak contained about 1,000 calories, and the vegetables, which had been stir-fried in oil, added another 250. The light beer had about 100 calories, making a total of 1,350 calories for dinner. Now let's add up the day's calories:

Breakfast   =   600
Muffin   =   350
Lunch   =   900
Dinner   =   1,350
Grand total   =   3,200

That is enough calories on a daily basis for a man to maintain a weight of about 267 pounds. But what if, as proposed, you weigh only 220 pounds? At 12 calories per pound, only 2,640 calories are required to maintain your weight of 220 pounds. Therefore, instead of a calorie deficit, you had a surplus of 560 calories for the day. If you were to consume that many calories consistently every day, you would have 3,920 excess calories each week. Since there are 3,500 calories in a pound, you would gain over a pound per week. Eventually, of course, your body mass would increase to a point that it would require the entire daily intake of 3,200 calories just to maintain that much weight. This would occur at around 267 pounds, at which weight you would stabilize.

Now let us suppose that you educate yourself about calories and their consequences. You begin to choose foods lower in fat and eliminate alcohol, thereby cutting calorie intake without compromising nutritional quality. For example, suppose that, on a typical day, you want a similar volume of food, but fewer calories. For breakfast you have shredded wheat with raisins instead of granola, and use skim milk instead of whole milk on your cereal. You also use skim milk in your coffee, instead of the powdered creamer. You add a slice of whole-wheat bread with a teaspoon of raspberry jam, but no butter or margarine. This revised breakfast would total about 460 calories, a savings of about 140 in comparison with your previous breakfast. For your midmorning snack, instead of the muffin, you eat two large pieces of fruit. They total 180 calories, saving you 170 calories in comparison to the muffin. For lunch a turkey-breast sandwich—made with mustard (only 15 calories per tablespoon) instead of mayonnaise, and on bread with lots of lettuce and a tomato slice—runs about 350 calories. The pickle and carrot strips you add have only 20 calories, and an apple for dessert is another 80. You choose mineral water instead of a wine cooler. So for lunch you consume only 450 calories, instead of the 900 you ate earlier. For dinner, instead of steak, you broil a large, 12-ounce serving of lean fish, seasoned with lemon and herbs, and steam your vegetables instead of frying them in oil. You have a salad with low-calorie dressing, a baked potato with a tablespoon of sour cream, and drink a glass of skim milk. A scoop of sherbet for dessert completes the meal. The entire dinner totals only 1,000 calories. Now let's add up the calories and compare them to the previous example.

$$
\begin{array}{rcl}
\text{Breakfast} & = & 460 \\
\text{Muffin} & = & 180 \\
\text{Lunch} & = & 450 \\
\text{Dinner} & = & 1,000 \\
\hline
\text{Grand total} & = & 2,090
\end{array}
$$

The combined savings for the entire day, as compared with the earlier total, was 1,110 calories.

You can calculate your calorie deficit by subtracting the calories you consume (2,090) from calories you need to maintain your current weight ($12 \times 220 = 2,640$). This gives a deficit of 550 calories. If continued daily, this calorie deficit would enable you to lose weight at the safe, reasonable rate of a pound a week. By adding a daily 15-minute walk to your current level of physical activity, you could lose more than a pound per week. Sustained consistently, this program would bring your weight gradually down to around 180 pounds.

Choices and substitutions like these are essential in a weight-reduction diet that is healthy and safe. When you restrict your intake of oil and fat, curtail alcohol, and increase your consumption of grains, vegetables, and fruits, you are on the right track. As we noted earlier, you also should consume sufficient protein, calcium, and other nutrients. It all adds up to eating a healthy diet with enough of all the essential nutrients, and enough calories to avoid the risks of too-rapid weight loss. Drinking more than a quart of water per day facilitates and further supports the process.

Not every meal or snack has to be balanced in terms of fat, protein, carbohydrate, vitamin, and mineral content; what matters is that one's diet generally should include all of these for adequate nutrition. For example, even though its calories are approximately 100 percent carbohydrate, with no appreciable protein, calcium, or fat, an apple still makes a good snack.

AN EXAMPLE OF SENSIBLE FOOD SELECTION

There are many ways to prepare tasty, low-fat meals that contain healthy nutrients. You can combine complex carbohydrates (from vegetables, fruits, and grains) and protein (from seafood, lean cuts of meat and poultry, skim milk, egg whites, and legumes) into a great variety of delicious soups, casseroles, snacks, and other dishes—all nutritionally adequate. Therefore, we do not recommend any single eating plan as the correct one. For purposes of illustration, however, we offer the following example of a healthy, low-calorie menu—one that is both appropriate and satisfying for someone who needs to control weight. These meals provide about 1,600 calories per day, and contain only about 20–25 percent of calories as fat. Combined with plenty of physical activity, they should be both enjoyable and enhance your health and vitality.

Healthy, Low-Fat Foods for a Week

Day 1	Day 2	Day 3
Breakfast	Breakfast	Breakfast
8 oz. skim milk Bowl of whole-grain breakfast cereal 1 oz. raisins 1 navel orange 1 small banana 1 slice whole-grain toast with 1 teaspoon of low-calorie raspberry jam	2 egg substitutes fried without oil on nonstick skillet with tomato, onion, and 1 oz. of skim-milk mozzarella cheese as "Spanish omelet" 2 slices whole-grain toast, 1 teaspoon of margarine, 1 teaspoon low-calorie jam 8 oz. skim milk	2 egg whites blenderized into a "tiger shake" with 8 oz. low-fat yogurt, 6 oz. orange juice, 1 banana, a dash of vanilla, 4 ice cubes, and ⅓ cup of oat bran
Snack	Snack	Snack
1 oz. string cheese	1 apple	12 animal crackers

Day 1	Day 2	Day 3
Lunch	**Lunch**	**Lunch**
Louis salad with 4 oz. shrimp or crab, ½ head of lettuce, large tomato, ½ cucumber, diced celery, 1 tablespoon low-calorie Thousand Island salad dressing 1 small French roll ½ cub sherbet	8 oz skim milk Sandwich of 2 oz. turkey breast, with lettuce, tomato, and mustard (no mayo) on whole-wheat bread Large pickle Several carrot sticks Peach	8 oz. split-pea or lentil soup made w/o animal fat Large tossed green salad, incl. tomato, ¼ cucumber, diced celery, 1 tablespoon low-calorie Italian dressing 1 slice French bread 1 scoop ice milk
Dinner	**Dinner**	**Dinner**
4 oz. chicken breast w/ seasoning to taste w/o skin or fat Lettuce and tomato salad 1 tablespoon low-calorie Italian dressing Small baked potato w/ 2 tablespoons nonfat plain yogurt 8 oz. skim milk	4 oz. broiled fish with lemon 1 cup steamed broccoli w/ 2 teaspoons margarine ¾ cup brown rice w/ mushrooms 1 slice angel food cake	1 cup spaghetti w/ 2 oz. lean ground beef in a tomato/onion sauce and 1 oz. Parmesan cheese 1 cup cooked carrots w/ lemon sauce 1 slice whole-grain bread 1 cup cooked Swiss chard or chopped spinach 8 oz. skim milk
Snack	**Snack**	**Snack**
8 oz. orange juice previously frozen, then half-thawed to a slush	8 oz. nonfat fruit yogurt	12 thin pretzels

Day 4	Day 5

Breakfast

½ cup orange juice
8 oz. skim milk
1 slice whole-wheat toast
1 teaspoon margarine

Snack

1 small banana

Lunch

Chicken salad sandwich w/ ½
  cup diced chicken breast, 2
  tablespoons celery, 1
  tablespoon low-calorie
  mayonnaise, ½ hoagie/hero
  bun
Carrot sticks
1 cup cantaloupe cubes

Dinner

Easy chili w/ 2 oz. ground beef,
  ½ cup kidney beans, ¼ cup
  chopped onion, ¼ cup salsa,
  and ¼ cup water
1 slice whole-wheat bread w/ 1
  teaspoon margarine
Salad w/ 1 cup chopped lettuce,
  ½ tomato w/ 1 tablespoon
  low-calorie Italian dressing
8 oz. skim milk

Snack

1 slice angel food cake w/ ½
  cup strawberries and 2
  tablespoons nonfat vanilla
  yogurt

Breakfast

1 orange
1 English muffin
1 poached egg
1 oz. mozzarella cheese

Snack

1 apple

Lunch

Salad w/ 2 cups chopped
  lettuce, ½ cup garbanzo
  beans, ½ cup sliced
  cucumber, ½ cup broccoli, ½
  tomato, ¼ cup grated carrot,
  ¼ cup peas, and 2
  tablespoons low-calorie
  Thousand Island dressing
1 roll
8 oz. skim milk

Dinner

3 cups lentil soup w/ lentils,
  tomatoes, carrots, and celery
1 slice French bread w/ 1
  teaspoon margarine
8 oz. skim milk

Snack

1 cup diced pineapple

Day 6	Day 7

Breakfast

½ grapefruit
1 bagel
2 teaspoons margarine

Snack

½ cottage cheese w/ 1 pear

Lunch

Tuna sandwich w/ 2 slices
  whole wheat bread, 1
  tablespoon low-fat
  mayonnaise, 2 oz. water-
  packed tuna, 1 tablespoon
  diced celery, slice of tomato,
  2 lettuce leaves
Carrot sticks and 2 cups
  broccoli flowerettes w/ 2
  tablespoons low-calorie ranch
  dressing as dip

Dinner

3 oz. lean sirloin steak
1 small baked potato w/ 2
  tablespoons plain nonfat
  yogurt w/ chives
½ cup butternut squash
Melon ball salad w/ ½ cup
  cantaloupe, ½ cup honeydew,
  ½ cup watermelon, and ½
  cup sorbet
8 oz. skim milk

Snack

3 cups air-popped popcorn

Breakfast

2 slices french toast
2 tablespoons low-calorie jam
8 oz. nonfat milk

Snack

1 cup strawberries

Lunch

2 cups beef noodle soup
1 roll
1 teaspoon margarine
Salad of ¼ cup kidney beans, 1
  cup chopped lettuce, ¼ cup
  sweet red pepper, ¼ cup
  garbanzo beans, ⅓ cup sliced
  cucumber, 1 tablespoon low-
  calorie French dressing
1 nectarine

Dinner

4 oz. salmon broiled with light
  butter/lemon sauce
½ cup brown rice
1 cup green peas
8 oz. skim milk
2 plums

Snack

2 graham crackers

These menus provide plenty of protein, calcium, and other nutrients, some roughage, and enough volume that one need not feel deprived. The foods included are generally low in fat and contain no alcohol, and therefore tend to be low in calories for the quantity of food eaten (i.e., they have low caloric density). As noted, each day's menu is approximately 1,600 calories. There is nothing unique or magical about these particular meals—you can concoct whatever pleases your palate from similar nutritious foods of low caloric density and do just as well. There is no necessity to eat three meals and two snacks; in the menus above, the snacks could as easily be combined with the meals. There is not even a need to observe any particular pattern or number of meals per day. A calorie is a calorie, whether at breakfast or bedtime. The point is that this is not a temporary guide to weight loss, but a model for a permanent style of eating.

FAD DIETS

Most Americans have been on a diet, and millions are dieting at any given time. Since we are a country well endowed with self-styled experts, the diets come from myriad sources—magazines, books, celebrities, Aunt Clara, dentists, chiropractors, and neighbors. Most of these diets feature gimmicks, and they come in countless varieties, from emphasizing a dietary constituent to claiming particular health and energy benefits, to ballyhooing geographic locations and support by respected authors and institutions with impeccable credentials, and on and on. In general, the more severe the calorie restrictions imposed by these fad diets, and the more deficient they are in supplying needed protein, minerals, and vitamins, the more likely they are to cause complications for the dieter. The number of these fad diets is too great for us to review them here comprehensively.

Richard lost 80 pounds on one of the most dangerous diets that we have learned about. He started this "lemonade fasting-and-cleansing diet" at a weight of 290 pounds. Each morning he drank two quarts of distilled water, to which two teaspoons of sea salt had been added— a so-called "salt-water flush." This induced diarrhea within 30 minutes. For the rest of the day, Richard consumed only the juice of three lemons, mixed with 12 tablespoons of grade-B maple syrup and one-tenth of a teaspoon of cayenne pepper. These ingredients were combined into a slurry that was then mixed with large volumes of water, and drunk. The book that proposed this diet recommended that it be followed only for ten days, but Richard was losing weight fast and decided to keep going. After 20 days his rate of weight loss slowed, so he cut the maple syrup to six tablespoons, and kept on going. He continued for a grand total of 42 days, during which he took no other food and lost 80 pounds. It is remarkable that Richard survived to tell about this adventure in malnutrition.

After completing the diet, Richard maintained his weight for two years by exercising and faithfully following a vegetarian diet. He felt healthy and energetic. Then he reverted to meat, burgers, french fries, and other fast foods, stopped exercising, and regained to a weight of 300 pounds. Now, years later, he weighs 265 pounds and is reducing on a nutritionally sound diet in the hope that weight loss will help relieve arthritic pains in his knees.

Although it was far more perilous than many, Richard's diet had features in common with a number of fad diets. It was simple, and its content differed greatly from normal food intake, characteristics that helped capture Richard's imagination and hold his attention. The necessity for choosing particular foods and determining portion size was eliminated. On the one hand, this narrowing of choice made the diet easier to follow, but on the other, it provided no preparation for its participants' return to normal eating. Worst of all, as stated previously, the diet was woefully inadequate in nutrition, with severe deficiencies of protein, minerals, and most vitamins.

More popular during the 1980s have been the high-protein, high-fat, low-carbohydrate diets that have attracted great attention in the media. Such diets have been called "ketogenic" because they advocate a generous intake of meat, fat, and/or alcohol in order to stimulate the production of ketones—breakdown products of fat and alcohol metabolism. They were based on the idea that high levels of ketones would be beneficial in two ways: ketones were supposed to suppress appetite; then they would escape in the urine and therefore carry calories out of the body, thus enhancing the calorie deficit.

These alleged benefits of ketogenic diets are illusory. First, studies have not confirmed the claim that high levels of ketones correlate with reduced hunger. Second, the amount of calories lost through the urine as ketones is negligible. Third, elevated levels of ketones set the stage for some of the dangerous complications of dieting, including gout, potassium depletion, and disturbances of heart rhythm. Fourth, a high intake of meat and fats tends to raise the blood levels of cholesterol—a poor outcome indeed for those who would lose weight to improve their health as well as their appearance. For these reasons, we deplore this approach to dieting and advise you instead to be guided by the eating habits we have outlined: limiting your fat and alcohol intake; substituting generous amounts of complex carbohydrates such as those found in grains, fruits, and vegetables; and choosing low-fat sources of protein, such as fish, white poultry meat, skim milk, and legumes.

Diets that overemphasize any particular food, or that attribute extraordinary powers to some specific facet of the diet, such as the timing or rotation of different nutrients, are playing upon the public's desire for a quick, magical cure for obesity. In so doing, they help guarantee short-term sales and success for their authors and publishers, but long-term disappointment for dieters.

COMPLICATIONS OF DIETING

Many of the complications of dieting relate to the rate at which a person loses weight. That is why it is so much safer to lose weight slowly rather than quickly, and why diets that produce a severe caloric deficit require medical supervision. With a cautious rate of weight reduction, most of the complications can be entirely avoided. What follows is a review of the complications of dieting, and the means of minimizing these problems.

Death

This, of course, is the ultimate complication, and it has occurred as the result of diets that severely restrict calories and are deficient in adequate protein content, such as the over-the-counter liquid-protein diets of the 1970s. When such severe or nutritionally unsound diets are undertaken without medical supervision for prolonged periods, consequent weakening and malfunction of the heart may lead to death. (Some deaths that occur during diets are, of course, coincidental. So many Americans are on diets at any given time that some dieters are bound to die of causes unrelated to their diet programs.)

Dizziness, Weakness, and Muscle Cramps

These symptoms are frequently experienced during a diet, especially during the first few days and weeks. They usually occur as a result of the loss of body water and salts.

When you go on a low-calorie diet, your body responds by eliminating salt and water. This is why the first week or two on any diet usually produces a remarkable weight loss—up to seven or ten pounds. Most of this weight loss is water, not fat. And as your body loses salt, troublesome symptoms of muscle weakness and cramps ("charley horses") can occur. Increased salt intake often relieves these symptoms.

Since our blood is mostly salt water, a reduction in body salt and water reduces our blood pressure. "Blood pressure" refers to the water pressure within our arteries, the vessels that carry blood from the heart to the rest of the body. Blood pressure often declines during a diet because of the loss of salt and water. This is not a problem if you have high blood pressure, but if your blood pressure is usually normal, a weight-reduction diet is likely to give you the symptoms of low blood pressure: weakness and faintness—sometimes described as "dizziness"—when sitting up or standing. Low blood pressure usually produces no symptoms while you are lying down. But when you sit up, or especially when you stand up, there needs to be sufficient blood pressure to drive your blood upward to your brain, against the pull of gravity. When your brain doesn't get enough blood, it responds by making you faint, or by making you feel faint. This is nature's way of making you lie down, so that blood flowing to the brain no longer has to go upstream against gravity.

These symptoms can be overcome by increasing the intake of salt and water. Consuming generous amounts of sodium-filled beverages such as bouillon, broth, chicken-noodle soup, or salty vegetable juices will do the trick. Or you can simply use more salt on your food, or eat salty, low-calorie foods such as pickles. Increased salt intake, with lots of water intake as well, usually will relieve the weak, faint feelings and muscle cramps brought on by low-calorie dieting.

If you have high blood pressure, of course, the fall in blood pressure brought on by dieting will be beneficial; it may allow your physician to discontinue the prescribing of medications for your high blood pressure. In these cases, the first blood-pressure medication to be discontinued is usually a diuretic, which is a substance that causes the kidneys to eliminate salt and water. Because low-calorie dieting itself leads to the loss of salt and water, diuretic medications can often be dispensed with during dieting. As weight loss continues, other blood-pressure medications may also need to be stopped in order to keep your blood pressure from going too low, and thereby causing weakness and faintness.

Some people protest about taking extra salt and water, because they *want* to lose fluid. They feel bloated and fat, and believe that losing fluid actually helps the pounds come off in a hurry. But most of us need salt to avoid the problems described above. Only if you have high blood pressure, heart failure, or severe fluid retention should you avoid salt while you are on a low-calorie diet. Besides, the real purpose of weight-reduction dieting, after all, is to lose *fat*. And the fat comes off only as a consequence of a calorie deficit. Since salt and water contain no calories, they do not affect the loss of fat.

In the long run, the body's powerful mechanisms for regulating fluid balance—the kidneys and the hypothalamus and adrenal glands—are going to regulate your fluid level. If you stop dieting, that fluid is going to come back anyway. So don't focus on the scales too much, and don't worry about these shifts in fluid. Remember instead that it is your shape and your fat mass that you are trying to improve. Instead of watching the scales, you can just as well monitor your weight loss by watching your belt size or dress size.

Potassium Depletion

Potassium is required for normal functioning of muscles and of many vital organs, including the heart and kidneys. We lose a certain amount of potassium every day, even when not dieting or losing weight. Our diet, especially the fruit, vegetables, and meats we eat, supplies potassium to make up for this normal daily loss. Weight reduction can deplete body potassium stores in two ways. First, dietary intake may be curtailed. Second, the body excretes potassium instead of sodium as it attempts to minimize the loss of salt and water (see above). Taking in adequate amounts of fruits, vegetables, salt, and water helps reduce the likelihood of potassium depletion during dieting.

Potassium depletion can manifest itself in weakness and irregular heartbeat, but often no symptoms are noticed as the condition is revealed by blood tests. Anyone who loses a significant amount of weight, such as 20 pounds, should have a blood potassium measurement. More-frequent monitoring is needed for people taking diuretics or laxatives, since these medications can accelerate potassium loss.

Depression and Irritability

Caloric deprivation is a stressful, uncomfortable experience for many people. Feelings of depression and symptoms of irritability are common. A high level of physical activity helps many people minimize such symptoms, and also promotes weight loss and maintenance of muscle mass and strength.

Unlike patients on conventional diets, patients on physician-supervised, very-low-calorie liquid diets often report feelings of elation during the weight-loss phase. This euphoria is probably due in part to excitement about the rapid rate of weight loss, and in part to the intensive support provided by weekly visits with the doctor, nurse, and behavioral-education group.

Hair Loss

This is a frequent complaint during weight loss. Fortunately, the hair loss induced by low-calorie dieting is not permanent, because the hair follicles are not destroyed. Hairs are formed by little nests of cells in the skin, called *hair follicles*. These follicles go through cycles of active hair growth. During the resting phase, the strand of hair stops growing and may easily fall out. Later, when the follicle goes back into a more active phase, hair growth resumes. If the hair strand has fallen out, it regrows, as long as the follicle is still healthy. A major metabolic stress, such as pregnancy or weight loss, can make many hair follicles go into a resting phase at the same time, but does not damage the follicles. Some of the strands fall out, and the hair seems to be thinning fast because not many strands are still growing to replenish the hair mass. Don't worry—the follicles are not dead, just resting. You can expect your hair to begin growing again at a later date—unless some other process, which actually damages the scalp and its hair follicles, is taking place in addition to the effects of dieting.

Dry Skin

This condition often occurs with dieting, and may relate to a reduced intake of oils. It is easily managed by the application of lotions and skin moisturizers.

Disturbances of Bowel Function

These include such symptoms as constipation and/or diarrhea, and they are common during low-calorie dieting. A generous intake of roughage usually solves both problems. It can be either in the form of vegetables, fruits, and grains, or of such bulk-forming preparations as those made of psyllium seed.

Occasionally, diarrhea will occur as the result of incorporating into your diet new foods that you don't tolerate well. The most frequent example of this occurs when someone is unable to digest milk sugar because of a deficiency of the necessary enzyme, *lactase*. Lactase deficiency is especially frequent among people with black, Asian, and Native American ancestry. It can be overcome by adding lactase, in the form of pills or drops, or by switching the source of protein in the diet from milk to something else.

Gallbladder Disease

This is the most serious of the common complications of dieting. It is especially likely to occur with the very-low-calorie diets, also known as protein-sparing, modified-fasting diets. The gallbladder is a sac attached to the liver, in the upper right part of the abdomen. It contains a digestive juice called bile. When crystals of cholesterol form in the bile, they can enlarge to form gallstones (see chapter 2). Ordinarily, the gallbladder empties much of its bile with each meal, so that cholesterol crystals and tiny stones get flushed into the intestine and eliminated in the stool. On a very-low-calorie diet, however, gallbladder emptying may be incomplete, allowing stones to be retained and to enlarge to the point that they cause inflammation and pain. Moreover, since the bile provides an exit route for cholesterol to leave the body, during weight loss the bile becomes more highly saturated with cholesterol, so that crystals and stones may form more rapidly.

A gallbladder attack is usually felt as pain in the abdomen, though sometimes the pain may be experienced in the chest, back, or right shoulder. It requires prompt medical attention. Surgery is sometimes required to remedy the situation, though some gallstones can be dissolved through the oral administration of the bile acid ursodiol (see page 189).

As noted in chapter 9, the increased risks of gallstone formation during weight reduction may be avoided by administration of ursodiol. This treatment reduces the rate of secretion of cholesterol into bile, rendering bile less likely to form cholesterol crystals. Further research trials are necessary, however, before this approach can be recommended as standard preventive therapy.

Other Abdominal Pain

Not all abdominal pain experienced during dieting is due to gallbladder disease. On a very-low-calorie diet, people who have ulcers may experience a reactivation of their pain and problems, because food normally helps buffer stomach acid. People who suffer chronic ulcer problems often make too much stomach acid, and without a normal amount of food to keep the acid neutralized, their ulcers can flare up. Other causes of abdominal pain, such as appendicitis or urinary infection, can of course occur during a diet by coincidence, even though the diet doesn't trigger them. Any severe abdominal pain requires prompt medical evaluation.

Chilliness

Many people on low-calorie diets report this symptom. It may relate to either a slowing of the metabolic rate, or to a decrease in circulation due to fluid depletion. It can also be caused by a loss of insulating fat. Increasing salt and fluid intake, and increasing exercise, often provide relief.

Skipped Menstrual Periods

This condition is common with weight loss, as it is with other severe stresses. The problem is usually temporary. After obesity has been corrected, menstruation is often more regular and predictable than it was prior to weight reduction. The possibility of pregnancy should not be ignored, however, especially since pregnancy requires not a calorie deficit, but extra nutrition.

DIETING IN PERSPECTIVE

It is one thing to climb to the top of Mount Everest. It is another to stay there and live happily ever after. As difficult as it is to achieve a reduced weight through dieting, it is even more difficult to keep the weight off happily ever after. Being at a reduced weight as a result of dieting is being in a very tenuous, unstable situation. One's natural tendency is to regain the weight. The only way to maintain a reduced weight is to permanently change calorie input and/or calorie output (see chapter 8). This means changes in habitual behavior, and it is why the behavior-modification approach with which this book concludes makes so much sense: your behavior must change or you will relapse into obesity.

In fact, if you make positive changes in your eating behavior and your physical activity, your weight will gradually change to its eventual maintenance level even without a temporary diet. If you are a woman who weighs 200 pounds, you require about 2,200 calories (11 calories per pound) to maintain your weight. Suppose that you intend to lose 50 pounds. When you get down to 150 pounds, you will require only 1,650 calories (11 × 150) to maintain your weight. If you make lasting life-style changes in diet and exercise that result in a net calorie balance of 1,650 calories, you will maintain your weight at 150 pounds; otherwise, you will regain. In fact, if you make those changes to a 1,650-calorie life-style when you still weigh 200 pounds, you will gradually lose weight. If you stick to those changes, the entire 50 pounds will eventually come off, even though you never go on a temporary weight-loss diet. A 200-pound woman eating only 1,650 calories per day will have a calorie deficit, and will consequently lose weight; she will keep losing weight until she reaches 150 pounds. Since 1,650 calories are required to maintain a weight of 150 pounds, she will stop losing when she gets down to 150 pounds because she will no longer have a calorie deficit. Therefore, a temporary, more severe, diet is not absolutely necessary and is not the main issue. What is critical is to make the life-style and habit changes that will keep her weight at 150 pounds. Those changes will bring her weight down to 150 pounds, even without temporary starvation.

People usually are in such a rush to change their weight that they focus in on the temporary diet that will make the reduction. But like a hiker racing to the top of a mountain without a tent or a sleeping bag, such people are unprepared to stay there once they arrive. The real challenge is to make *lasting* shifts in food choices and activity levels, since these are what eventually determine weight. If you need to reduce your weight, your attention should be directed toward building new habits of healthy eating and generous physical activity, and sustaining them. Temporary reducing diets are of no use in achieving permanent weight reduction unless they are combined with other approaches, including new eating habits, exercise, and behavior modification.

11

Exercise

Throughout this book, we use the terms *exercise* and *physical activity* interchangeably. From the perspective of fat storage, it makes no difference whether the activity is something we commonly think of as exercise—such as playing tennis or doing aerobics—or something we do without being conscious of caloric expenditure—such as sweeping out the garage. By physical activity, or exercise, we mean all activities requiring energy expenditure except for the essential, automatic body functions that keep us alive and warm even when we are resting.

EXERCISE AND THE OBESITY EQUATION

Exercise and obesity are inescapably linked. The amount of fat our bodies store is the difference between calorie intake and calorie output:

Fat storage equals calorie intake minus calorie output.

In other words, the energy in the food you eat will be stored as fat unless you use it up. Calories are used up (see chapter 6) in three ways: (1) basal metabolism, or resting energy expenditure; (2) thermogenesis, i.e., the production of heat, including that which results from the intake and processing of food; and (3) physical activity.

At present, we do not have safe and effective ways to manipulate our rates of basal metabolism or of thermogenesis. Therefore, in order to increase caloric expenditure, our efforts must focus on physical activity.

Most weight-control programs consist of diets, and are directed only at calorie consumption. This is understandable, since food is tangible, and more visible than calorie expenditure. But diet represents only half of the necessary weight-loss picture.

Dr. Jean Mayer, former professor of nutrition at Harvard, and currently president of Tufts University, was one of the first to realize that inactivity contributes as much to the problem of obesity as food intake, and sometimes more. In studies of teenage girls, he found that overweight subjects actually ate fewer calories than those who were thin, but were much less active. Other studies have shown this same pattern, even in infants; the thinnest infants eat more, but are more active. For many overweight people, therefore, increasing physical activity means getting to the heart of their problem: not enough calorie expenditure.

THE BENEFITS OF INCREASED PHYSICAL ACTIVITY

The benefits of exercise go far beyond weight control. By improving fitness and strength, exercise enhances our performance and enjoyment of a wide range of athletic and recreational activities. It increases our capacity for accomplishment of everyday work tasks. Most important, being physically fit protects us against coronary heart disease, stroke, and high blood pressure. Exercise is a vital tool for treating not only obesity, but also diabetes and depression.

Many people find that exercise fosters feelings of energy, optimism, and self-esteem. Not only does physical activity relieve tension and frustration; it often produces a sense of physical vitality and inner well-being that inspires many of us to make it a regular part of our lives.

Exercise promotes cardiovascular health in several ways. It lowers blood pressure and heart rate, and improves the circulation of the blood. It also reduces total blood cholesterol levels while increasing HDL-cholesterol—the kind of cholesterol that helps prevent heart attacks. In addition, research shows that physical activity protects against heart disease even more than can be explained by its beneficial effects on blood pressure and cholesterol. While medical investigators have long believed that strenuous physical activity—strenuous enough to get the heart beating fast—protects the heart, more recent data show that even gentle forms of exercise, such as walking, also confer cardiovascular protection.

Exercise carries special benefits for people with diabetes mellitus. It helps reduce the characteristic elevations in blood sugar and blood fats in diabetes. Among overweight diabetics, weight reduction through diet and exercise makes the diabetes much easier to control, and it sometimes eliminates the need for medication.

In terms of weight reduction, the benefits of exercise are threefold. First, exercise maintains muscle mass. It keeps your muscles bigger than they would be if you didn't exercise. Bigger muscles mean more calories expended in basal metabolism, because lean tissue is metabolically more active than adipose tissue. The 150-pound runner who is lean, trim, and muscular has more lean body tissue than a 150-pound person who is flabby and out of shape; in addition to the calories expended by running, the runner's resting energy expenditure will be higher. Second, the exercise itself expends calories, contributing directly to weight loss. Third, the calorie expenditure of strenuous physical activity extends beyond the calories burned during the exercise itself. For several hours after strenuous exercise, the body busily burns calories as it repairs the muscles used in exercise, replenishes their glycogen stores, and disposes of the waste products generated during exercise. You probably have noticed a feeling of warmth for several hours after prolonged, vigorous exercise, a feeling produced by the process of the calories as they are being expended in these "clean-up" activities. In athletes who are undergoing very vigorous training, such as football and basketball players, the effect has been shown to last as long as 24 hours after extreme exercise. For those of us who are overweight dieters and not athletic, the effect is more modest, though it is still helpful in achieving weight control.

Some investigators have described this post-exercise burning of calories as a temporary enhancement of the basal metabolic rate, or resting energy expenditure. We prefer the above interpretation, however, since the effect lasts only for a matter of hours; there is no lasting revision of your basal metabolic rate as a result of exercise, except insofar as it maintains muscle mass. The total energy expended by an individual during and after exercise can be compared to the total energy expended in a stadium during and after a football game. Most of the energy is expended during the game, by the athletes running around on the field and the fans walking around in the stands. Afterwards, however, there is a period during which the janitorial crew expends energy to clean up the place, before the stadium returns to its resting state.

Still other weight-control benefits accrue to those who exercise. Particularly in overweight persons, exercise appears to decrease appetite. This has been seen in steel-mill workers, athletes, the elderly, and even children enrolled in "head-start" programs. Children who were given a ten-to-fifteen-minute recess to play before eating lunch ate less food at lunch than did those children whose play period followed lunch.

EXERCISE AND CALORIES

"How many calories is exercise worth?" This is a common question with a complex answer. Many factors go into a precise calculation of caloric expenditure, including the weight of the person exercising, the efficiency and coordination with which the activity is performed, resistance to the exertion, such as the presence of an uphill incline or of headwinds in a race, temperature, and so on. For practical purposes, however, you can use rough estimates of the caloric costs of exercise to get an idea of how many pounds of fat a particular activity consumes. In making such calculations, remember that 3,500 calories go into one pound of fat, whether the calories are entering as food or exiting as exercise.

A 150-pound person expends about 100 calories in traversing a mile on level ground. This approximation holds whether one walks, jogs, or runs the mile, because the efficiency with which a person moves his or her body along does not change appreciably with speed. Running the mile burns calories more quickly than walking, of course, so you finish the mile sooner and get more out of breath. But the amount of energy you expend is about the same, whether you traversed the mile while running or walking. So if you don't feel up to jogging, don't worry. You can walk that same distance and burn up approximately the same number of calories as if you had jogged; it will just take you longer.

To estimate how many calories you burn in walking one mile, simply multiply your weight by 0.67. Or you can look it up on this table:

Table 11.1

My Weight in Pounds	Calories I Burn Walking One Level Mile
100	67
110	73
120	80
130	87
140	94
150	100
160	107
170	114
180	121
190	127
200	134
210	141
220	147
230	154
240	161
250	168
260	174
270	181
280	188
290	194
300	201
310	208
320	214
330	221
340	228
350	235
360	241
370	248
380	255
390	261
400	268

To calculate the calories burned for higher weights, find two weights in the table that add up to your weight, and add their calories together. For example, if your weight is 550 pounds, add the calories for 300 pounds (201) and the calories for 250 pounds (168), and you get a total of 369 calories for walking one mile.

If the mile is uphill instead of level, it will require more energy, because you will be lifting your body upward against gravity. The steeper the grade, the more calories will be burned in covering the mile.

Knowing how many calories you burn with each level mile walked is helpful in two ways. In the first place, walking is the most practical, convenient, inexpensive, and widely used form of exercise. Most people who consistently expend lots of calories in physical activity are walkers. Knowing how many calories you consume in walking helps you relate your walking to your weight. For example, someone who weighs 180 pounds will expend about 240 calories a day by walking two miles every day. That is enough to maintain a 20-pound weight loss (see chapter 8).

A second benefit of knowing how many calories you expend in walking one mile is that you can use that information to estimate the caloric value of other forms of exercise. Here's how it's done: Suppose that one of your favorite forms of exercise is working out on your rowing machine for 20 minutes each day while you watch the TV news. Count your pulse rate at the end of walking one mile in 20 minutes. Then count your pulse rate at the end of your 20-minute rowing workout. Divide your rowing pulse rate by your walking pulse rate, and multiply that by the number of calories you expend in walking one mile. This estimation is based on the assumption that calories expended are proportional to oxygen consumed, which is proportional to the rate of blood flow, which is proportional to the pulse rate. It is simply the solution to the following equation:

$$\frac{\text{Pulse rate walking}}{\text{Pulse rate other exercise}} = \frac{\text{Calories expended walking}}{\text{Calories expended other exercise}}$$

You can use this method to estimate the calorie expenditure of any exercise.

Another way to estimate roughly your calorie expenditure with other exercises is to realize that walking one mile on level ground in 20 minutes, which is a rather leisurely three miles per hour, expends calories at approximately the same rate as leisurely bicycling on level ground, playing tennis or racquetball at a recreational level, dancing, or doing light calisthenics or aerobics.

You could expend calories at about twice that rate through vigorous swimming, cross-country skiing, or playing singles tennis or racquet-ball on a competitive level.

Gardening and housework usually consume calories about half as fast as walking three miles per hour.

Walking upstairs is extremely intense exercise, and most people cannot keep doing it for even five minutes without stopping. A 150-pound person burns about one calorie for each five steps. A 300-pound person, of course, expends energy at twice that rate, since he is propelling twice as much weight up the stairs. If your time is very limited, stairs are available, and you want to burn calories in a hurry, stair-climbing is a great way to expend energy.

Many patients who seek medical advice about exercise are surprised to learn that they burn as many calories walking as in a recreational-level tennis game. But remember that a good deal of the time during a tennis game is spent standing around while one's opponent is re-trieving a ball between points. Standing there crouched over with your hands on the racquet while awaiting the next serve, you may feel tense, but you are burning very few calories. The same is true of downhill skiing. Most of the work is being done by gravity on the way down and by the tow rope on the way up, and not much energy is being expended.

Some people believe that calisthenics and downhill skiing expend calories faster than walking, because they feel more sore and tired afterwards. This feeling usually results from heavily straining a few muscles involved in the exercise. The beauty of walking is that it constantly employs very large muscle groups, so that a lot of work is being done, and lots of energy is being expended, without straining any particular group of muscles. Pull-ups, sit-ups, and downhill skiing leave people feeling quite sore not because they have expended great amounts of energy, but because they have been straining a few muscles that they don't often use. Likewise, five minutes of heavy weight lifting can leave you stiff and sore, but it doesn't expend very many calories.

Many people think that exercise doesn't "count" unless it is fast and vigorous enough to raise the pulse rate. This is not true, however, when it comes to weight management. Calories burned off gently, without cardiovascular strain, weigh as much and count the same as calories expended with sweat, sound, and fury. When you go for a walk or engage in some other physical activity, you do not need to feel you are in a race. The tortoise who takes three hours and the hare who takes 30 minutes will burn approximately equal numbers of calories if they weigh the same and cover the same distance. By exercising strenuously, a person may lose an extra pound or two of sweat, but this water weight will come right back with the next stop at a water fountain.

Vigorous, strenuous exercise does improve cardiovascular conditioning, if done regularly and safely. On the other hand, gentle walking or other activities that do not raise the pulse rate do improve health, strength, and endurance, and do consume calories. And a benefit of gentle exercise is that it doesn't leave you too sore to go out and do it again the next day. After all, it is consistent, regular exercise that will pay off with reduced weight in the long run.

Exercise involving the repeated contraction of large muscle groups against low resistance has been called *aerobic*. Walking, dancing, running, playing basketball, cross-country skiing, and jumping rope are examples of aerobic exercise. Aerobic activities tend to burn lots of calories, and are thus helpful in weight loss.

Another type of exercise involves contracting muscles against high resistance, with much less movement than aerobic activities demand. This kind of exercise has been called *isometric,* and is exemplified by lifting heavy weights. It tends to build big muscles, and is difficult to continue for long because the muscles being used become fatigued. Although isometric exercise doesn't burn calories as fast as aerobic exercise, it is a valuable part of a weight-reduction program, because it maintains muscle mass. As noted earlier, bigger muscles mean that more calories are expended in basal metabolism. A well-balanced exercise program will therefore include both high-resistance, muscle-building activities as well as low-resistance, aerobic exercise.

NOT BY EXERCISE ALONE, OR OCCASIONALLY

To use exercise as the exclusive basis of a weight-loss program is to invite failure. The weight reduction brought about by exercise is relatively small, and it can easily be overwhelmed by food intake unless this, too, is somehow managed. People who take exercise as a license to gorge on high-calorie foods will find themselves gaining body fat, not losing it.

As you look at Table 11.1, you may feel a bit discouraged that it takes so much walking to equal a few bites of burger. Again, the key here is in adopting and *sustaining* new habits. A single spasm of exercise does next to nothing for long-term weight control; it is as worthless as a brief burst of dieting. For example, a 240-pound man burns about 480 calories in jogging three miles—less than one-seventh of a pound of fat, and fewer calories than are in one Big Mac. He would have to run over 21 miles—more than three miles every day for a whole week—just to burn off a single pound of fat. The payoff comes, however, when the exercise becomes habitual. Three miles walked or jogged every day will take off about 40 pounds in a year for a person of his size, and keep it off indefinitely. As noted in chapter 8, about 12 calories are required to maintain each pound of a man's weight. By eliminating 480 calories each day from his total amount through a daily three-mile walk, he would therefore subtract about 40 pounds from his fat stores in a year. So the caloric payoffs of exercise are considerable, but only if the exercise is continued on a habitual basis.

PRECAUTIONS

Certain medical conditions need to be considered before you start an exercise program. If you use drugs, such as blood-pressure or heart medications, stimulants, or antidepressants, you should consult with your physician before you undertake an exercise program. If you are significantly overweight or out of shape, you should have a physical examination and receive specific approval from your doctor before you embark on exercising. People over 40 years of age should have an electrocardiogram (EKG) and receive their doctors' standard blood and urine tests before beginning.

Previously sedentary people with cardiac risk factors (such as being 20 percent or more overweight, being over 40, smoking, suffering from hypertension, diabetes, cardiovascular disease, or having a strong family history of heart attacks) may require exercise testing, such as the "treadmill EKG" test, to determine how hard they should push themselves and how rapidly they can safely increase the intensity of their exercise. Patients with known cardiovascular disease and who are taking medications must be carefully monitored, with the degree of exercise specifically approved by their physicians.

Supervised exercise programs, for those who need them, can usually be found through local YMCAs, YWCAs, and community centers, as well as through the physical education departments of local educational institutions. Your local American Heart Association chapter is another resource for locating programs that provide cardiac rehabilitation through exercise.

For people who are overweight and out of shape, it's important to go slowly when beginning an exercise program. Not only is their cardiovascular system deconditioned and in need of a long, slow reconditioning program, but their musculoskeletal system is often in a weakened condition. This makes them prime targets for muscle strain, joint problems, tendonitis, shin splints, and even stress fractures. Non-weight-bearing exercises, such as swimming, are often an excellent way to get started. The most practical starting point for most people is simply walking.

People with chronic respiratory conditions such as asthma or emphysema, especially those who exercise in locations with excessive air pollution, humidity, or particularly high or low temperatures, need to adjust their program accordingly, under the guidance of a physician. This will usually include engaging in less activity, and less intense aerobic activity, when it is hot, smoggy, or very humid. It may include rescheduling the exercise to a safer time of day. If the smog is at the level of an alert, it may be better to forgo aerobic exercise that day and do stretching instead.

WHY IT'S HARD TO STICK WITH EXERCISING

If exercise makes us feel so good, and is so good for us, why is it so difficult to sustain it as a routine? The number of people who stay with an exercise program is disappointingly small—a fact that has not escaped the notice of entrepreneurs who establish health spas. They know that many of their enrollees will drop out before a year of membership has expired. The spa keeps the membership fees of the dropouts, and the spa operator is free to oversell his or her facility by 300 to 400 percent of capacity.

Even among the high-risk cardiac population, there is a 50-percent dropout rate from prescribed exercise. In a study in Scotland, only one-third of such patients were following prescribed exercise programs after six months. In a long-term Swedish study of patients who had had heart attacks, 70 percent dropped out over three years. Not surprisingly, the dropout rate for people who are simply overweight is even worse, since they are not motivated by the immediate fear of death or by the painful memory of a heart attack. Even in a program as simple as walking, after a one-year follow-up, only 32 percent of an experimental sample continued to take walks on a regular basis.

Sticking to it is probably the most difficult part of an exercise program, and despite the benefits to health and self-esteem, many people simply don't sustain the routine. People who start at too high an exercise level often injure themselves and drop out. Others, who choose too low an exercise level, may become bored or begin to feel they're making insufficient progress, and drop out. People who unrealistically anticipate a "runner's high," a major transformation in attitude, or a sense of being ready for the Olympics are rapidly disappointed and drop out.

HOW TO SUCCEED

Many exercise programs have had some success in motivating their participants with such devices as monetary refunds, information about the benefits of exercise and the risks of dropping out, keeping graphs of miles walked or minutes of activity per day, or posting weekly records of blood pressure, heart rate, and endurance. In general, joining a group seems to enhance motivation more than exercising alone, especially if the group shares a sense that "we're all in it together."

With family or group support, motivation and persistence are higher. Cardiovascular fitness training programs, for example, have shown that spouse involvement, particularly when the spouse is highly enthusiastic, produces far greater success than when the spouse is not involved. Workplace exercise programs have also shown great success, particularly when a certain esprit de corps can be developed to the point that nonparticipants feel excluded.

Recognizable exercise, such as athletic performance and taking walks, is not the only way to increase one's calorie expenditure. For many, a more significant expenditure of calories can be achieved by becoming "inefficient." Routinely answering a phone that is farther away, using a more distant bathroom, or getting off the bus one stop earlier all introduce extra calorie expense and help eliminate weight. Parking across the parking lot and walking to the supermarket spends more calories than driving around the lot for five minutes looking for a closer parking spot. Standing when you could sit, sitting when you could be lying down, climbing stairs when you could take the elevator or escalator, are all ways to burn more calories. These types of activities can be systematically introduced into almost every aspect of anyone's day.

Working on your total energy output in this way carries a number of bonuses. First, you can dramatically increase your calorie expenditure. Second, the increased activity and exercise breaks up otherwise dull routines and can relieve some of the boredom that leads certain people to unnecessary eating. Third, this kind of "inefficient" exercise maintains appreciable physical activity even on those days when schedule conflicts prevent engaging in the usual formal exercise routine.

When you start to exercise, don't expect miracles. A useful way to judge a beginning exercise program is not by the intensity you bring to it, but simply by the minutes per day that you devote yourself to it. Figure 11.1 shows a graph you can keep of the minutes per day you spend on any type of exercise. The goal should be to increase the minutes per day. What type of exercise you choose matters less than the time you spend actually doing it, since a calorie is a calorie, no matter how you burn it.

Using a graph is an easy way to follow your progress and maintain your motivation (see Figure 11.2). Plot the miles per day that you walk (measure them with a pedometer or with your car's odometer) and the minutes you exercise each day, and try eventually to double both. The act of graphing your activity on a daily basis will help keep you motivated—especially if you keep your graph in a highly visible place, such as on the refrigerator door in the kitchen.

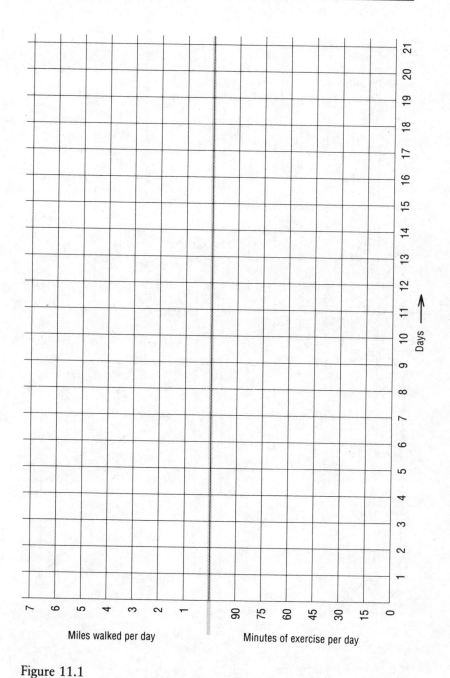

Figure 11.1

Typical chart for tracking progress in developing behavior patterns of increased physical activity.

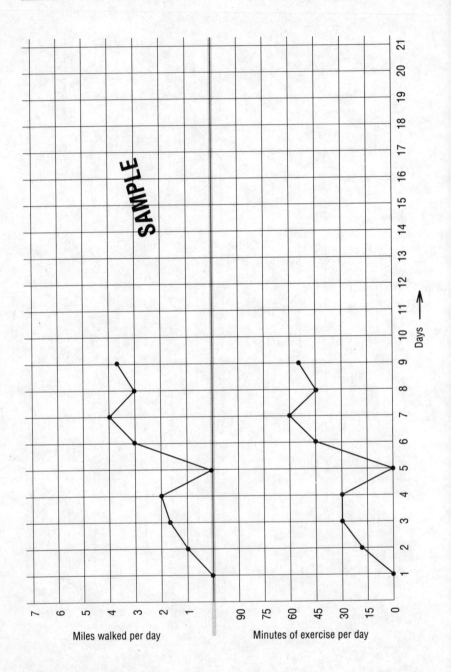

Figure 11.2

Exercise graph, partially filled in.

12

Pills, Potions, and Shots

Throughout history, we humans have sought magical cures for unwanted conditions, and it is hardly surprising that the search for effortless weight loss dates back to antiquity. Certainly it continues with us today. A walk through any drugstore, health-food emporium, or supermarket turns up a tremendous variety of products that promise to remove excess weight, including preparations to suppress the appetite and to let you lose weight while you sleep. While such magic seems ever in demand, it still doesn't exist.

REDUCING POTIONS

In the third century B.C., Philon the Byzantine busily promoted a hunger- and thirst-checking pill composed of sesame, honey, oil, almonds, and sea onion. In 1694 a person desirous of losing weight would rub his or her skin with vinegar and then apply a "reducing ointment" composed of fuller's earth, white lead, henbane (a poisonous plant of the nightshade family) juice, and myrtle oil. By 1907 a similar-minded person might apply "Absorbid Reducing Paste," which included ox bile, beeswax, lard, oil, and perfume, or a substance called "Fatoff," which was composed of 90 percent water and 10 percent soap. Many recipe books of the 1800s contained reducing formulas, including combinations of vinegar, lemon juice, and soap. The struggle against obesity reached the White House in the late 1880s, when Mrs. Grover Cleveland, whose husband weighed more than 250 pounds, lent her prestige to the promotion of "sulfur bitters," a digestive medicine to aid in weight loss.

Around the turn of the century, the popular patent and prescription medicines for weight loss included laxatives and cathartics (to produce diarrhea), emetics (to induce vomiting), and diuretics (to increase urination). In theory, these substances were intended to dissolve or expel fat from the body. "Russell's Anti-Corpulent Preparation" was composed chiefly of citric acid. "Every Woman's Flesh Reducer" was bath powder with citric acid, Epsom salts, camphor, alum, and baking soda. "Densmore's Corpulency Cure" was brewed from sassafras, and "Kimball's Powder" was a combination of soap, Epsom salts, and baking soda. Arsenic was added to some weight-loss preparations because it was claimed to speed up the system. Perhaps the most toxic preparation among these purported remedies was a combination developed by one Dr. W. W. Baxter. He produced a tablet containing pokeberry (the poisonous seeds of the pokeweed, or phytolacca, plant), caffeine, and a strychnine derivative called Phytoline, which he claimed would "restore vital cellular physiological action, and upgrade fatty tissue to muscle, while sweeping away all of the waste." Although these preparations were marketed in the days prior to laws requiring that side effects be reported to the Food and Drug Administration, many people were undoubtedly made ill by these "cures."

HCG Shots

HCG stands for *human chorionic gonadotropin*, a hormone produced in the placenta and extracted from the urine of pregnant women. In the middle of the century, injections of this hormone became popular as an adjunct to the dietary treatment of obesity. Dr. Albert T. Simeons first used it in India in the mid-1930s to treat young boys suffering from a condition called Froelich's syndrome, characterized by obesity and small genitals. Dr. Simeons developed a 500-calorie diet to accompany the shots, and established a weight-control practice in Rome in 1949. In 1954 he announced to the medical profession that daily HCG shots facilitated the process of drastic curtailment of caloric intake. The diet itself was very strict; the 500 calories were to be accompanied by at least eight glasses of water per day, and nothing more. After HCG had been in use for 20 years, the U.S. Food and Drug Administration concluded that no adequately controlled scientific study had established its safety or efficacy in the treatment of obesity. Controlled clinical trials showed that shots of sterile water worked as well when the patients thought they were receiving HCG. The program's effectiveness derived from the daily contact with a nurse for a shot and a weigh-in, plus the 500-calorie-per-day diet. The HCG itself was merely an expensive placebo.

CONTEMPORARY OVER-THE-COUNTER PREPARATIONS

Regimen

Perhaps the most popular weight-reduction pill of the twentieth century was invented by John T. Andreadis in the early 1950s. According to the diet historian Hillel Schwartz, Andreadis established the Wonder Drug Company, and sold a pill called Regimen, which contained *benzocaine* (a local anesthetic), *ammonium chloride* (an acid-forming salt with diuretic effects), and *phenylpropanolamine hydrochloride* (an adrenaline-like compound used as a decongestant). A box of Regimen cost 30 cents to manufacture and sold for five dollars. These green, pink, and yellow pills were promoted for "no-diet reducing." In 1959 the product's advertising campaign included 218,000 one-minute TV commercial spots and 1,064,000 lines of newspaper advertising in which clinical reports were touted and actresses testified about lost weight. Unfortunately, the clinical reports on Regimen were invented. The actresses in the testimonials had been on their own diets of coffee and phenobarbital.

Phenylpropanolamine

After twenty years of investigating Andreadis for suspected fraud and misrepresentation, the Food and Drug Administration agreed that one of the ingredients in his combination pill, phenylpropanolamine (the adrenaline-like compound used as a decongestant), was safe and mildly effective as an appetite suppressant. Andreadis was partially vindicated when a variety of preparations containing phenylpropanolamine hit the market, including Anorexine, Appedrine, Ayds, Dexatrim, Dietrim, Prolamine, and Spantrol. Each shares common features: they are cheap to produce, expensive to buy, safe for most people if taken in small doses, and little better than placebos in long-term effectiveness. The benefits disappear as soon as the drug is discontinued. Taken in doses larger than approved for over-the-counter sale, they can cause high blood pressure. People with heart disease, hyperthyroidism, or high blood pressure should avoid the drug entirely, since even approved dosages may exacerbate these conditions. Because of its potential for side effects, and because its benefits persist only as long as the drug is taken continually, we advise against the use of phenylpropanolamine for purposes of weight loss.

Amino Acids, Anesthetics, Dietary Supplements, and Vitamins

A variety of health-food and weight-loss gurus periodically claim to have discovered the answer to the problem of obesity. *Tryptophan* and *phenylalanine* are amino acids, the basic building blocks of protein. Alone or in combination with other amino acids, they have been promoted as remedies for obesity. Only tryptophan has been shown to have a small effect in some people in reducing craving for carbohydrates. The Food and Drug Administration recently banned tryptophan supplements because some people who take it develop a serious illness characterized by muscle pain and abnormal blood counts. Proof of the effectiveness of amino-acid supplements in producing weight reduction does not exist; such supplements are most accurately described as an overly expensive form of dietary protein. Moreover, when taken as large doses of tryptophan, they can be dangerous.

Vitamins are often touted as weight-loss supplements. Their sole effectiveness, however, is in supplying missing nutrients when one is on a very strict diet, or when one is deficient in a certain vitamin. Whether in megadoses or minute, physiologic quantities, vitamins are otherwise of no use in weight control.

Local anesthetics temporarily numb the tongue and taste buds, making swallowing unpleasant. Most of these products can be recognized by the suffix *-caine* in their names, such as *benzocaine, xylocaine,* or *novocaine.* Despite their wide availability, there is no evidence that they are even mildly effective in controlling weight.

Many specialized food preparations and dietary supplements, including herbs, lecithin, and extracts of grapefruit or eggplant, have been touted as helpful in controlling weight. Convincing evidence to support such claims is nonexistent.

Bulk-producing Agents

A more benign and mildly effective weight-loss treatment is the use of generous amounts of fiber. The fiber can be supplied as wafers, capsules, powders, or in cereals. Some of the fibers, such as pectin and oat bran, are soluble in water. Others are visible in breakfast cereals made from the hulls of grains. The theory behind these agents is that if the stomach is filled with bulky fiber, hunger will decrease. Although the effect on weight loss is mild, fiber does have an additional mild effect in lowering cholesterol, and in treating constipation. While these bulk supplements have little effect on the sensations of hunger, with regular use they do have a modest effect in promoting weight loss. A wise way to take advantage of this effect would be to include plenty of whole grains, fruits, and vegetables in your diet, thus seeing to it that you ingest the fibers in their natural form.

Sugar Substitutes and Fat Substitutes

Aspartame (Nutrasweet, Equal) and saccharine have been used for years in a variety of "diet" drinks and foods. One might assume that these sugar substitutes would be effective in promoting weight loss since they do reduce the caloric density of foods, but they do not appear to be effective cures for obesity.

In 1990 the makers of Nutrasweet won approval from the Food and Drug Administration to market a fat substitute known as Simplesse. The FDA approval signifies the safety of the product, not its effectiveness as an aid in weight reduction. Another fat substitute, Olestra, has been developed by Procter & Gamble and is awaiting FDA approval at the time of this writing. Neither Olestra nor Simplesse has been proven effective as treatments for obesity. Their health benefits, if any, remain to be determined.

Weight-loss Pills

A variety of weight-loss pills for self-prescribed use are widely advertised under various names, particularly in the Sunday supplements of many newspapers. Most are little more than ineffective placebos, or combinations of bulk, phenylpropanolamine, and/or benzocaine. Many are sold by companies that go out of business as soon as authorities begin to make inquiries based on consumer complaints. These cruel hoaxes are endlessly perpetrated on people who are desperate to lose weight. The names of the products seem to change each month, but the sales pitch remains the same. Look for the words "miracle," "breakthrough," "revolutionary," "magic," "no effort," and "easy." But remember, there is no magic, and no quick fix, only a quick buck.

Money-back guarantees do not ensure that a product will work, and most purchasers are too embarrassed to ask for their money back.

MIRACLE CURES

Opportunists exploit and misrepresent fragments of scientific fact, weaving a thread of truth into a fabric of falsehood. For example, the "Medical Council on Weight Loss" in Florida announced that the supplements of amino acids and fatty acids they promoted would "switch on the fat-burning powers of your own body." The following quotation from their advertising brochure epitomizes this sort of misleading hype:

> Today's space-age research into the body's most complex chemical processes has finally discovered the special substance that triggers fat burn-off and literally pierces through the fat barrier to break up and slough away fat.
>
> What's even better, we now know how to get your body into that special chemical state with organic fat-burners called lypolites, like linolenic acid, arginine, ornithine, and lysine, technical medical terms for natural (and safe) stimulants that can spontaneously convert fat into energy. . . .
>
> With the NO-FAULT System you have to forget about everything you've ever learned about dieting. Simply take the NO-FAULT System supplements as directed, and wait for weight loss to happen.
>
> Some people lose 2–3 pounds in the first night! Most people lose 3–5 pounds a week.
>
> Rest assured, once you've realized that it's not your fault that you're fat, the NO-FAULT System puts your body back into its natural, healthy state of leanness.

No doubt, many salesmen would like to have an address list of those gullible enough to nibble at this kind of bait.

PRESCRIPTION REMEDIES

Perhaps no area in the treatment of obesity is as controversial among physicians today as the use of prescription medications to treat obesity. In general, society has responded by limiting their use, which is appropriate, but for the wrong reason. There is a widespread belief that weight-control pills "don't work." In fact, clinical data in animals and humans have repeatedly demonstrated that the weight-control pills listed in Table 12.1 (see below) do work. But they work only *temporarily*, and at a high cost in side effects. In our view, the side effects of these drugs outweigh their benefits for the treatment of obesity. We therefore believe that they should not be used for weight reduction.

Table 12.1
Prescription Drugs Used to Treat Obesity

Brand Name	Chemical Name	Manufacturer
Adipex-P	phentermine	Lemmon
Anorexin	phenylpropanolamine, caffeine, and vitamins	SDA
Bacarate	phendimetrazine	Tutag
Biphetamine	dl-amphetamine	Pennwalt
Bontril PDM	phendimetrazine	Carnrick
Desoxyn	methamphetamine	Abbott
Dexedrine	d-amphetamine	Smith Kline & French
Didrex	benzphetamine	Upjohn
Fastin	phentermine	Beecham
Ionamin	phentermine	Pennwalt
Mazanor	mazindol	Wyeth
Melfiat	phendimetrazine	Reid-Provident
Obe-Nil	phendimetrazine	Thera-Medic
Obetrol	d-amphetamine and dl-amphetamine	Obetrol
Plegine	phendimetrazine	Ayerst
Pondimin	fenfluramine	A. H. Robins
Prelu-2	phendimetrazine	Boehringer Ingelheim
Preludin	phenmetrazine	Boehringer Ingelheim
Sanorex	mazindol	Sandoz
Statobex	phendimetrazine	Lemmon
Tenuate	diethylpropion	Merrell-National
Tepanil	diethylpropion	Riker
Trimtabs	phendimetrazine	Mayrand

All of the drugs listed in the table have produced consistent weight loss of one-half to one and a half pounds per week, for as long as a year. This weight loss, however substantial, is almost always tempo-rary. In addition, most of the drugs listed in Table 12.1 cause euphoria.

When they are discontinued, patients tend to become depressed, and they usually eat to counteract this depression. Many also experience a "rebound hunger" when the restraint imposed by the medication is removed. As a result of both these responses, an almost inevitable return or even an "overshoot" of obesity takes place when the drug is stopped. It should also be noted that some clinicians believe that the use of amphetamine-like drugs during teenage years actually increases the probability of obesity in middle age.

Several difficulties accompany the use of medication in a weight-control program. The most important is a tendency to attribute all of one's weight loss to the pill—that is, to give the pill all the credit. But when the pill is stopped, what remains to "hold back" one's drive to eat? Dieters who rely upon medication learn little about controlling their eating from their experience of losing weight. They learn only to put their appetite "on hold" with a chemical for a few weeks or months. One study showed that even in a comprehensive treatment program, those who received medication had a greater tendency to relapse than did those who lost weight on their own in a behavior-modification program (see Figure 12.1). Furthermore, it is simply fool-hardy to take medications all of one's life unless the benefits clearly outweigh the side effects. Although continuing medication is medically appropriate for some diseases—for example, high blood pressure, gout, and diabetes—the long-term prescription of weight-control medications is inappropriate, given the side effects of the currently available drugs.

Many drugs used for weight control have a high potential for addiction and a wide variety of side effects. Many are stimulants, similar to dextroamphetamine, with side effects that include mood elevation and euphoria, sleeplessness, jitteriness, psychosis, depression, weight gain, addiction, and withdrawal symptoms. They seem to work by decreasing the subjective experience of hunger, or by making hunger more tolerable through a sense of euphoria or "speediness" and dis-tractibility. Even though some of these drugs have been on the market for up to 50 years, their exact mode of action is not clear.

Appetite-suppressing Drugs

As shown in Table 12.1, a variety of appetite-suppressing medications are available by prescription for weight control. All currently available weight-control drugs, including amphetamines, are chemically related to their parent compound, phenylethylamine. This mol-

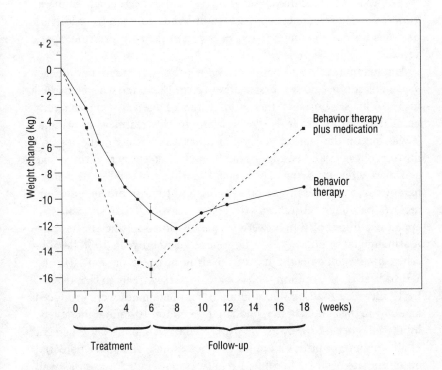

Figure 12.1 Weight Change Chart

Impact of medications in the treatment of obesity. Two groups of overweight patients both lost weight in a six-week treatment program emphasizing behavior modification for better habits of eating and exercising. One of the groups, however, received weight-reducing medications in addition to the behavior therapy. This group lost weight more rapidly than did the group getting behavior therapy alone, without drugs. But they also regained more weight, and did so more rapidly. Twelve weeks after the completion of the treatment, the group who had taken medications had regained more weight, and were still regaining at a faster rate, than the group who had not taken the medications. Obviously, the benefits of medication did not last.

ecule is also the basis of the neurotransmitters (substances within the brain that provide communication among brain cells) *norepinephrine* and *dopamine.* All of these drugs have powerful effects on the body's regulatory systems, and many are potentially addictive. By altering the molecule, chemists have created a variety of compounds that range from the highly stimulating (and highly addictive) drugs *Methedrine* and *Dexedrine* to the mildly sedating (sleep-inducing) compound *fenfluramine*. The tendency of these compounds to produce addiction parallels their stimulant activity, rather than their suppression of appetite.

Amphetamine. Most commonly known by the trade name *Benzedrine,* this compound was first synthesized in 1887, and was researched in 1927 by scientists at the Smith Kline & French drug company because they thought it would be useful in the treatment of asthma. It was put on the market in 1932 as a nasal inhalant to relieve stuffy noses. College students soon began using it to keep themselves awake and alert while studying. Physicians began to prescribe it to control narcolepsy, exhaustion, and depression, and to promote mental alertness. A physician, Abraham Meyerson, reasoned that since loss of appetite and loss of weight were frequently noted as side effects, Benzedrine might be effective as a treatment for obesity. In 1938 he published his findings on the use of the drug in obese patients. During World War II, 180 million tablets were dispensed freely to U.S. troops. By 1952, more than 60,000 pounds of amphetamines were produced annually in the United States, enough for 3 billion 10-milligram tablets. By the summer of 1970, at the peak of the Vietnam War, 8 percent of all drug prescriptions were for amphetamines. The abuse potential of amphetamines had become a reality in the United States, as well as in Japan and in much of Europe. Subsequently, its dangers and therapeutic limitations were investigated more thoroughly. In order to control its prescription and use, it was then reclassified with other drugs that have high potential for abuse, such as morphine. Although amphetamine is still available, it is rarely prescribed today for weight control. Awareness of its social cost and its overall limited effectiveness have combined to curtail its use and abuse.

Dexedrine (dextro-amphetamine). This is a potent form of amphetamine, and *Methedrine* (methamphetamine) is very similar in structure and effects. The federal government has classified these more stimulating compounds as Schedule II drugs, requiring special triplicate prescription forms, as with other highly addictive drugs, including narcotics. The less stimulating compounds, such as *Tenuate* (diethylpropion), and *Pondamin* (fenfluramine) are less addictive, carry much less abuse potential, and can be prescribed with fewer controls.

The exact action of these agents is not clear, but their effect appears to lie in their ability to block the initiation of the process of eating. In experiments with these drugs, animals showed less interest in food, had a shorter attention span, and, when eating, tended to be more easily distracted. Humans report similar effects. On the other hand, if you have your heart set on eating a piece of chocolate cake, a pill will not stop you. In other words, while these medications can enhance or act in concert with a decision to curtail food intake, they will not *replace* it.

Nonstimulant appetite-suppressing drugs. These substances, including fenfluramine, operate through a different mechanism within the central nervous system. They primarily affect the neurotransmitter *serotonin.* When the amount of this compound in brain tissue is increased, animals become sated more rapidly, and stop eating. This appears to be particularly true when the meal consists of carbohydrate-rich foods such as sweets, breads, and pasta, and less so for proteins and fats. Research is currently being conducted in this area, stimulated by the recent discovery that the new antidepressants *fluoxetine* and *sertraline,* which change brain serotonin levels, help curb runaway appetite in people with bulimia, and help others to lose weight. The research on a series of drugs in this category is still in its early stages, but side effects appear to be mild. No long-term studies have been completed. The use of these particular appetite-suppressing drugs, as with other medicines, probably will be as temporary short-term therapy, and probably will not revolutionize the treatment of obesity. Unless those for whom they are prescribed change their eating and exercise habits, they will regain lost weight when the medicine is stopped.

METABOLIC STIMULATORS: THERMOGENESIS

Another pharmacologic approach to treating obesity tries to enhance the expenditure of calories by accelerating the body's metabolism. These drugs have been called *thermogenic* (heat-producing) agents. They speed up the rate of metabolism, causing the body to burn more calories per hour than otherwise might be expected. Several potent agents have this effect, and as a result they have been found in experimental studies to cause weight loss. However, as one might expect from drugs affecting the basic life processes involved in metabolism, their side effects are significant.

Thyroid Hormone

In 1883, a researcher named Baron found that giving an extract of sheep thyroid glands to overweight people made them lose weight.

Over the next century, the use of this hormone to treat obesity has been a topic of study and debate. We now know that apart from its use in replacement therapy for people who are truly deficient in thyroid hormone, it has no place in the treatment of obesity.

Thyroid hormone is a natural chemical substance produced in the thyroid gland and released into the bloodstream, which carries it throughout the body. So dispersed, it affects the function of virtually every tissue in the body, setting the pace of metabolism. Too little thyroid hormone (hypothyroidism) results in abnormally slow metabolism, with consequent slowing of calorie expenditure. This often leads to weight gain, though most cases of obesity are not due to hypothyroidism.

The diagnosis of thyroid hormone deficiency has been difficult until recently, and some doctors are still not aware of an improved test that allows reliable determination of whether a person is truly hypothyroid. A pituitary hormone detected by a blood test is elevated in hypothyroidism. The hormone, called TSH for *thyroid-stimulating hormone*, accurately detects more than 95 percent of cases of hypothyroidism.

Truly hypothyroid patients should be treated with thyroid hormone—just enough to restore their metabolism to normal. But many overweight people have been given thyroid hormone without a firm diagnosis of hypothyroidism ever having been made. The side effects of excess thyroid hormone make this practice unwise.

Too much thyroid hormone causes abnormally rapid metabolism and increases caloric expenditure. Although this sometimes leads to weight loss, most of the weight lost is muscle and fluid, not fat. The research results displayed in Figure 12.2 demonstrate this unfortunate fact. In addition to depleting the muscles, excess thyroid hormone also causes osteoporosis—a weakening of the bones which can eventually lead to devastating fractures of the spine, hips, and other bones. Too much thyroid hormone also causes nervousness, tremors, sweating, intolerance of warm weather, weakness, and rapid heartbeat. Worse, too much thyroid hormone strains the heart, above and beyond the increased cardiac load imposed by obesity. Giving an obese person more thyroid hormone than his or her body requires for normal metabolism is therefore risky, and can even be fatal.

Dinitrophenol

A second metabolic stimulator, dinitrophenol, illustrates again the need for caution in adopting miracle cures for obesity. This drug came

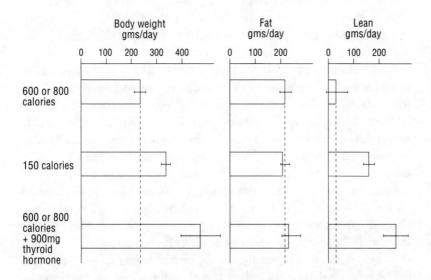

Figure 12.2 Impact of Adding Thyroid Hormone Treatment to Calorie Restriction

Obese volunteers were treated with a liquid formula diet of 600–800 calories per day. Their losses of weight, fat mass, and lean body mass were compared with those of subjects on the same diet but with thyroid hormone added, and to subjects on a very low 150-calorie liquid formula diet. On the 600–800 calorie diet, subjects lost an average of about 220 grams of body weight per day, most of which was fat. On only 150 calories per day, subjects lost weight more rapidly, but the additional weight loss was lean tissue such as muscle, not fat. On 600–800 calories per day plus thyroid hormone, subjects also lost very fast—almost 500 grams of body weight per day. Once again, however, the additional weight loss was lean tissue, not fat. Thyroid hormone should not be taken for purposes of weight reduction because it wastes lean tissue without improving the rate of fat loss.

out of the German textile industry in the 1800s. It is related to the aniline dyes, which provide brilliant colors such as mauve and "shocking pink." Aniline chemicals were also important constituents of explosives during World War I. In the 1920s one of these compounds, *dinitrophenol* (DNP), was found to increase the human metabolic rate by 50 percent. Dieters who used this compound lost two to three pounds per week, and DNP seemed to hold the promise of being a miracle drug. As with many new drugs, the initial burst of enthusiasm was followed by the discovery of increasingly severe side effects. People who used DNP felt warm, perspired heavily, and got rashes. Some lost their sense of taste, others went blind from cataracts, and some died.

DNP, which can be absorbed through the skin or inhaled as a dust or in fumes, had been noted as an industrial toxin as early as 1889. Research eventually would show that the higher the concentration of DNP in the body, the more the metabolic rate would be increased, until fatal overheating occurred. In the popular press of the 1930s, however, DNP was hailed as safe and effective. *The New Republic* magazine in 1933 welcomed it not only as a treatment for excess weight, but as part of the solution to the Great Depression, saying, "Those who now suffer from obesity will be able to work harder and be more productive than before." In 1938 the use of DNP was finally stopped, but only after many hopeful dieters had been injured or killed.

Today, with equally deadly results, many people rationalize their use of *tobacco* on the grounds that they will gain weight if they stop smoking. Cigarette smoking produces a 10-percent increase in 24-hour energy expenditure as measured by oxygen consumption. This effect accounts at least in part for the common observation that people who give up smoking may gain five to ten pounds. Studies do show that smokers tend to weigh less than nonsmokers, but the distribution of fat in smokers tends to be more abdominal than in nonsmokers, and fat in the abdomen (see chapters 2 and 6) is associated with increased risk of heart attack, stroke, gallbladder disease, high blood pressure, high blood cholesterol, and diabetes. Thus, although cigarette smoking does reduce total body fat somewhat, it does so in a most unhealthy way.

Other, apparently less harmful preparations are also widely used in weight control today. *Caffeine* stimulates the metabolic rate, and has long been included in over-the-counter diet preparations. *Ephedrine,* a decongestant and bronchodilating agent initially extracted from a Chinese herb used to treat asthma, has produced weight loss in some studies. This compound, plus caffeine and phenobarbital, constituted the active ingredients in the Elsinore pill, developed by a Danish general practitioner in 1972. The medication was very popular in Europe until 1977, when it was withdrawn from the market because of side effects of nervousness, insomnia, perspiration, cardiac irregularity, and occasional psychosis. It appeared to enhance weight loss about as much as the prescription medication Tenuate (an appetite suppressant described earlier in this chapter), but with less abuse potential. Although once widely prescribed, the Elsinore pill proved to be yet another "flash in the pan," with marginal benefits outweighed by unacceptable side effects.

Many major drug companies continue in their efforts to develop such metabolic-enhancing agents. Preliminary animal research data often demonstrate effectiveness with apparent safety, but it is difficult to predict the outcome of these medications in humans, since the human body is not designed to run in a constant state of "overdrive." The track record for thyroid hormone, DNP, tobacco, and the Elsinore pill make it doubtful that safe and effective agents to accelerate metabolic rate will be developed in the foreseeable future.

ABSORPTION INHIBITORS

Theoretically, one might reduce caloric intake by preventing the bloodstream from absorbing food from the intestine. After all, only food that is absorbed can contribute to obesity. If one could eliminate food from the intestines before it was absorbed, one could eat as many calories as desired without gaining weight. This presumption is carried to its extreme, of course, by bulimic patients, who gorge and then regurgitate. It was also the concept underlying the commercial sale of tapeworms for weight control in the last century.

The first attempt to use a drug to inhibit the absorption of food was made with the use of laxatives, and they remain today the most widely abused substances for promoting weight loss. For centuries, misinformed folk wisdom has indicated that "a good cathartic" will wash out extra calories along with other impurities. We observe this thinking today in some bulimic patients who take up to 200 laxative tablets, or a quart of milk of magnesia, *per day* to speed calories through their bowels. Studies show, however, that even in extreme cases of laxative abuse, almost 90 percent of the calories become absorbed despite the laxatives. Nearly all the weight loss caused by laxative use is from the water in the diarrhea fluid, and even it is gained back promptly with the next glass of water. This is a dangerous and severely mistaken approach to weight control. Laxative abuse produces serious biochemical disturbances, especially potassium depletion, as well as symptoms of weakness, faintness, and cramps.

"Starch blockers" were used in another popular attempt to block calorie absorption. Scientists found that a substance found in beans inhibits *amylase*, the enzyme that digests starch. When amylase is inhibited, the starch in the intestine is not broken down into absorbable molecules. Instead, it passes into the colon, and out of the body in the feces. Bacteria in the colon attack the undigested starch, and convert it to gas—a well-known side effect of eating beans.

Based on what they had learned about beans, scientists reasoned that perhaps these substances, which block the digestion of starch, could be taken in pill form, making it possible to eat pasta, bread, and other starches without their being absorbed. Despite wide cele- bration in the media, these compounds produced pain, gas, and diar- rhea instead of weight loss, and they were withdrawn from the market. Current research continues to seek ways to inhibit the enzymes in- volved in the digestion and absorption of both carbohydrates and fats. Despite its theoretical appeal, this approach is not likely to provide safe, comfortable weight loss. Diarrhea, gas, abdominal pain, and malabsorption of vital nutrients can be anticipated as side effects.

DIURETICS

Medications that interfere with the function of the kidneys by causing them to release more salt and water into the urine are called *diuretics*. Since the excreted fluids have weight, taking a diuretic will temporarily reduce your weight. It will not, however, get rid of fat.

Fluid and salt loss occurs naturally as a person loses weight through diet and exercise (see chapter 9). Too much fluid loss causes muscle cramps, dizziness, weakness, and cardiovascular problems. Taking diuretics only makes the problem worse. In the absence of another condition that may require diuretics (such as heart failure or hyper- tension), obese persons on a diet would do well to avoid these drugs.

DIGITALIS

Digitalis (sold most often in the form known as *digoxin*) is a long- established and potent drug, useful in the treatment of heart failure. Digitalis improves the circulation in some cases of heart failure, en- abling the kidneys to get rid of excess fluid. As a consequence, many patients with heart failure have lost weight taking digitalis. But the weight they lost was the excess edema fluid of heart failure. Digitalis does not get rid of fat.

Symptoms of digitalis overdosage include nausea and loss of ap- petite. Unfortunately, digitalis has been included in many quackish medical treatments for obesity, in hopes of creating this nausea and thus interfering with appetite. This is a dangerous and foolhardy way to try to treat obesity. Too much digitalis can cause lethal heart malfunction.

Digitalis, or digoxin, can be safely used, under proper medical supervision, in the treatment of certain heart problems. For this purpose, its use can be beneficial. As a treatment for obesity, however, digitalis has no place.

THE FUTURE STILL LIES AHEAD

Spurred by intense consumer demand for effortless weight loss, and by demand from the medical profession for effective forms of treatment, pharmaceutical companies continue the search for compounds to cure obesity. Researchers are actively investigating a variety of hormones, brain neurotransmitters, metabolic enhancers, compounds that prevent fat production, and synthetic, no-calorie fat substitutes. At present, however, the safety and usefulness of these substances in humans is unproven.

It is conceivable that scientists will one day discover a safe and effective drug to cure obesity. A substance to suppress appetite safely seems the most likely possibility. For the present, however, the marginal, temporary benefits of available drug treatments do not compensate for their side effects, risks, and expense. As physicians who treat many obese patients, we do not recommend any such medications for purposes of weight control.

Sensible treatment for obesity still centers on changing one's behavior and life-style. Increasing your physical activity and curtailing your intake of fat and calories remain indispensable. No pill in the world can do these for you.

13

Surgery

Wouldn't it be wonderful if you could go to a surgeon, have an operation, and be cured of obesity? In hopes of such a cure, thousands of patients have submitted to surgical procedures. Some of these operations remove excess fat directly; others reduce food intake by making it difficult to eat much. Still others prevent food from being absorbed after it is eaten. The results of these operations have been favorable in some instances. In others they have been disastrous, and even fatal.

So many problems have occurred with weight-control surgery that the surgeons who perform it continue to modify the procedures in their efforts to improve outcome and reduce complications. Consequently, most current operations in the field have been widely used for less than ten years. The newness of present surgical treatments for obesity makes it impossible to evaluate fully their long-term risks and benefits. As with dieting, short-term success in losing weight is easy enough to come by. It is the long-term outlook that is crucial.

Keeping in mind that this surgery is still evolving, let's take a look at the operations in recent and current use. The surgery is of three main types:

---

1. Surgical removal of fat. The medical term for this is *lipectomy.*
It includes *suction lipectomy,* or *liposuction,* as well as the excision
of fat with a scalpel.

2. Surgical constriction of the alimentary canal—the passageway
of food from mouth to anus. This constriction can take place at the
level of the jaws, which can be wired shut, or farther down, at the
level of the stomach.

3. Surgical bypass of portions of the alimentary tract involved in
food absorption, intended to reroute the food's journey so that some
of the calories eaten pass through the body without being absorbed.

Some operations, such as *gastric bypass,* combine elements of the
second and third kinds of surgery listed above.

SURGICAL REMOVAL OF FAT

It would seem that the obvious way to correct excessive fatness would
be to cut it off. Since too big a nose can be corrected permanently
with plastic surgery, why not treat too big a belly in the same way?
The problem with this approach is that unless the patient also permanently changes calorie intake and/or output, the fat will grow back.

After the surgical removal of fat, the remaining fat cells enlarge and
multiply to store the excess calories still being consumed. But, one
might ask, what if the surgeon removes *all* the fat in an area? This
strategy has been tried in experiments, by removing specific fat pads
from rodents. The outcome is that the fat grows back in other body
areas. The same occurs in humans.

One 50-year-old woman decided to have liposuction to remove
several pounds of fat on her lower abdomen. At first she was pleased
with the results of the operation, but then she found that her weight
was returning to its previous level. (This was to be expected, since her
diet and physical activity had not changed.) The fat that came back
returned not so much to her abdomen as elsewhere, so that her arms,
back, and shoulders now were visibly heavier than they had been. She
feels that the only lasting effect of the surgery was to redistribute her
excess fat tissue.

Since subcutaneous (superficial) fat is the most accessible to the
surgeon, the regrowth of fat that takes place after lipectomy is likely

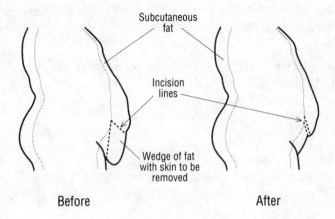

Figure 13.1 Dermolipectomy

Subcutaneous (superficial) fat, with overlying skin, is surgically removed. Fat lying deeper within the abdominal cavity is not removed by this procedure.

to occur in deeper sites, such as within the abdominal cavity. This intra-abdominal obesity is the type that is most harmful to health (see chapter 6), and it is thus possible that lipectomy will lead to an intensification of the medical risks of obesity, unless the patient's eating and exercise habits change to maintain the reduction in weight.

During the 1970s, a theory propounded by researchers at the Rockefeller Institute in New York gave credence to lipectomy as the logical way to cure obesity. The theory held that some people cannot lose weight because they have too many fat cells. According to this theory, fat cells send messages to appetite centers in the brain, stimulating food intake until they become adequately filled with fat. The implication of this theory was that lipectomy—cutting out fat cells—should cut down appetite. Unfortunately, however, lipectomy does not alter appetite. Lipectomy makes no more lasting a change in body weight than does a crash diet, for it does not solve the $64,000 question of how to *maintain* a reduced weight.

Two principal approaches to lipectomy have been used. The first is simply to remove a wedge of fat, along with the overlying skin, as diagrammed in Figure 13.1. This procedure is called *dermolipectomy,* because skin (*dermo-*) as well as fat (*-lip-*) is removed (*-ectomy*). Although it is useful in contouring the body, as in plastic surgery, dermolipectomy is not a practical treatment for obesity. First, the excess weight will be regained unless calorie intake is permanently curtailed, or physical activity is permanently increased. The regain occurs throughout the remaining areas of fat tissue. Second, fat tissue often heals poorly. Fluid may accumulate in the wound, infection may occur, and/or the incision may pull apart before healing is complete.

A much more popular approach is suction lipectomy, or liposuction. This technique involves a small incision in the skin, through which is passed a suction tube. (A photograph of several such instruments is shown in Figure 13.2.) The tube is passed back and forth through the area to be reduced. It cuts fibrous bands in the adipose tissue, and suction draws the fat out through the tube—hence the nickname "fat-sucking."

Suction lipectomy is very much in vogue. Dermatologists, ear, nose, and throat specialists, plastic surgeons, and general surgeons all have employed this lucrative procedure. Before-and-after photos show the disappearance of "saddlebag" fat deposits on the outer hips, double chins becoming single, and fat, lumpy bottoms becoming less so. But although the initial cosmetic results are often quite good, the weight loss is no more lasting than after a temporary diet-and-exercise program. Complications of liposuction include infection, hollowed-out areas, and lumpy ridges. If too much fat tissue is removed at once, shock—a dangerous condition of circulatory collapse—can occur.

Suction lipectomy should not be regarded as treatment for obesity. As with dermolipectomy, in order to remove a significant amount of fat, the surgeon would have to operate all over the body. Like facelift or cosmetic breast surgery, this is a cosmetic, "touch-up" procedure for sculpting specific parts of the body. It is not a way to lose a significant amount of weight. In experienced hands, however, the aesthetic results of liposuction are often quite satisfactory—at least for a short time.

SURGICAL CONSTRICTION OF
THE ALIMENTARY CANAL TO REDUCE FOOD INTAKE

For centuries, fishermen in China have used the cormorant, a web-footed, long-necked seabird, as a means of catching fish. To keep the birds from swallowing the fish they catch, the fishermen place a strap, or a metal ring, around the birds' necks. This is essentially the approach used by surgeons to constrict or partially obstruct human anatomy to

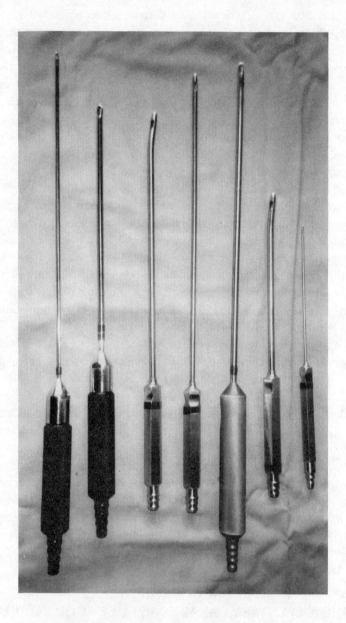

Figure 13.2 Suction Lipotomes

These instruments are like vacuum-cleaner attachments. The surgeon passes the slender portion through subcutaneous fat tissue while suction is applied to the handle. Fat is broken up and sucked out through the tubes.

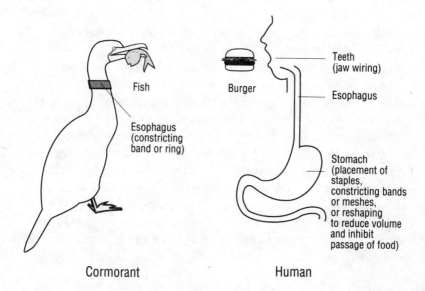

Figure 13.3 Levels of Surgical Constriction

Reducing calorie intake by constricting the passageway of food.

interfere with food intake and thereby treat obesity (see Figure 13.3).

For purposes of weight control, surgical constriction of the alimentary canal in humans is currently carried out at either of two levels: the jaws or the stomach.

Jaw Wiring

A rather direct approach to stopping someone from eating too much is to wire his or her jaws shut. This technique was developed in England by Dr. John S. Garrow as a safer alternative to intestinal bypass procedures for the treatment of severe obesity, described later in this chapter. The procedure involves tying wires or nylon sutures around the upper and lower teeth, and then tying these to each other. This technique effectively prevents the eating of solid foods, but permits the drinking of liquids. After the jaws are wired, one sips a nutritious liquid formula diet through a straw in controlled amounts. Cow's milk, with vitamins and iron supplements in liquid form, makes a suitable and inexpensive formula. Sometimes a dentist must remove a tooth to accommodate the straw. Typically, patients lose 70 to 90 pounds in this manner, although some have been known to avoid weight loss by drinking several chocolate milk shakes per day.

The procedure is relatively painless; the primary risk is that if physical illness causes one to vomit while the mouth is wired shut, the vomit is forced into the lungs. Patients usually carry wire cutters with them at all times to undo the jaw wiring should they become ill.

The major drawback to this method is the familiar one. After the dental wires are removed, weight is regained, just as it is after more conventional dieting, unless fundamental changes in eating or exercise habits take place. As with dieting, long-term studies have shown relapse rates of 95 percent or more. Because weight is regained after removal of the wires, jaw wiring by itself is not an adequate treatment for obesity.

The Garrow Belt or Waist Cord

Dr. Garrow, who pioneered jaw wiring at St. Bartholomew's Hospital Medical College in London, has recently added an ingenious technique to help patients maintain their reduced weight after the wires come off. A keen observer of human behavior, he had among his patients a model who wore a golden chain around her waist. When he inquired about it, she replied that it had been given her by a lover and soldered permanently closed by a jeweler, so that it could not be removed without cutting it. Whenever she felt it to be tight, she knew she had eaten too much and would decrease her food intake. With this in mind, Dr. Garrow devised a thin, soft plastic cord to be snugged around the waist of patients who had just lost weight with jaw wiring. After tying the cord, he melted the knot with a cigarette lighter so it could not be removed and replaced surreptitiously. He then checked the waist cord at subsequent follow-up visits. The cord remained comfortable until or unless the patient regained weight, in which case it began to pinch, providing a reminder of the need to curtail food intake and/or to exercise more.

Dr. Garrow reported on 14 patients who used this combined technique of jaw wiring followed by the waist cord. They lost an average of 92 pounds with jaws wired, then had the wires removed and waist cords applied. Three years later they were still an average of 73 pounds lighter than they had been before treatment. No significant complications occurred. These results compare favorably with operations involving general anesthesia and surgical alterations of the stomach and/or intestines. Moreover, jaw wiring and waist cords involve much less risk and expense than gastrointestinal surgery. Since long-term follow-up data are not available, however, the jaw-wiring/waist-cord method still must be viewed as experimental.

Of interest in Dr. Garrow's report was his mention of three patients who were treated in the same way except that they did not have their jaws wired. Instead, they simply sipped the same milk, iron, and vitamin formula as though their jaws *were* wired. They also lost an average of 92 pounds each, then were fitted with waist cords. Two years later, they too had successfully maintained an average of 73 pounds lost. In other words, the benefits of jaw wiring are available without actually having to tie your teeth together, if you follow the prescribed diet.

We describe the jaw-wiring/waist-cord method first in this section because it is relatively cheap, and is safe and effective in selected patients who are willing to maintain regular follow-up—the same sort of patients often selected for surgery. Those contemplating gastrointestinal surgery for treatment of obesity should consider this as an alternative. In making the comparison, note that undoing the wires is a simple matter: the patient can clip the wires, and a dentist easily removes the entire appliance. Undoing an operation on the stomach and intestines, on the other hand, requires hospitalization, general anesthesia, surgical risks such as infection and bleeding, and considerable expense.

Stomach Surgery

Besides the jaws, the stomach has been the other main target site for constricting the alimentary tract to curtail food intake. Several operations for obesity constrict the stomach. To understand them, let's look first at normal stomach function and anatomy (see Figure 13.4).

The stomach is a reservoir, or holding tank, for food. It is located in the upper abdomen, at the end of the esophagus, or "food pipe." Swallowed food, liquid, and saliva proceed from the throat, down the esophagus to the stomach. There they mix with powerful acid secreted by glands in the stomach wall. The stomach wall also secretes a factor necessary for the absorption of vitamin B_{12}. The exit from the stomach is a muscular ring called the *pylorus,* which is usually closed, preventing the dumping of more food into the intestine than can be

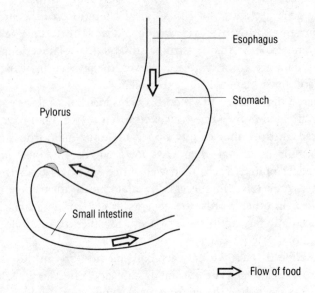

Esophagus

Stomach

Pylorus

Small intestine

Flow of food

Figure 13.4 Stomach Anatomy

The stomach is a food reservoir located in the upper abdomen. As indicated by
the bold arrows, swallowed food flows from the throat through the *esophagus*
(commonly called the "food pipe") to the stomach. The stomach secretes
digestive juices that mix with the swallowed food and saliva. The exit valve of
the stomach is called the *pylorus*. It opens intermittently, allowing small
amounts of food and digestive juices to pass into the small intestine, where
absorption takes place.

comfortably digested and absorbed at once. Intermittently the pylorus
opens and the stomach contracts, propelling small amounts of food
downstream into the small intestine, where absorption takes place.

Some surgeons have tucked and sewn a big fold into the stomach,
thereby reducing its volume (see Figure 13.5). The idea is to create a
feeling of fullness after only a small amount of food has been eaten.
To prevent compensatory expansion of the stomach, some surgeons
have then wrapped the stomach with a fabric mesh, sewn in place.
This requires a great deal of tissue dissection, and adds risks of bleeding, damage to the spleen (an important organ located beside the
stomach), perforation of the stomach, and infection, which can accompany the placement of any foreign material within the body.

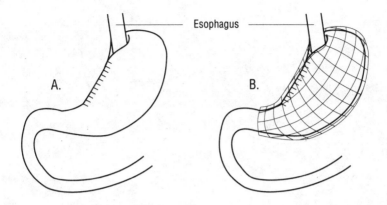

Figure 13.5 Constricting the Stomach

(A) Stomach folded over and sewn down to reduce its reservoir capacity, with the intent of making the patient feel full after eating only a small amount of food. (B) Same, with silicone-mesh wrap added to prevent distension.

Stomach Stapling

This procedure constricts the stomach with staples; the surgeon staples the front wall of the stomach to the back wall. Just as you can't put many groceries into a paper bag if its opposite sides have been stapled together, you can't put much food into a stomach that is constricted by staples connecting the front and back walls. (Figure 13.6 diagrams some of the configurations used for placing the staples.)

Stomach-stapling techniques have evolved as surgeons have learned how better to place the staples in double, triple, or quadruple rows. With earlier techniques, staples tended to pull out, especially at the edge of the passageway for food. Once the passageway was thus enlarged, the effectiveness of the obstruction was lost. Recent improvements in technique appear to have reduced the rate of staple loosening.

Vertical Banded Gastroplasty

After much trial and error and hard-won experience, surgeons have developed a currently popular procedure that appears to avoid many previous problems: *vertical banded gastroplasty*.

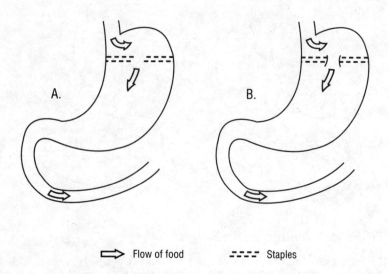

Figure 13.6 Stomach Stapling

Stomach stapling leaves a small receiving pouch, so that the eater feels full after consuming small amounts of food. A narrow exit passage allows food to progress slowly downstream. The staples attach the front and back sides of the stomach to each other. In diagram A, a few staples have been left out to create the exit passage. In diagram B, the staples completely block the stomach, but a narrow detour passage has been created surgically.

This procedure does not interfere with the absorption of food that has been eaten, since it preserves the usual anatomical flow of food and digestive juices. By leaving a small pouch of only one ounce or less, the surgery curtails calorie intake in most people. Surgical risks and time are less than for other procedures, and in experienced hands the likelihood of death during hospitalization for the procedure is now under 1 percent. The extent of weight reduction following this operation has been reported as around 60 pounds on the average, though some reports claim as much as 79 pounds lost in the first year by patients who had been at less than twice normal weight, and 119 pounds for patients who had been at more than two and a half times normal weight. At two years after the operation, weight loss is often well maintained. Long-term follow-up data are difficult to find, how-

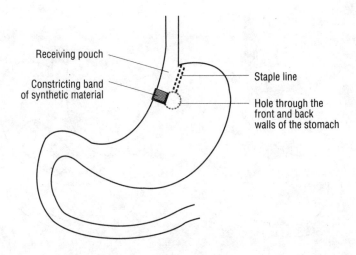

Receiving pouch

Constricting band
of synthetic material

Staple line

Hole through the
front and back
walls of the stomach

Figure 13.7 Vertical Banded Gastroplasty

Vertical rows of staples extend to a surgically created hole that, like a doughnut
hole, passes all the way through the front and back of the stomach. A band of
synthetic material passes through the hole, encircling and constricting the exit
passage from the small vertical pouch.

ever, due to the newness of the operation. Some patients report that
they have difficulty eating meat unless it is pureed, and some have
difficulty with vegetables. Some patients resort to drinking many milk
shakes, with resultant poor nutrition as well as poor maintenance of
weight loss. Immediate complications of surgery are fewer than with
many other kinds of gastrointestinal operations performed for weight
loss, and the fewer than 1 percent of patients who die before leaving
the hospital is a relatively excellent figure. Late complications, such
as erosions of the constricting mesh through the stomach wall, intestinal obstruction due to adhesions, or loosening of staples, appear to
be uncommon. Over the coming years, follow-up studies of this relatively new procedure should clarify its long-term risks and benefits.

The Garren-Edwards Bubble

A glowing exception to the general lack of properly controlled trials
is found in the saga of the "gastric bubble"—a widely used device for

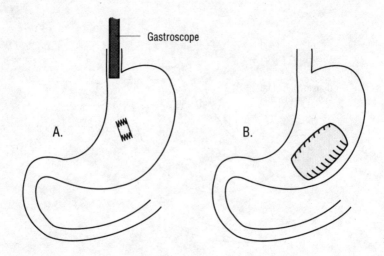

Figure 13.8 Gastric Balloon

Gastric balloon, inserted into the stomach via a gastroscope, then inflated with
the intent of reducing the reservoir capacity of the stomach and creating a
feeling of fullness.

producing weight loss by reducing the reservoir capacity of the stomach.

In 1984, Dr. L. R. Garren reported successful weight reduction by
means of a balloon (or "bubble") that he passed through the esophagus
of a patient and then into the stomach. Once in the stomach, the
balloon is inflated (see Figure 13.8).

The hope was that the bubble would cause a feeling of fullness,
thereby reducing appetite, food intake, and weight. Early reports
looked promising, so the U.S. Food and Drug Administration approved
the device in late 1985 despite the absence of scientifically controlled
studies. FDA approval was met with enthusiasm by both health-care
providers and overweight patients.

Between November 1985 and December 1986, an estimated 20,000
Garren-Edwards Gastric Bubbles were inserted into individual patients, at an average cost of $2,000 to $4,000 for a three-to-four-
month treatment period. This calculates out to about $60 million spent
on this treatment in its first year.

Dr. Reed Hogan, in Jackson, Mississippi, then initiated a controlled study of the device, wanting to test whether, used properly in conjunction with standard weight-loss therapy, it was any better than standard weight-loss therapy alone. He recruited 60 patients who were at least 50 pounds overweight, informed them fully of the nature and purpose of the study, then randomly allocated them to receive either a Garren-Edwards Gastric Bubble or else an otherwise identical sham procedure in which no bubble was inserted. The patients, and those who evaluated and treated them for the following three months, were not informed as to who actually received the bubble and who had the sham procedure.

Of the 59 patients who completed the study, 34 received the bubble and 25 had sham bubble placements (in other words, no bubble was placed in their stomach). All patients met weekly with a dietitian, an exercise physiologist, and a clinical psychologist to help them lose weight through diet and exercise. After three months the bubbles were removed and weight loss results were analyzed.

The results showed no statistically significant difference between the treatment group and the control group in the amount of weight lost, the percentage of weight lost, or the amount of nausea, vomiting, or abdominal pain. Both groups lost an average of about 18 pounds, or 8 percent of body weight. Even though doctors and patients all over the United States were extolling the device as a major aid to weight reduction, evidently, these patients' success in losing weight was due to the diet and exercise rather than to the placement of a bubble within the stomach. Subsequent studies have confirmed Dr. Hogan's conclusion that this device is essentially useless as a treatment for obesity.

Although the Garren-Edwards Gastric Bubble does not help control weight, it is possible that a device designed or used somewhat differently might indeed work. The uselessness of this particular device does not disprove the theory that obstruction or constriction of the stomach might produce permanent weight control. Next time, however, we hope that patients (and the FDA) will insist on better evidence of efficacy.

All procedures designed to restrict the flow of food from the mouth to the small intestine (such as jaw wiring or vertical banded gastroplasty) have one element in common: they can easily be defeated by a determined patient. By consuming "soft" calories, such as milk shakes and chocolates, patients can—and indeed, many do—maintain or even gain weight despite the constriction of their alimentary canals.

For this reason, some surgeons choose to interfere deliberately with normal food absorption by rearranging part of the small intestine.

SURGICAL BYPASS OF THE INTESTINE TO INTERFERE WITH FOOD ABSORPTION

What dieter hasn't wished that food would simply go straight through the body, without being absorbed, so that he or she could eat cake and not have to wear it, too? Bypass operations for weight reduction were developed in the hope of creating just such a situation. To understand this approach to weight loss, let's look at the normal anatomy of the intestine, where calorie absorption occurs (see Figure 13.9).

The intestine is a long, muscular tube extending from the stomach to the rectum. Considered in the direction of food flow, the first part of the intestine, attached to the stomach, is called the *duodenum*. Iron and calcium are absorbed here. This is also where important digestive juices are added to the food to promote its emulsification and chemical breakdown in preparation for being absorbed. These juices include bile, entering from the gallbladder and liver, and powerful enzymes from the pancreas.

Downstream from the duodenum is the *jejunum*, where most of the calories in a normal meal are absorbed. The jejunum then blends into the *ileum*, which contains specialized cells for the absorption of specific substances such as vitamin B_{12} and bile acids—detergent molecules secreted in bile (see chapter 5). The duodenum, jejunum, and ileum together make up the small intestine, where almost all calorie absorption takes place. After the small intestine comes the large intestine, or colon, in which water and salts are extracted from the intestinal contents as they solidify into stool. The formed stool then passes through the rectum and out of the body.

Weight-control surgery aimed at the intestines employs two strategies for impairing food absorption: (1) bypassing parts of the small intestine to reduce the opportunity for absorption, and (2) delaying the mixing of food with digestive juices, so that food is not absorbed because it is still undigested. Several different anatomic rearrangements of the intestines have been used to implement these two strategies. Some of these maneuvers are combined with stapling or other procedures to reduce the size of the stomach to a small pouch that admits only a very small meal.

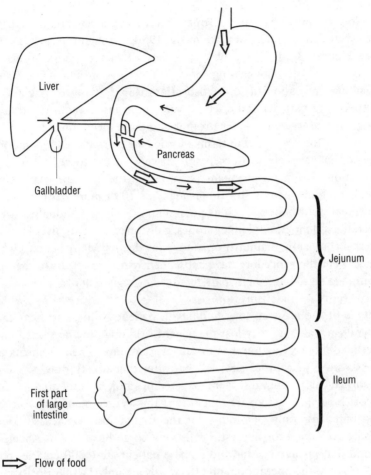

Liver

Gallbladder

Pancreas

Jejunum

Ileum

First part
of large
intestine

⟹ Flow of food

→ Flow of digestive juices from pancreas, liver, gallbladder, and stomach

Figure 13.9 Normal Gastrointestinal Anatomy

Normal gastrointestinal anatomy and function. Food (bold arrows) passes from the stomach into the first part of the small intestine, known as the *duodenum*. There food mixes with digestive juices (slender arrows) from the pancreas, liver, and gallbladder, and the chemical breakdown of food continues. Absorption of digested food begins in the duodenum, continues in the *jejunum* and then the *ileum*. The residue then passes into the large intestine, where water is extracted as intestinal contents are compacted into feces, which eventually pass out of the body via the rectum.

Jejunoileal Bypass

Now virtually obsolete, this operation was performed on thousands of overweight people from late in the 1950s through the early 1970s (see Figure 13.10). Done with a variety of minor modifications in design, it involved bypassing most of the jejunum and ileum, with resulting prevention of food absorption. Rapid, massive weight loss ensued, and patients and doctors were enthusiastic about the results as gross obesity came under prompt and permanent control.

At first, the price paid in terms of side effects from these operations seemed manageable and acceptable in view of the successful weight reduction. The main problems perceived in the first few years were frequent, foul-smelling stools—as many as 20 or more per day—and chemical disturbances, such as potassium depletion. Gradually, however, the toll mounted: kidney stones, gallstones, arthritis, liver failure, mental confusion, malnutrition, and many deaths. Many patients who underwent the procedure have subsequently had to return to the operating table to have the bypass removed or revised in order to reduce the severity of malabsorption.

One of the most curious findings in patients who underwent this operation was *how* they lost the weight. Although the presumed and intended mode of action was malabsorption, direct measurements of the wastage of calories showed that after the surgery only 593 unabsorbed calories per day were excreted in stool, as compared to 131 calories per day before the operation; this degree of malabsorption accounted for only one-fourth of the weight lost. Decreased food intake accounted for the rest. Professor George Bray, in Los Angeles, found that his average morbidly obese patient ate 6,300 calories per day prior to the operation, and afterwards ate only 1,200 calories per day. At an 18-month follow-up, after an average of 140 pounds of weight loss, his patients were still eating an average of only 3,500 calories per day. This decrease in food intake accounted for 60 to 70 percent of the lost weight. The food wasn't malabsorbed; it wasn't being eaten. Studies showed that many patients adopted a more normal eating pattern, with less snacking, slower eating, and an earlier sense of fullness. An unexpected benefit of this procedure, then, was improved eating behavior. Some of this change in eating was doubtless due to the fact that in many patients the intake of sugar and fats caused cramps, bloating, and diarrhea. Some of the behavioral changes may relate to psychological effects that became apparent after the operation.

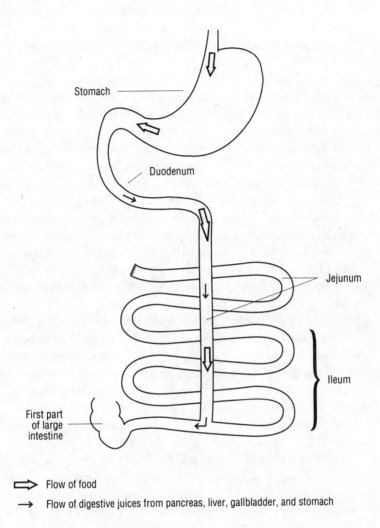

Figure 13.10 Jejunoileal Bypass

Food and digestive juices bypass most of the small intestine, where most food is normally absorbed into the bloodstream. Only the duodenum and small portions of the jejunum and the ileum remain available for food absorption.

Many patients demonstrated improvement in their psychological status after jejunoileal bypass. While severe dieting often produces depression and anxiety, these patients demonstrated improved self-esteem, less depression, increased daytime activity, better body image,

a greater sense of effectiveness, and in many cases better marital relationships. The operation seemed to bring new hope, breaking the
cycle of discouragement and failure so common in extremely obese
patients.

Although jejunoileal bypass produced weight loss, with attendant
medical and psychological benefits, it also produced many severe complications. Immediate operative complications, including stroke, infection, hemorrhage, kidney failure, and death, were not uncommon.
In one series of 2,500 patients, 3 percent died before getting out of
the hospital. In other hospitals, where only a few such operations were
performed, mortality rates were even higher. The most common complication of the operation was diarrhea. Patients lost essential nutrients, such as calcium, magnesium, potassium, and several important
vitamins. The malnutrition, kidney stones, gallstones, and arthritis all
occurred as delayed complications. Moreover, many people found that
within 18 months they were regaining weight because the bowel gradually adapted to its shortened length, with less malabsorption and less
diarrhea.

It is the combination of these complications and risks that has ren-
dered jejunoileal bypass largely obsolete. Even those few patients for
whom consideration of surgery might be appropriate—more than 100
pounds overweight, with life-threatening medical complications and
proven inability to lose weight on more conservative treatment programs—will find that better and safer operations are available.

Most bypass operations in current use create malabsorption that is
milder than that produced by jejunoileal bypass. Presumably, therefore, the long-term side effects will be slower to appear. Again, long-
term results and well-controlled trials are not available to help us
weigh the benefits and risks of these operations, but we remain concerned that problems may emerge because of the malabsorption which
they purposely entail.

Should all intestinal-bypass operations be condemned because of
the bad track record of the jejunoileal bypass? Probably not. Each
must stand or fall on its own merits, once it has been studied and
followed in a scientific manner over a long period of time. Until then,
we consider these operations still experimental.

Gastric Bypass

For many years, surgeons have bypassed the duodenum in operations for ulcers, with known complications of impaired iron absorption

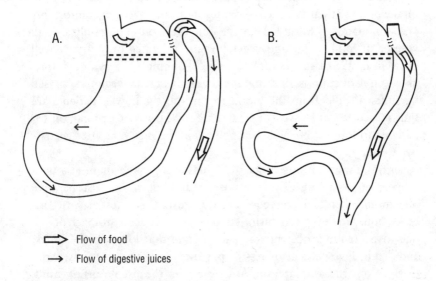

Flow of food
Flow of digestive juices

Figure 13.11 Gastric Bypass

Two types of gastric bypass. In both versions, the stomach is completely closed off, leaving only a small pouch of stomach accessible via the esophagus. The stomach pouch has a volume of only one to two ounces. It is connected directly to the jejunum, bypassing most of the stomach, the pylorus, and the duodenum. In the "loop gastrojejunostomy" (a), the intestine is left intact, whereas the "Roux-en-Y" arrangement (b) prevents bile and pancreatic juices from irritating the stomach pouch. It also delays the mixing of these digestive juices with food until more of the absorptive area of the intestine has been passed. Therefore, the farther downstream the two segments of bowel are connected in this Roux-en-Y arrangement, the greater the impairment of food absorption. By varying the distance "downstream" where the two segments of bowel are joined, the surgeon can vary the degree of malabsorption introduced by the operation.

and long-term depletion of bone calcium. Another common, unwanted side effect of such ulcer operations was weight loss. With the intent of making this side effect into a virtue, gastric-bypass operations were devised for the treatment of obesity.

Pioneered by Dr. Edward Mason at the University of Iowa, gastric-bypass operations combine a short intestinal bypass with constriction of the stomach. Several variations of this operation have been developed (see the two diagrammed in Figure 13.11). All have in common the fact that most of the stomach, the pylorus, and the duodenum are bypassed.

After undergoing one of these operations, patients reduce their food intake because their stomach and intestines can no longer comfortably accommodate much food. They feel full after consuming only a small volume of food. Meat and vegetables are tolerated only if very well chewed. Intake of sugars often causes "dumping," a very uncomfortable feeling of cramps, flushing, rapid heartbeat, and weakness, caused by shifts of fluid from the bloodstream into the bowel. Patients are thus forced to eat slowly, in small amounts. It is not uncommon for patients to lose as much as 100 pounds in the first year after gastric-bypass surgery.

Serious complications of gastric-bypass surgery occur in less than 10 percent of patients. These include wound infections, postoperative pneumonia, hemorrhage requiring transfusion, strokes or heart attacks, injury to the spleen during surgery, rupture of the stomach pouch due to overeating, obstruction, blood clots that lodge in the lungs, and death. Five percent or less of patients develop ulcerations, strictures, or obstructions later on. As time passes, the discomfort of eating subsides, and weight loss slows and then stops. Eventually, many patients begin to regain the weight they have lost.

As we look now at an actual case history in which surgical treatment appears to have worked out fairly well, keep in mind that other patients have had serious, even fatal, complications.

A CASE HISTORY

Helen was 56 when she had gastric-bypass surgery. Like many overweight women, she had first started gaining excess weight with her first pregnancy. By age 30, she had become seriously overweight and had already tried a variety of weight-loss programs. By the time she was 56, she was more than 100 pounds overweight.

Helen had taken off, and put back on, approximately 1,000 pounds over the years since she started fighting her obesity. Diets, including liquid-protein formulas, exercise programs, and even hypnosis, had produced no lasting benefit. Some diets had resulted in as much as 60 pounds of weight reduction, only to be followed by regain. Helen also had participated in a variety of support groups, including Overeaters Anonymous, TOPS (Take Off Pounds Sensibly), and Weight Watchers.

Obesity took a heavy toll on her, physically and psychologically. She developed high blood pressure and diabetes, and despite taking medications for these conditions, her blood pressure and blood sugar remained elevated. Concerned and compassionate physicians had repeatedly counseled weight reduction, and Helen had truly done her best to reduce.

Now she was discouraged. She felt deep concern about her apparent lack of willpower as well as her deteriorating health. Complications of diabetes plagued her, especially a relentless, burning pain in her feet and ankles that prevented sleep. Bell's palsy—a temporary paralysis of half of her face—was attributed to her poorly controlled diabetes. But diabetes, high blood pressure, and obesity were not all that Helen coped with. Marital and family stresses contributed to her difficulty in dieting. At times she responded to stress and deteriorating self-esteem by eating. On the other hand, she was—and continues to be—a psychologically resilient individual. She copes with her problems with apparent grace and good humor.

When Helen first heard about surgery for the treatment of obesity, she was skeptical. She admired and respected her own physician, but she had doubts about medical professionals who touted quick or easy cures for obesity. She studied information about the kinds of operations available, and then spoke to patients who had been through gastric-bypass surgery. She looked into insurance coverage for the procedure. Here, in her own words, is why she decided to have the operation:

> My decision to try the surgery was made after many years of despair and too much depression. I couldn't and didn't believe it would work for me. I didn't fully understand that only I could make it work in the long run. Surgical intervention was my way of interrupting the ultimate in discouragement.
>
> In retrospect, I see that the surgery helped me regain that critical element I had lost: hope. Maybe instead of "hope" I should say faith in my ability to manage my own self and life, or belief in my own worth.
>
> Overeating is a serious reflection of the lack of control—the lack of positive belief in oneself and one's future and joyful life expectancy. I read large highway billboards proclaiming hospital-sponsored intervention for the drug addict or alcoholic, but the message didn't include other addictive-obsessive personality problems. The AA philosophy is that you have hit bottom when you can start back up. I had reached a bottom that was beyond dreary. Knowing and having experienced this place makes me wonder how I can ever knowingly ingest anything other than a carrot stick. But surgical intervention, while severe, does not remove this

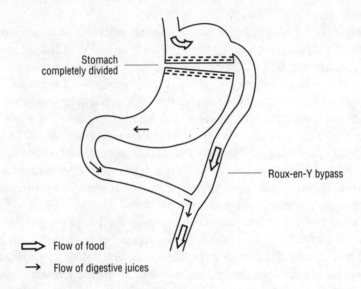

Stomach completely divided

Roux-en-Y bypass

⇨ Flow of food

→ Flow of digestive juices

Figure 13.12 Helen's Gastric Bypass

Diagram of Helen's gastric-bypass operation, which promotes weight loss in two ways. First, the small stomach pouch creates discomfort if much food is eaten at once. Second, absorption is impaired by the delayed mixing of food and digestive juices, and by the detour around part of the intestine. Unfortunately, calcium and iron are normally absorbed in the duodenum, which is bypassed, but most fat is absorbed downstream, in the jejunum and ileum, which are not bypassed.

basic responsibility of choosing food wisely, and getting exercise.

So basically I tried the surgery because it offered hope, and I felt I had to try something to get out of the physical and psychological mess I was in.

Helen's operation is diagrammed in Figure 13.12. It is a variation of the "Roux-en-Y" bypass shown in Figure 13.11. Her stomach was stapled and divided, leaving a small receiving pouch attached to the esophagus, which connects the mouth to the stomach, thus creating discomfort unless only small amounts of food are consumed. Her small intestine was also divided at the first part of the jejunum, which was then brought up and sewn to the small stomach pouch, delaying the mixing of food and digestive juices and thus impairing absorption.

The small passageway from the stomach pouch lets food pass directly into the jejunum, bypassing most of the stomach, all of the duodenum, and the first part of the jejunum. This rearrangement delays digestion, impairs absorption, and sets up the patient to experience the cramps and weakness known as "dumping" if more than small amounts of sugar are eaten.

Helen came through her surgery with no major complications. For the first several months her stomach hurt whenever she ate more than the prescribed few ounces of food. She lost weight steadily, and within ten months she was 70 pounds lighter than before surgery.

Twelve months after the operation she reached her lowest weight in more than 40 years—85 pounds less than she had weighed before surgery. She felt and looked much better. She was no longer noticeably obese, and she no longer required medications for blood pressure or diabetes. Her blood sugar and blood pressure were both normal, although her foot and leg pains persisted. She felt good about herself and about her decision to have the operation.

Two years after the surgery, Helen began gradually to regain some of her weight. She no longer found it uncomfortable to eat, and stress often triggered unnecessary eating, especially of sweets. She regained about ten pounds, and felt a return of her previous concern. Her blood glucose levels crept upward to abnormal levels. Once again, her doctor counseled her to diet and exercise.

Helen decided she "was not going to blow it." She set some firm guidelines for herself about eating and exercise. She believes now that reaching this moment of inner decision and determination was as crucial to her long-term success as was the operation itself. With support from her doctor, she implemented a daily walking program, and consciously worked on controlling her portion sizes and her intake of high-calorie foods. Her weight stabilized at 70 pounds less than it had been before the operation.

Then Helen developed an infected foot ulcer as a result of diabetic nerve damage. This required her to stay off her feet as much as possible for almost a year. It effectively eliminated her exercise program, and consequently she gradually regained another 20 pounds.

Now, four years after her operation, Helen's weight is about 50 pounds less than it was before her surgery. Her doctor would like her to lose 25 pounds. She has mildly elevated blood sugar, but takes no medication. She allows herself an occasional piece of chocolate. She is learning not to treat fatigue with food. She attends monthly meetings of a support group for persons with compulsive and addictive behavior problems. The meetings keep her conscious of the role of compulsions in overeating, and she believes that they help her with weight control.

Helen is glad she had gastric-bypass surgery. She realistically understands that it did not cure her obesity, and that the long-term outcome of her weight problem still depends on her exercise and eating behavior.

We include Helen's story because it demonstrates that, despite our own serious reservations, many individuals are pleased with the results of surgery for obesity. On the other hand, we wish to sound three loud notes of caution. *First,* the surgery's long-range benefits in terms of maintaining a reduced weight are unknown, both for Helen and for everyone else who has had this relatively new operation. If Helen's weight is back up to preoperative levels within six to eight years, one would have to question the benefit of the surgery. *Second,* not everyone does as well as Helen did. Complications, even occasionally fatal ones, can and do arise. *Third,* the long-term benefits and complications of this and similar operations are still unknown. What, for example, if the operation were to cause subtle impairment of calcium absorption, and if, as a result, in 15 years Helen suffers devastating osteoporosis, with fractures of the spine and hips, and years of painful disability prior to a premature death? Would that not change our assessment of the risks and benefits of her surgery? Or suppose she gained back all her weight within ten years. Would the pain, expense, and risks of anesthesia and surgery have been worth the temporary relief she obtained?

For these reasons we consider gastric-bypass surgery as still in an experimental phase. Well-controlled scientific studies to define its risks and benefits are needed. As we noted earlier in reference to the "gastric bubble" procedure, doctors and patients can be firmly and enthusiastically convinced of the great benefits of a procedure that is subsequently shown to be worthless.

If you have had gastric-bypass surgery for weight control, or if you are considering it, take the following cautions into account:

- Medical and surgical procedures must be regarded as experimental until their long-term side effects are known. Gastric-bypass surgery still presents the possibility of the later subtle malabsorption of trace elements, vitamins, and minerals such as calcium. Such malnutrition could conceivably have devastating effects on health in years to come. This is only one example of the potential for long-term negative results.

- Careful, lifelong medical follow-up is mandatory after such surgery to detect possible side effects, especially malnutrition. Because most of these operations bypass at least part of the duodenum, where iron and calcium are absorbed, it is imperative that your physician continue to monitor bone mineralization and blood content of iron and calcium.
- Because many of the procedures eliminate part of the stomach, which produces the factor necessary for vitamin B_{12} absorption, it is imperative that your physician watch regularly for gradual depletion of that essential vitamin. Anemia, nerve damage, and brain malfunction can all result from B_{12} deficiency.
- Surgery that involves a reduction in stomach-acid production, or a bypass of swallowed food and secretions around the acidic environment of the stomach, may predispose the patient to tuberculosis. Stomach acid appears to be an important defense mechanism in preventing the activation of tuberculosis infection.
- Remember that you cannot rely on such bypass surgery to "take care of" your weight problem. Any of these procedures can be defeated by eating lots of soft, easily absorbed calories. You'll have to control your food intake to some extent, and exercise regularly.

The very advantage of the bypass operations in terms of weight loss—i.e., malabsorption—is also their greatest liability, since it may expose the patient to long-term complications. For this reason, we favor those procedures that are purely obstructive, rather than malabsorptive, such as jaw wiring and waist-cord attachment, or vertical banded gastroplasty.

On the other hand, no surgical procedure for obesity should be regarded as a "cure." These procedures do not correct the cause of obesity; they are simply one aspect of individualized patient management, to be employed in a few, carefully selected patients, along with other modes of therapy, including exercise, dietary restraint, behavior modification, and group support.

Who, then, should consider surgery for obesity? Only those for whom other, safer methods have failed, and whose obesity is so severe that it clearly poses a greater threat to life and health than do the known complications of the contemplated procedure.

ACUPUNCTURE

Acupuncture is the Chinese treatment of inserting thin needles into special points on the body to produce anesthesia or relieve pain. In many demonstrations, the effects have been dramatic. Some acupuncturists have extended the method to the treatment of obesity, claiming that there is a feeding center that can be activated by inserting needles, or staples, in the ear. In a scientific test, staples were placed by an acupuncturist where he believed the feeding center was, while in a control group of subjects staples were placed in another part of the ear that was thought to have no effect on appetite. Predictably, all patients lost weight to the extent that they stayed on their diets. There was, however, no significant difference in weight loss between those who had been stapled in the "hunger center" and those who had been stapled elsewhere.

14

Behavior Modification

The words *behavior modification* conjure up a mass of images that range from simply changing one's habits to cruel experiments in which animals are shocked or children are tormented. Many books and movies have depicted behavior modification as a menacing, diabolical force with which experimenters change the personalities of their "subjects." This depiction is largely a myth, the province of the fiction writer's trade. In fact, negative conditioning, with the prompt imposition of unpleasant consequences for calorie consumption, tends to be counterproductive in the long run. Most people steer away from unpleasant methods. The approach to obesity that comes closest to this negative conditioning is gastric-bypass surgery, described in the previous chapter, since it leads to cramping, vomiting, weakness, and pain when large meals, especially of sugar, are consumed.

New habits—new and enduring patterns of eating behavior and physical activity—are the key to permanent weight reduction. Weight loss lasts only as long as calorie intake is curtailed and/or energy expenditure is enhanced. To make lasting changes in eating behavior and physical activity is the aim of behavior-modification treatment for obesity.

To achieve a lasting solution to obesity, behavior-modification therapy teaches people to:

- eat in a controlled way
- continue to exercise and stay physically active
- eat food that is not calorically dense (has low fat and alcohol content)
- assert themselves in eating situations
- enlist peer support or family support, and maintain it
- change their thoughts and attitudes about food, appetite, and hunger
- free themselves from environmental cues to eat
- avoid eating for emotional reasons
- use problem-solving techniques to eliminate excessive eating
- contract with themselves to achieve both short- and long-term goals
- enjoy being thinner
- take responsibility for monitoring their eating and exercise behavior for a long period of time, long after they have achieved a normal body weight

If you can learn to do these things, you are likely to succeed at long-term weight control.

Behavior modification, like surgery and other forms of obesity treatment, is still evolving. New strategies to improve eating and exercise behavior are constantly being tried. Although some of the techniques are successful for some overweight people, more research is still needed to determine which strategies are most helpful, and to what extent success depends on the qualities of particular therapists.

Behavior modification is neither magic nor a panacea. It is simply a systematic, problem-solving approach to changing calorie intake and output. Much of it could be called "common sense"—that uncommon quality which enables you, for example, to keep cookies out of the house if you can't resist eating them and need to lose weight.

All of the techniques of behavior modification depend upon becoming aware of one's own eating patterns and consciously trying to alter them. Underlying the approach is the fact that the cerebral cortex of the brain (see chapter 7), through thought and deliberate decision, can and does affect eating behavior and energy expenditure.

HOW IT WORKS

Behavior modification approaches the task of changing eating and exercise habits in a manner similar to a mathematics problem involving three numbers, or factors. The three factors are A (antecedents), B (behaviors), and C (consequences, or payoffs). Behavior-modification therapy assumes that the frequency and intensity of behaviors (B) are influenced by everything that sets the stage for the behaviors (A), and by the consequences (C) resulting from the behaviors. This framework applies to any behavior, such as doing homework, eating a doughnut, or throwing a tantrum. In the context of obesity, the behaviors include eating (calorie intake) and physical activity (calorie output).

The antecedents (A) of eating behavior include the availability of food, the type of food available, and the presence or absence of hunger or other feelings, such as nervousness, loneliness, or sleepiness. Antecedents to eating also include "cues," or reminders, that trigger the desire to eat, such as advertisements or the sight and smell of food. In other words, the antecedents of eating encompass everything that sets the stage for eating greater, or lesser, amounts. The power of behavior modification lies in the fact that these antecedents can be modified. For example, if having snack food available in the house leads to more impulsive eating, then removing it and leaving only low-calorie snacks will cause you to consume fewer calories, and eventually to weigh less.

Two types of events set the stage for any behavior. One type is *overt,* and includes tangible environmental signals or cues, such as an advertisement, someone saying that it's time for lunch, or the smell of freshly baked bread. The other type is *covert,* or internal—for example, a feeling of loneliness, anger, or depression that sets one scavenging through the refrigerator.

If something in your environment is stirring up your hunger at the wrong time, like the smell of food cooking or the sight of a co-worker eating a snack, then changing or eliminating this cue, or trigger, or signal, will lead to less eating on your part. If the antecedent can be eliminated, the behavior is less likely to occur. Similarly, if a feeling, like anxiety, is an antecedent to extra eating (nervous nibbling), then reducing or eliminating the cause of the anxiety will lead to less inappropriate food intake. Psychologists have developed a number of techniques to alter the overt and covert antecedents to behaviors.

The consequences (C) of a behavior also help determine whether and how frequently it is repeated. If a behavior pays off, we tend to repeat it, and the behavior increases in frequency. The casinos in Nevada and New Jersey are founded on this principle. There, visitors engage in a certain behavior, i.e., pulling a lever on the side of a machine. Once in a while a flood of quarters rewards that behavior.

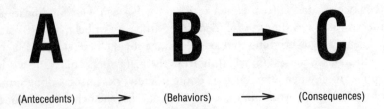

Figure 14.1

The likelihood of any particular behavior (B) is influenced by its antecedents (A)—literally, the things that go before—and its consequences (C).

The lever-pulling is then repeated, usually until all their quarters are gone. Behavior-modification treatment of obesity simply applies such facts of human nature to the problem of weight control.

If a yummy snack soothes you when you are anxious, you will probably reach for a snack the next time you feel nervous. Why not? It works. You feel better, and what are a few calories compared with feeling nervous? If you get food poisoning from the corner deli, you will tend not to buy lunch there again. If a certain food—a potato chip, for instance—tastes good, the positive consequences of snacking (a good taste) may undo the knowledge that the food is almost 60 percent fat and loaded with salt.

Like antecedents that set the stage for behavior, consequences can be both internal (such as the feeling of a job well done, or a feeling of being in control), and external (such as a dozen quarters, congratulations, or a chocolate-chip cookie). The behavior-modification treatment of obesity seeks to structure consequences that promote positive habits of eating and physical activity.

THE HISTORICAL BACKGROUND OF BEHAVIOR MODIFICATION FOR OBESITY

Charles Ferster, a psychologist, is often considered the father of contemporary behavior modification. He suggested a "learning" approach to weight control in 1962. Ferster proposed that fat and thin people had different styles and habits of eating, and that overweight people might be able to "relearn" how to eat, in a style similar to that of

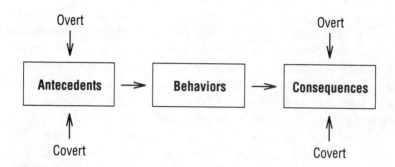

Figure 14.2

Antecedents as well as consequences can be both *overt* (external or environmental) and *covert* (internal).

thin people. Although his own treatment program based on these concepts was not successful, it planted a seed of scientific inquiry. The seed sprouted in 1967 with the work of Richard Stuart, a social worker at the University of Michigan.

Stuart developed a more effective treatment program than Ferster's. He began by treating ten overweight women on an individual basis for a year. Two dropped out, but the remaining eight each lost more than 25 pounds, and four of them lost more than 40 pounds. Although the patients had been carefully selected, and Stuart's treatment was intensely individualized, his results were dramatically better than any that had been previously published for the outpatient treatment of obesity. He later used these and other techniques to design the behavioral treatment program used by Weight Watchers.

The principle that behavior is influenced by antecedents and consequences formed the basis of Stuart's 1967 work. At about the same time, other researchers began looking into the effect of environment on the eating behavior of obese people. It had been suspected on the basis of casual observation that overweight people were more responsive to the taste, smell, sight, and other sensory aspects of food than were thin people. In other words, they appeared to be more susceptible to certain antecedents than did thin people. For example, many of us have had an experience like this: After finishing a perfectly ample meal and feeling satisfied, we might go for a walk, and, smelling the aroma of freshly baked bread coming from a bakery, walk inside and have still something more to eat. Other examples of environmental triggers include seeing a vending machine and feeling a sudden craving for candy, or watching TV and becoming aware of being hungry during a commercial for food. The common notion was that overweight people were more likely than thin people to respond to such environmental cues as the aroma and availability of food.

One of those who suspected that the environment affected overweight people differently from slender people was Stanley Schachter, a psychologist, who designed a series of elegant experiments to explore the possibility. One of his experiments was designed to find out whether a specific environmental cue—the time of day—affected food intake in fat people differently from that in slender people. Schachter set up a pair of rooms, each with a peculiar clock. In one room the clock ran at half-normal speed, and in the other the clock ran at twice-normal speed. The experiments began at 5:00 P.M. After their watches were removed and five minutes were spent getting them settled, the subjects were left alone in a room with one of these special clocks on the wall. The experimenter returned 30 minutes later. In one room—the one with the slow clock—the clock read 5:20. In the other room, the fast clock read 6:05. In each case, however, the time was really 5:35. The experimenter entered the room nibbling crackers from a box, set the box down in front of the subject, invited the subject to help himself, and gave the subject a written personality test to reinforce the illusion that the experiment had to do with something other than appetite. The subject was left alone to take the test, and asked to drop it off at the office on the way out of the building.

What Dr. Schachter actually measured was the weight of the crackers consumed. There were two groups of subjects; one was of normal weight and one was overweight. The overweight subjects ate almost twice as much when they thought the time was 6:05 as when they thought the time was 5:20. The thin subjects ate fewer crackers at 6:05 than at 5:20 because they didn't want to spoil their dinners. The study showed that environmental time cues affected the eating behavior of both overweight and normal-weight subjects, but in opposite directions.

Other psychological experiments concentrated on visual cues, such as the sight of food, or food-related items. These included studies done in cafeterias, in which ice cream, for example, was placed in a closed freezer versus an open freezer. Overweight people were more likely than thin people to overlook the ice cream if it was out of sight. They were also more likely to take the ice cream if it was visible. Desserts on the back row of a cafeteria display were taken at the same frequency as those on the front row by thin patrons of the restaurant, while overweight patrons tended to ignore those desserts on the back row.

These and a multitude of similar experiments showed that many overweight people react to food cues differently from normal-weight people. Whether such a cue is directly associated with food (such as a dessert on display), or indirectly (such as dinnertime on a clock), they seemed to respond more quickly to the cue and by obtaining more food than those of normal weight.

Many weight-control techniques evolved from these early experiments. Most of them confirmed what was already common knowledge: for example, that food out of sight is out of mind. This led to a number of behavioral modification techniques that came to be known as "environmental control." Although subsequent research casts some doubt on some of the experiments that helped form many of these behavioral techniques, a number of obese people find them effective in weight control.

MAKING AND BREAKING BEHAVIOR CHAINS

A basic notion of behavior modification is that antecedents often occur sequentially, in chains. Even the behaviors themselves, as well as the antecedents and the consequences, are usually a series of individual actions or circumstances. These chains present many opportunities for intervention—that is, a number of stages at which a desired behavior may be promoted, or an undesired behavior prevented. Let's examine, for example, the behavior chain of a dieter who ate some leftover cheesecake (see Figure 14.3).

Unfortunately for this dieter, the leftover cheesecake had been stored in the refrigerator after dinner. He ate an ample meal, after which he sat in his favorite chair, watched a dull television program, felt restless, bored, and sleepy, started arguing with his spouse, and then got up and walked aimlessly around the house. Eventually he entered the kitchen, opened the refrigerator, and discovered the leftover cheesecake. He ate the cake, felt guilty, and wished he had more.

Each of the steps in this chain is closely linked to the behavior that precedes it, and in turn leads to the next step toward the act of eating. Each link is also susceptible to modification. Although much of our snacking behavior feels "spontaneous," very little of it actually is.

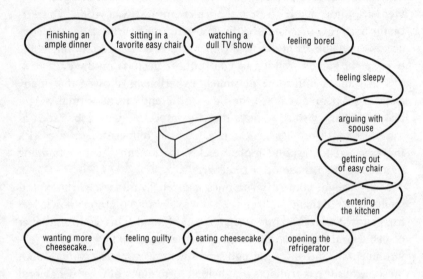

Figure 14.3 Behavior Chain

Undesired behaviors (such as overeating) as well as desired behaviors (such as
getting exercise) occur often in chains. Each link of a behavior chain may be
susceptible to change, and may therefore present an opportunity to avoid an
undesired behavior, or to promote a desired behavior.

Examining our eating behaviors, especially the chains of related behaviors that lead up to eating, allows us to plan strategies to interrupt
the chain.

For example, what if the dieter just described decided that instead
of watching TV after dinner, he would do something else, such as
taking a bath or a walk around the block? Or suppose he read an
exciting book? Suppose that he decided to go to bed when he felt
sleepy, instead of heading for the kitchen? Suppose that when he
opened the refrigerator, instead of immediately seeing the cheesecake,
there had been a bowl of carrots and celery in front, and no lightbulb
in the refrigerator, and that the cheesecake had been hidden in back,
under aluminum foil? Any of these strategies could have been implemented with a little planning. And any one of them might prevent the
behavior of eating the cheesecake.

Some of the strategies suggested above might sound useless to you, but they could appeal to—and work for—someone else. Behavior modification takes an individualized approach to formulating strategies to influence a particular person's actions. By its very nature, it involves tinkering and trial and error. It is a practical, problem-solving approach that enables people to follow Ben Franklin's advice in *Poor Richard's Almanack:* "Labor in the first place to bring thy appetite into subjection to reason."

Behavior modification does not try to increase your "willpower." On the contrary, it aims to stack the cards in your favor, and make it easy and practical to avoid weight gain. If there is no cheesecake in the refrigerator, you don't need as much willpower (or "won't-power") to avoid eating it. If you like a lower-calorie food, such as fresh melon, why not put it in your refrigerator, instead of testing your willpower against the mating call of a chocolate mousse?

Just as negative behaviors follow antecedents, so do positive behaviors, such as taking a walk. Examining antecedent chains allows us to plan strategies to enhance the likelihood of such behavior. Developing antecedent strategies to enhance a desired behavior is as important a part of behavioral therapy as finding ways to avoid unwanted behavior. You can start a chain of behavior by phoning your friend and making a date to go walking or jogging early tomorrow morning. It's easier to make that decision at 9:00 P.M. than at 6:00 A.M., when you are warm and comfy in bed. Consequently, your strategy of committing the night before may make the difference in getting you out the door in the morning to exercise. Another link in that chain might be buying a more comfortable pair of walking shoes. Another might be to get some warm gloves or a sweatsuit. With a little forethought, you can initiate a behavior chain that leads to your expending more calories.

Consequences, as well as antecedents, can be restructured. If our dieter who ate the cheesecake had made any of the several interventions suggested above, he'd have been less likely to eat the cheesecake, taste how good it was, feel guilty, and gain weight. In that example, the multiple antecedents were all susceptible to change. Likewise, the consequences, or payoffs, could have been changed. Instead of eating the whole thing, our dieter might have taken one bite and said, "That's enough," or he might have put the cheesecake in the garbage, or he might have reminded himself that he was watching his calories, and patted himself on the back for shutting the refrigerator. He also could previously have enlisted the help of his wife to remind him, "George, wouldn't it be better to go to bed now rather than have a snack?" as soon as she heard the refrigerator door open.

The multitude of techniques that make up behavior modification are most easily conceptualized by arranging them according to their place of action in the behavioral chain (see Figure 14.4). The first set of techniques affects the antecedents, the events that precede eating. The second set affects the behavior directly—for example, dietary instruction that changes our knowledge and understanding of what we are eating. The third set of techniques affects consequences, both positive and negative. Establishing negative consequences—making the act of eating result in some physical, mental, emotional, or financial pain—is little used and seldom effective.

Note that self-monitoring, or self-awareness, is in the middle of the diagram as a technique that affects behavior directly. Self-awareness, however, acts throughout the behavior chain to set the stage for deliberate change.

THE FOOD DIARY: BE AWARE—EAT WITH CARE!

All the techniques of behavior modification are based on *awareness*. Those who are unaware of their snacking, or of their habit of taking seconds and thirds, or of borrowing a bite from the person sitting next to them at dinner, will have no identifiable behavior to modify. Just as people cannot improve their grammar until they become aware of their own speech patterns, people who eat inappropriately need to become conscious of their eating patterns. Once aware, they can lay worthwhile plans to eat otherwise.

Until you are aware of your behavior and its antecedents, you are not in a position to set the stage for better behavior next time. A food diary is the easiest way to become aware (see Figure 14.5).

To keep a food diary, write down a description of each eating episode, when it occurred, where it occurred, how long it lasted, whether it was a meal or a snack, and how much antecedent hunger you felt on a scale from 0 (none) to 5 (a lot). Keeping such a diary will make you keenly conscious and aware of your eating patterns in a way that may surprise you at first. The process of keeping the diary, and the information you record, will offer a number of possibilities for intervention, using techniques to be described in what follows.

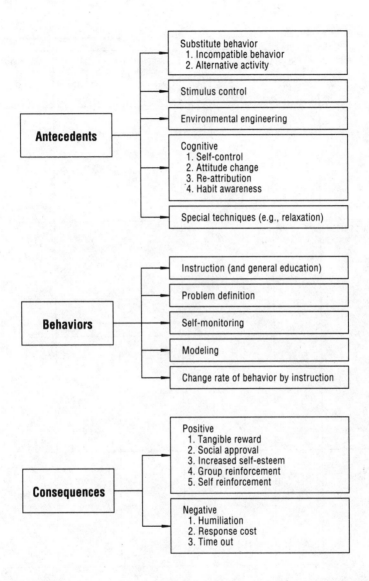

Figure 14.4

Techniques employed in behavior modification, related to the antecedents and the consequences of individual behaviors, and to the behaviors themselves.

Day of the week _____ Date _____

Time	Minutes spent eating	M/S	H	BP	Activity while eating	Location of eating	Kind of food
6:00							
11:00							
4:00							
9:00							

M/S: Meal or snack
H: Degree of hunger (0=none, 1=some, 2=normal, 3=good healthy hunger, 4=ravenous)
BP: Body position (1=walking, 2=standing, 3=sitting, 4=lying down)

Figure 14.5 Food Diary

Example of a food diary. Although this diary focuses on certain specific aspects of eating (where, when, how long, how much, and how hungry), diaries can be designed to monitor other aspects of eating behavior, such as calorie content, antecedent feelings and events, and so forth.

Day of the week _Wednesday_   Date _April 2._

Time	Minutes spent eating	M/S	H	BP	Activity while eating	Location of eating	Kind of food
6:00							
7:30 – 7:40	10m	M	1	3	Paper	Kitchen	eggs toast coffee
8:15 – 8:30	5m	S	0	2	Talking	Work	banana
11:00							
12:15 – 12:30	15m	M	3	3	Reading	Rest-aurant	hamburger fries shake cherry pie
4:00							
6 – 7	1 Hr	M	2	3	T.V.	Dining room	Fish pasta salad ch. cake
9:00							
10:30 – 10:45	15m	S	0	4	T.V.	Living room	pepsi pretzels

SAMPLE

M/S: Meal or snack
H: Degree of hunger (0=none, 1=some, 2=normal, 3=good healthy hunger, 4=ravenous)
BP: Body position (1=walking, 2=standing, 3=sitting, 4=lying down)

Figure 14.6 Food Diary

Sample food diary, filled in.

TECHNIQUES FOR CHANGING BEHAVIOR ANTECEDENTS

Alternative Behaviors

The first technique for change is substitution—do something else. If you are aware that you have an urge to open a box of cookies, what can you do other than eat? Well, you can throw the cookies over the back fence, step on them, walk around the block, call a friend, or take a shower. If you have worked out in advance a list of behaviors that will interfere with that cookie-box-opening behavior, the chances are greater that you can avoid those extra calories. The list must be thought out in advance; otherwise you won't have time to think, and the urge to eat the cookie will win. It's best to select alternative behaviors that are incompatible with eating.

In searching for such alternative behaviors, think of four categories of substitute behaviors. The first category consists of those activities that are *pleasant,* such as taking a nap, or watching a movie. The second category comprises *necessary* activities, and includes balancing your checkbook or doing the laundry. The third category consists of alternative activities that are *useful or healthful,* such as gardening, taking a shower, jogging, or going for a walk. The fourth is simply to *interpose time.* For example, you can set a timer for ten minutes, after which, if the urge to eat is still present, you can plan to have a small but, it is to be hoped, satisfying snack that you control—as opposed to being the passive receptor of a longer chain of increasingly intense events that propel you to eat without that control.

Figure 14.7 is an example of the type of list you might make to help you combat the urges to eat that pop up in everyday life. Another good time to use this type of list is when you have identified a behavior chain (Figure 14.3) and need to have some "chain-breaking" alternatives on hand. It is not a list to make and then put away in the drawer, but one to be carried with you into the "heat of battle" with calories and temptations.

Stimulus Control

We are all surrounded by reminders to eat: advertisements, the sight of other people eating, the smell of food, or a chocolate on the bedside table of a hotel room, to name only a few. Stimulus control for obesity treatment is based on the premise, described earlier in this chapter, that many overweight people are easily influenced by stimuli, cues, or

Before snacking I will...

Pleasant	1. Call a friend 2. Take a bath 3. Read a magazine
Necessary	1. Go shopping 2. Do the vacuuming 3. Wash the dishes
Useful or healthful	1. Go for a walk 2. Water the garden 3. Write a thank-you note
Interpose time	1. Set timer for ten minutes 2. Drink ten ounces of water

Figure 14.7 Alternative Activity Sheet

A list of alternative behaviors can be helpful in breaking unwanted behavior chains.

reminders in the environment that say, "Eat!" Becoming aware of these stimuli or cues is a difficult but necessary step in learning to control them. A food diary gives clues about these stimuli and how you respond to them. By looking at the events in the environment immediately prior to excessive eating, you can often figure out cause and effect. Sometimes they are surprising. One woman found that each time she walked through the front door of her house she wound up snacking, but not after she entered through the *back* door. For years she had brought her groceries in through the front door, taken them to the kitchen, put them away, and in the process had eaten one or two goodies that she had bought in the market. Since she rarely brought her groceries in through the back door, it held no association with eating or snacking. Similarly, many people have learned that a coffee break is a time to eat snack foods, like a cheese Danish. They have been trained by the arrival of the doughnuts or the lunch wagon that it's time for a short meal at 10:00 A.M., even though they aren't really hungry.

Cues can be mental as well as environmental. In the case of mental cues, patterns sometimes persist long after they have served their usefulness. For example, it is not unusual to overeat after the loss of a loved one. A woman who is recently widowed or divorced is used to cooking for herself and her husband. In all the sadness, it is possible to both cook the extra portion and consume it, continuing one's long-established buying and cooking habits. Unless the grieving process and associated eating behaviors come to an end, however, this pattern will lead to weight gain.

Anxiety is another potent mental cue. Many students, for example, respond to the stress of exams by increased intake of chips, cookies, and anything else that will "help them concentrate," or "sleep," or "relax," or "remember."

Whether the cues, or stimuli, that trigger your eating are external or internal, the first step toward controlling them is to become aware of them and their connection to your eating behavior. The second step is to plan and implement ways of avoiding or eliminating the stimulus, or changing your response to it. The third step is to monitor your success in altering the chain of behavior, and the fourth step is to evaluate and improve your interventions.

Environmental Engineering

Environmental engineering is a fancy term for a simple concept: working with the environment to get rid of appetite "triggers," or reminders to eat, by removing them or changing them. If food is stored prominently in the kitchen, put it in opaque containers. If commercials for food are troublesome when they come on television, walk out of the room. If passing the bakery shop increases your appetite, drive to work a different way. If the snack wagon at work is a signal to eat, try substituting the diet drink you brought to work with you.

Removing "advertisements" for food from your environment can help you decrease your calorie consumption. Over the years, industry has learned subtle and sophisticated ways to create desire by inserting such reminders into our daily lives. It is our challenge to be aware of and get rid of them, since, after all, it is our environment.

On the other side of the calorie equation, environmental engineering includes introducing into your environment some triggers to increase your level of physical activity. This could range from erecting a basketball standard in your driveway to not getting a new TV set, or not subscribing to cable TV. Or it might include buying a bicycle, or keeping a pair of good walking shoes handy at the office.

Cognitive Behavior Modification

This is the process of changing the way you think or feel. Cognition, or thinking, precedes most types of behavior. Here is an example of a cognitive antecedent of eating: remembering how the boss spoke to you crossly, reliving this negative experience in fantasy, experiencing tension, and then turning to the solace of a sugar doughnut. A number of techniques have been developed to modify these cognitive processes, or thoughts. By identifying the thoughts and feelings that precede activities associated with eating, the probability of consequent eating can be decreased. Cognitive techniques fall into four categories:

Self-instruction. This technique consists of looking at one's irrational thoughts and statements about food (often accepted without criticism), and changing them. For example, "I have a headache. I would feel so much better if I had something to eat." In reality, aspirin would be a more efficient remedy. The self-instruction might be: "Who am I fooling? I have a headache, not a hunger ache. Why don't I get an aspirin instead of a doughnut?" The more you can practice substituting such "thin" thoughts for "fat" rationalizations, the more easily you can control your weight.

Attitude change. This similarly involves observing your internal state or internal dialogues. Once you have identified your attitudes, you can modify them. For example, if someone who is attempting to increase his exercise has the habit of telling himself, "I really hate jogging," he can remind himself each time this thought pattern crosses his mind to say something new—such as adding the thought that "everyone at work is jogging, and it would be fun to join them," or "I enjoy getting outdoors and seeing the trees and flowers and birds in the neighborhood." It is surprising but true that gradually the new thought pattern displaces the old chronic excuses, and the attitude toward the behavior (jogging, in this case) will change.

Reattribution. This is another mental technique for changing the focus of one's attention—in this instance, by relabeling. For example, if you are instructed to lose weight, and you begin to feel hunger pains on a 1,200-calorie diet, you might remind yourself that "hunger is the feeling of losing weight," or the gratifying feeling of fat being burned off your body. If you were an athlete, your coach would be saying,

"No pain, no gain." If you were in an aerobic conditioning program, you might tell yourself, "It doesn't hurt—I didn't work hard enough" (or "feel the burn"). The same is true of dieting. For many people, hunger is an unavoidable part of weight loss. They might as well welcome the hunger with a positive attitude by attributing virtue to it. This mental rearrangement—realizing the value of the sensation of hunger—can be simultaneously a cue, a reminder, a pat on the back, and a milestone on the way to losing weight.

Habit awareness. This technique is related to the direct observation of behavior and self-monitoring. The more one is aware, the more one tends to change behaviors that might, with close scrutiny, appear absurd. Much of our everyday behavior is automatic, especially our eating. We follow routines unconsciously. For example, if you drive, it probably would be difficult for you to name all the highway exits between your home and work, even though you may have passed them a thousand times. The same phenomenon exists with food. We eat in an automatic, thoughtless way. At the end of the day, most people can't even remember those three jelly beans on the receptionist's desk, the sweet rolls their officemate brought to work, or the leftover piece of Johnny's peanut-butter sandwich they found on the counter and ate while doing the dishes. Being intensely aware of food habits helps many people decrease their calorie consumption.

Special Techniques for Emotional Antecedents

Many emotional states can lead to excess eating. Nervous nibbling is something most of us experience at times. Depression, anxiety, frustration, anger, happiness, sadness—the whole gamut of emotions—can trigger eating. But there are more helpful (and healthful) ways to deal with emotions. For example, it is more appropriate—and far more helpful—to discuss anger and its source than to feed it with food. A telephone call is a less caloric response to loneliness than is a hot-fudge sundae. There are several techniques to help people deal with stress-related feelings such as nervousness, frustration, and tension. These include *progressive muscle relaxation,* in which one consciously relaxes muscles, one group at a time; *autogenic training,* similar to self-hypnosis, in which one concentrates on feelings of calm, peace, and relaxation while deliberately letting go of tense feelings; and *positive imagery,* using brief, one-minute mental "vacation" interludes of imagining yourself far from food, relaxed and serene in a quiet setting.

Low self-esteem and poor self-image contribute to problems of excess eating in many people. To achieve and maintain thinness, it helps to start *feeling* thin and to enjoy that feeling. Techniques such as visualization of what it will be like to be thin, and how one's social and family life might be improved, help motivate some people toward that goal. (Such a technique is not to be confused with mounting grandiose expectations about how being thin will miraculously transform one's life—a scenario that sets the stage for potential depression.)

Dealing with Family and Friends

Family and couple interactions often weigh heavily in the caloric equation. Research shows that couples who lose weight together keep it off longer, and that treating a child for obesity when overweight parents do not participate in treatment is usually a waste of time. The family should work together, not necessarily eating separate foods, but with portions scaled to individual dietary needs. "Modeling" within the family—whether positive or negative—influences eating behavior strongly, and will be discussed further in the next section. Many people need training in assertiveness, in which they learn to refuse, easily and graciously, unwanted high-calorie food pressed upon them in social situations.

TECHNIQUES FOR CHANGING BEHAVIOR DIRECTLY

Nutritional Education

This is a cornerstone of motivating behavioral change for weight control. Knowing the caloric and nutritional content of food is fundamental to the task of losing weight. Few people have lost weight aided only by a calorie counter, but it makes the task far easier if one knows that a potato chip contains over 60 percent fat, a cracker can be 40–50 percent fat, but bread contains less than 10 percent fat. Health education, along with dietary education, encourages better eating and exercise behavior, but, unfortunately, knowledge alone does not make anyone healthy. If it did, there would be no overweight doctors who smoke and don't exercise. Nevertheless, knowledge does help set the stage for better behavior.

Problem Definition

It is easier to make a small change in behavior than a great big one. *Problem definition* is the process of clearly stating behavior problems so they can be broken down into small steps to be taken one at a time. Problems and plans should be clearly stated in defined, measurable terms. For example, compare these two statements: "I'm going to lose some weight by summer," and "I'm going to lose a half-pound every week between now and July 14." Or these two statements: "I've got to start exercising more," and "By bringing a light sack lunch every day to work, I can skip the cafeteria and walk for 30 minutes on my lunch hour." Which approach is more likely to lead to losing weight?

Self-monitoring

This is such a fundamental part of any behavioral modification that we described it at the outset of the chapter, in terms of keeping a food diary. Until you know what, when, how much, and why you are eating, it's very difficult to change. Writing down your self-observations enables you to appreciate your progress as well as plan further change. Keeping a food diary keeps you conscious of your eating, and this awareness in itself helps eliminate some snacking.

Modeling

Personal examples around us, especially within our original families, are a powerful influence on our eating and exercise behavior. We tend to eat as our parents ate, choose the same types and amounts of food, cook it in the same way, and eat it with the same speed and table manners. These patterns pass from generation to generation more through custom than by way of acquired taste or instruction.

In seeking to establish a new dietary pattern, the effects of modeling and family style should be taken into consideration. Johnny and Suzie, for example, are unlikely to lose weight if Mom and Dad don't change their own ways of eating. Changes that can be made include eating more slowly, leaving serving dishes off the table, and purchasing and preparing foods with plenty of bulk but not many calories (low calorie density), such as vegetables, fruits, and grains. Second helpings can be made less available. Conversation can replace television-watching at mealtime. Popcorn (air-popped, as opposed to oil-popped) and apples can replace nuts, crackers, and cheese as readily available snacks. Myriad other small behaviors that go into the "simple" act of eating can be altered in the direction of consuming fewer calories.

Physical activity is also a good candidate for example and modeling. Does the family go out for hikes or walks together, or mostly just for drives in the car? Do they walk to church, for example, or go by car? Does the family play ball in the backyard, or watch it from the couch? Do the parents hire a gardener, or do they work in the yard with the kids? If the video rental store is five blocks away, do you rent the videotape by taking a family walk to get it, or does someone drive? If pizza is planned, do you phone in your order for delivery, or walk to the store for it? Do the children walk or bicycle to school, or does Mom or Dad drive them? Does either Dad or Mom walk or bicycle to work, or at least to the train station? There is no substitute for example and group participation.

Direct Instruction

As children grow up, we shape their eating habits and styles through instruction. For example, "John, don't eat the spaghetti with your fingers," or "Sally, slow down. You can't leave the table until everyone has finished," or "Mark, put that second dessert back." To some extent, adults can be instructed in new eating habits that slow the intake of calories. They might practice putting down the fork between bites and taking smaller servings on small plates, for example. These methods have helped some people slow their rate of calorie intake and control their weight. However, just as one can know all about calories and still eat fattening foods, one can know all about slender styles of eating and not practice them. Changing people's habits and styles of eating in ways that reduce calorie intake remains a difficult problem, still partly unsolved by current behavior-modification therapy of obesity.

TECHNIQUES FOR CHANGING CONSEQUENCES

Positive Consequences

One reason why weight control is so difficult is that food intake provides immediate positive payoffs. Food shares attributes of many addictive drugs: it tastes good, feels good, and it's quick to satisfy. When you consider prompt motivational consequences alone, food wins out every time over exercise and dieting.

As if its qualities of almost instant gratification weren't enough, overeating's negative consequences are delayed. For any single episode of overeating, the negative consequences may even be imperceptible. The same is true of neglecting physical activity on any given day. The positive rewards of being slim, athletic, and healthy may be a year or more off and may be preceded by months of deprivation, exercise, and hard work on changing one's behavior patterns.

Positive consequences can be added to the scales, however, tipping the balance in the direction of change. For example, money can be set aside, with its access contingent upon one's accomplishing a certain amount of weight loss. Or the accomplishment can be defined as a certain degree of exercise, or as the consistent keeping of food records, or of adopting some other positive behavior.

Rewards should be accompanied by praise and social reinforcement whenever possible. Although you can provide yourself with positive consequences, very often the rewards provided by others are more powerful. This is why group support is essential to many people in controlling their weight. Members of a group—whether it be a family, a neighborhood, a behavior-modification class, or a group at a weight-loss center or at Overeaters Anonymous—can provide important rewards that make a decisive difference.

Social approval is a vital agent for change in the area of eating habits. Many of us feel that if no one notices, why bother? For some of us, health, fitness, and even cosmetic improvements aren't strong enough rewards in themselves without that external reinforcement. A pat-on-the-back compliment from a friend or loved one can be a powerful motivator.

Given that it is important for people to notice a change we've strived for, it helps for them to know we are *trying* to change, and why. Members of a weight-control group, working together, understand each other's struggles and motivation. This combination of understanding and social approval is one reason why group weight-loss programs succeed. It feels especially good to get a pat on the back from someone who really knows what you are going through. For many dieters, this reward comes only from fellow group members in the same program, because family and neighbors may not care or notice. Ideally, someone seeking to lose weight would arrange for, or receive, reinforcement from family members, friends, and/or co-workers. Food deprivation and regular exercise are much more tolerable when you know someone else cares.

Self-reinforcement

Self-reinforcement is psychological jargon for patting yourself on the back, giving yourself a compliment for a job well done. If positive rewards are not forthcoming from others, it is vital that the individual provide them for himself or herself. Unless the effort to control weight is made worthwhile on some level, the siren call of food will lure one onto the rocks of obesity.

Self-reinforcement also builds self-esteem. Enhanced self-esteem contributes to weight control, through a greater sense of self-control. One should give oneself real credit for accomplishing small behavioral steps, such as not snacking at 10:00 A.M., or not nibbling despite frustration, or finally getting started on a daily walking program.

Aversive Consequences

For many people, behavior modification is associated with negative consequences, or punishment. These particular techniques are generally not useful for controlling one's weight. If you expect to be punished, for example, why should you show up for appointments with your weight-control therapist? If you expect to be made fun of, or humiliated, the net consequence will be escape or avoidance rather than self-confrontation and behavior change. Dunce hats, public announcements of weight regained, and similar such negative consequences only promote the feelings of failure and discouragement that perpetuate overeating. Groups that have tried such an approach, such as TOPS (Take Off Pounds Sensibly), have generally abandoned it in favor of more positive methods.

Attempts also have been made to apply to obesity control the aversive conditioning used in alcohol treatment programs. For example, alcoholic patients were given a drug that induced nausea and vomiting, such as ipecac, then encouraged to drink their favorite alcoholic beverage until the chemical effect of the drug made them retch. The drug Antabuse, which causes severe illness if followed by a drink of alcohol, is currently used to treat alcoholism, with a similar rationale. Parallel attempts to apply these approaches to obesity treatment, however, have failed, and not surprisingly. While one can go through life without ever drinking alcohol again, one still needs to eat food every day.

FINDING A GOOD PROGRAM AND A GOOD THERAPIST

In practice, the specific techniques of behavior modification are usually woven into a general therapeutic program without clear-cut distinctions made as to whether they apply to antecedents, behaviors, or consequences. All of the aspects described here, however, would be included in a comprehensive behavioral program for the control of obesity. The outline for a typical one might look like this:

Lesson 1. Introduction to the behavioral control of weight—habit awareness.

Lesson 2. Home decalorization—what you don't have, you won't eat.

Lesson 3. Cue elimination—the signals that lead you astray.

Lesson 4. Being active—the difference between success and failure.

Lesson 5. Being active, continued—fitness versus fatness.

Lesson 6. Maintenance—keys for survival.

Lesson 7. Behavior chains and alternate activities—one thing leads to another.

Lesson 8. The act of eating—changing your style.

Lesson 9. Preplanning—heading off the urges.

Lesson 10. Cue elimination, part two—switching more signals.

Lesson 11. It's time to eat out—how to do it.

Lesson 12. Practice week—you deserve it.

Lesson 13. How we think is how we eat—think before you buy.

Lesson 14. Dealing with feelings—think before you bite.

Lesson 15. Stress—the soft underbelly of fat.

Lesson 16. Couples—is your family fattening?

Lesson 17. Behavioral analysis and problem-solving—the key to self-help.

Lesson 18. Maintenance week number three—more survival.

Lesson 19. Living in the world: personal goals—how to cope.

Lesson 20. Snack cues, and holidays—how to celebrate.

Lesson 21. The end and the beginning—here's to a new life, and a new life-style.

The skills and changes covered here take time to implement. Ideally, one would work with a therapist for a year or more to solidify new habits of thought and action. Most patients, however, do not participate in a program for that long.

As in all such endeavors, behavior-modification programs to control obesity vary widely in terms of the methods used and the expertise of the teachers and therapists who lead them. One essential ingredient for success is a therapist's willingness to *individualize* the program according to each person's needs and situation. As we have observed, what triggers eating in one person may or may not trigger it in another, and what helps one person to avoid overeating, or to keep active, may or may not be effective for another. What's essential isn't the presentation of the subject matter, but its practical application in the lives of each class member. Otherwise, the course is simply being offered in a vacuum, and only chance will make it work for you. Although books and videotapes can convey the concepts and techniques of behavior modification, they exist in a vacuum until you use them to improve your own specific habits. A good therapist will help you adapt and apply the principles of behavior modification to solve your individual problems.

The overall strategy in treating overweight people through behavior modification is *not* to train them all to eat at only one place, chew for a longer period of time, or learn other such simplistic, short-range behavior; it is to change the habit *patterns*—of eating and of physical activity—that led to obesity in the first place.

Successful programs typically feature weekly weighing, frequent reinforcement, frequent analysis of individual behavior patterns, and frequent goal-setting to modify behavior in small, attainable steps. By changing a person's eating habits so that fewer calories are consumed, and modifying a person's activity patterns so that more calories are expended, day after day, weight will inevitably be lost.

In a well-run program, one can expect to lose approximately one pound per week. The average total amount of weight lost is often around 20 pounds. You can and should, however, inquire about what the program's own experience has been. For example, you might ask:

1. What percentage of people who start the course actually complete it?

2. What is the average rate of weight loss?

3. What is the average total amount of weight lost for everyone entering the program, including those who drop out before completing the course?

4. What data can you supply regarding success in maintaining weight loss after the course has been completed?

Since the weight loss in these programs is relatively modest, and takes a great deal of time, people who need to lose more than 50 pounds may need a more intensive approach, such as a physician-supervised modified fasting program, *in addition* to behavior-modification training.

In choosing a program, look for a leader who knows the material well, and who is both a stern taskmaster and a caring therapist. The sternness may be needed to help people confront the tendency to rationalize and avoid real change. The leader must care enough to give truly personalized attention to individual differences in behavior problems, so that strategies are tailor-made to each person's needs.

Choosing a leader is often difficult, particularly in commercial programs. The people in charge of signing up clients are often not those who will be leading the behavioral treatment, so that a client might not meet the instructor/therapist until after having paid for the program. If possible, interview the group leader beforehand. Ask the leader such questions as these:

1. How long have you been leading these groups? (The longer the better.)

2. How did you learn to do this? (If only from an instruction manual, watch out.)

3. Were *you* ever overweight? (Yes—good; no—OK; still overweight—watch out.)

4. On the basis of your own experience, what success do you expect people to have after one month, six months, and one year after the program ends? (Note: This is not the same as the success for the nationwide chain. You need to find out a therapist's *own* success rate.)

5. Can I sit in on a group, or talk to former clients?

In making your decision, you should most of all ask yourself, "How do I feel about this person? Is this someone I can work with and relate to?" If you feel even slightly intimidated or pressured to buy, be careful. If a long-term contract is involved, take it home to read through.

If guarantees or special incentives are offered, make sure you understand them. Finally, use your intuition: If you feel uncomfortable, interview the instructor of another program. There are plenty to choose from.

Some programs, such as Jenny Craig and The Diet Center, use videotapes to present behavioral material. Depending on the particular program, skilled leaders to help individuals problem-solve their own behavior may or may not be provided. Evaluate carefully, on the basis of the information here as well as your own instincts.

Unfortunately, among the good programs of every kind are also the bad, some of which are led by well-meaning but untrained or incompetent therapists. Many weight-reduction programs pay lip service to behavior modification only so they can sell their products—preprepared food, protein powders, vitamins, counseling, health-spa memberships, and even cosmetics. Their proprietors know that "behavior modification" sounds good and sells well.

Behavior therapies that are presented solely by written instruction and videotape have been tried with mixed success. After all, you can buy a book yourself, or send in personally for a series of tapes and written materials. The limiting factor for this approach seems to be compliance, or "sticking to it." On the other hand, when you work with a skilled leader and a group with which you are able to develop an affinity, your behaviors may change far more quickly and more permanently than when you work alone with written or taped instructions. Some people, however, do succeed in working on their own, so this method should not be dismissed.

THE METHOD IN PERSPECTIVE

Among the various treatment approaches to weight control, behavior modification focuses on forming the new habits that are necessary to *maintain* a reduced weight. Although the method's original researchers envisioned its use as a cure for obesity, what evolved through methodical research was instead a method for modest weight loss and weight maintenance.

The promise of behavior-modification techniques is that they may produce lasting results. A study that compared behavior modification to drug treatment showed that people treated with drugs lost more weight, but that those treated with behavior modification succeeded in keeping more of the weight off.

Few studies, unfortunately, give long-term results. A five-year follow-up of 36 overweight people treated with behavior modification showed virtually all the lost weight regained. Perhaps newly evolving strategies, better techniques, and more effective therapists can produce more lasting benefits, but this hope is still unrealized.

Sources

Abraham, S., M. D. Carroll, M. F. Najjar, and R. Fulwood. "Obese and Overweight Adults in the United States." *Vital and Health Statistics* 11, No. 230 (1983).

———, M. F. Najjar, and C. L. Johnson. "Trends in Obesity and Overweight Among Adults Ages 20–74 Years: United States 1960–1962, 1971–1974, 1976–1980." *Vital and Health Statistics* 11, No. 288 (1984).

American Heart Association. *Dietary Treatment of Hypercholesterolemia: A Manual for Patients.* American Heart Association, 1988.

American Psychiatric Association. *Diagnostic and Statistical Manual of Mental Disorders,* Third Edition Revised. Washington, D.C.: American Psychiatric Association, 1987.

Andres, R. "Mortality and Obesity: The Rationale for Age-Specific Height-Weight Tables." In *Principles of Geriatric Medicine and Gerontology,* 2nd edition, edited by W. R. Hazzard, R. Andres, E. L. Bierman, and J. P. Blass. New York: McGraw-Hill, 1990.

———. "Effect of Obesity on Total Mortality." *International Journal of Obesity* 4 (1980): 381–86.

Aristimuno, G. G., T. A. Foster, A. W. Voors, S. R. Srinivasan, and G. S. Berenson. "Influence of Persistent Obesity in Children on

Cardiovascular Risk Factors: The Bogalusa Heart Study." *Circulation* 69 (1984): 895–904.

Ball, M. F., L. H. Kyle, and J. J. Canary. "Comparative Effects of Caloric Restriction and Metabolic Acceleration on Body Composition in Obesity." *Journal of Clinical Endocrinology* 27 (1967): 273–78.

Barrett-Connor, E. L. "Obesity, Atherosclerosis, and Coronary Artery Disease." *Annals of Internal Medicine* 103 (1985): 1010–19.

———, and K. T. Khaw. "Cigarette Smoking and Increased Central Adiposity." *Annals of Internal Medicine* 111 (1989): 783–87.

Bennion, L. J., and S. M. Grundy. "Risk Factors for the Development of Cholelithiasis in Man (Part 2)." *New England Journal of Medicine* 229 (1978): 1221–27.

Berry, E. M., S. H. Blondheim, H. E. Eliahou, and E. Shafrir, eds. *Recent Advances in Obesity Research: V.* London: John Libby, 1987.

Björntorp, P. " 'Portal' Adipose Tissue as a Generator of Risk Factors for Cardiovascular Disease and Diabetes." *Arteriosclerosis* 10 (1990): 493–96.

Blair, D., J. P. Habicht, E. A. Sims, D. Sylwester, and S. Abraham. "Evidence for an Increased Risk of Hypertension with Centrally Located Body Fat and the Effect of Race and Sex on This Risk." *American Journal of Epidemiology* 199 (1984): 526–40.

Bouchard, C., A. Tremblay, J.-P. Després, A. Nadeau, P. J. Lupien, G. Thériault, J. Dussault, S. Moorjani, S. Pinault, and G. Fournier. "The Response to Long-Term Overfeeding in Identical Twins." *New England Journal of Medicine* 322 (1990): 1477–82.

Bray, G. A. "Complications of Obesity." *Annals of Internal Medicine* 103 (1985): 1052–62.

———, ed. "Obesity: Basic Aspects and Clinical Applications." *The Medical Clinics of North America*, Vol. 73, No. 1 (January 1989): 1–269.

Bray, G. A., and D. S. Gray. "Obesity, Part I—Pathogenesis." *Western Journal of Medicine* 149 (1988): 429–41.

———. "Obesity, Part II—Treatment." *Western Journal of Medicine* 149 (1988): 555–71.

Bjorntorp, P. "Regional Patterns of Fat Distribution." *Annals of Internal Medicine* 1103 (1985): 994–95.

Blankenhorn, D. H., R. L. Johnson, W. J. Mack, H. A. El Zein, and

L. I. Vailas. "The Influence of Diet on the Appearance of New Lesions in Human Coronary Arteries." *Journal of the American Medical Association* 263 (1990): 1646–52.

Build Study 1959, Vols. I, II. Chicago: Society of Actuaries, 1960.

Build Study 1979. Chicago: Society of Actuaries and Association of Life Insurance Medical Directors of America, 1980.

Clauw, D. J., D. J. Nashel, A. Umhau, and P. Katz. "Tryptophan-Associated Eosinophilic Connective-Tissue Disease: A New Clinical Entity?" *Journal of the American Medical Association* 263 (1990): 1502–06.

Codellas, P. S. "The Epimonidion Pharmacon of Philon Byzantine." *Bulletin of the History of Medicine* 22 (1948): 630–34.

Cohen, A. W., and S. G. Gabbe. "Obstetrical Problems in the Obese Patient." In *Obesity*, edited by A. J. Stunkard. Philadelphia: W. B. Saunders Company, 1980.

Collipp, P. J. "Obesity in Childhood." In *Obesity*, edited by A. J. Stunkard. Philadelphia: W. B. Saunders Company, 1980.

Committee of Principal Investigators. "A Co-operative Trial in the Primary Prevention of Ischaemic Heart Disease Using Clofibrate: Report from the Committee of Principal Investigators." *British Heart Journal* 40 (1978): 1069–1118.

Committee On Diet and Health, Food and Nutrition Board, Commission on Life Sciences, National Research Council. *Diet and Health: Implications for Reducing Chronic Disease Risk*. Washington, D.C.: National Academy Press, 1989.

Consensus Development Conference. "Lowering Blood Cholesterol to Prevent Heart Disease." *Journal of the American Medical Association* 253 (1985): 2080–86.

The Coronary Drug Project Research Group. "Clofibrate and Niacin in Coronary Heart Disease." *Journal of the American Medical Association* 231 (1975): 360–81.

Craighead, L. W., A. J. Stunkard, and R. M. O'Brien. "Behavior Therapy and Pharmacotherapy for Obesity." *Archives of General Psychiatry* 38 (1981): 763–68.

Crisp, A. H. "Epidemiology and Natural History." In *Anorexia Nervosa: Let Me Be*. New York: Grune and Stratton, 1980.

———, R. S. Kalucy, J. H. Lacey, B. Harding. "The Long-Term Prognosis in Anorexia Nervosa: Some Factors Predictive of Outcome." In *Anorexia Nervosa*, ed. by R. A. Vigersky. New York: Raven Press, 1977.

Després, J.-P., S. Moorjani, P. J. Lupien, A. Tremblay, A. Nadeau, and C. Bouchard. "Regional Distribution of Body Fat, Plasma Lipoproteins, and Cardiovascular Disease." *Arteriosclerosis* 10 (1990): 497–511.

Dustan, H. P. "Obesity and Hypertension." *Annals of Internal Medicine* 103 (1985): 1047–49.

Ekelund, L. G., W. L. Haskell, J. L. Johnson, F. S. Whaley, M. H. Criqui, and D. S. Sheps. "Physical Fitness as a Predictor of Cardiovascular Mortality in Asymptomatic North American Men: The Lipid Research Clinics Mortality Follow-up Study." *New England Journal of Medicine* 319 (1988): 1379–84.

Felig, P. "Editorial Retrospective: Very Low Calorie Protein Diets." *New England Journal of Medicine* 310 (1984): 589–91.

Ferguson, J. M. *Habits Not Diets.* Palo Alto, Calif.: Bull Publishing Company, 1989.

———, and J. P. Feighner. "Fluoxetine-Induced Weight Loss in Overweight Non-Depressed Humans." *International Journal of Obesity* 11, Supplement 3 (1987): 163–70.

Ferster, C. B., J. L. Nurnberger, and E. B. Levitt. "The Control of Eating." *Journal of Mathetics* 109 (1962): 87–109.

Frick, M. H., O. Elo, K. Haapa, O. P. Heinonen, P. Heinsalmi, P. Helo, J. K. Huttunen, P. Kaitaniemi, P. Koskinen, V. Manninen, H. Maenpaa, M. Malkonen, M. Manttari, S. Norola, A. Pasternak, J. Pikkarainen, M. Romo, T. Sjoblom, and E. A. Nikkila. "Helsinki Heart Study: Primary-Prevention Trial with Gemfibrozil in Middle-Aged Men with Dyslipidemia: Treatment, Changes in Risk Factors, and Incidence of Coronary Heart Disease." *New England Journal of Medicine* 317 (1987): 1237–45.

Friedman, R. M., ed. "The Continuing Search for Low-Fat Cheese." *University of California, Berkeley Wellness Letter* 4 (1988): 2.

Frisch, R. E., ed. "Adipose Tissue and Reproduction." *Progress in Reproductive Biology and Medicine, Vol. 14.* Basel, Switzerland: Karger, 1990.

Fujioka, S., Y. Matsuzawa, K. Tokunaga, and S. Tarui. "Contribution of Intra-abdominal Fat Accumulation to the Impairment of Glucose and Lipid Metabolism in Human Obesity." *Metabolism* 36 (1987): 54–59.

Garfinkel, P. E., and D. M. Garner, eds. *The Role of Drug Treatments for Eating Disorders.* New York: Brunner-Mazel Publishers, 1987.

Garner, D. M., P. E. Garfinkel, D. S. Schwartz, and M. Thompson. "Cultural Expectations of Thinness in Women." *Psychological Reports* 47 (1980): 483–89.

Garrison, R. J., and W. P. Castelli. "Weight and Thirty-Year Mortality of Men in the Framingham Study." *Annals of Internal Medicine* 103 (1985): 1006–09.

Goldblatt, P. B., M. E. Moore, and A. J. Stunkard. "Social Factors in Obesity." *Journal of the American Medical Association* 192 (1965): 97–102.

Griffen, W. O. Jr., and K. J. Printen, eds. *Surgical Management of Morbid Obesity.* New York: Marcel Dekker, Inc., 1987.

Haffner, S. M., M. S. Stern, B. D. Mitchell, H. P. Hazuda, and J. K. Patterson. "Incidence of Type II Diabetes in Mexican-Americans Predicted by Fasting Insulin and Glucose Levels, Obesity, and Body-Fat Distribution." *Diabetes* 39 (1990): 283–88.

Hartz, A. J., D. C. Rupley, R. D. Kalkhoff, and A. A. Rimm. "Relationship of Obesity to Diabetes: Influence of Obesity Level and Body Fat Distribution." *Preventive Medicine* 12 (1983): 351–57.

———, D. C. Rupley, and A. A. Rimm. "The Association of Girth Measurements with Disease in 32,856 Women." *American Journal of Epidemiology* 119 (1984): 71–80.

Hirai, A., T. Terano, H. Saito, et al. "Eicosapentaenoic Acid and Platelet Function in Japanese." In *Nutritional Prevention of Cardiovascular Disease,* edited by W. Lovenburg and Y. Yamori. New York: Academic Press, 1984.

Hoebel, B. G. "Pharmacologic Control of Feeding." *Annual Review of Pharmacology and Toxicology* 17 (1977): 605–21.

Hoeg, J. M., R. E. Gregg, and B. H. Brewer. "An Approach to the Management of Hyperlipoproteinemia." *Journal of the American Medical Association* 255 (1986): 512–21.

Kern, P. A., J. M. Ong, B. Saffari, and J. Carty. "The Effects of Weight Loss on the Activity and Expression of Adipose Tissue Lipoprotein Lipase in Very Obese Humans." *New England Journal of Medicine* 322 (1990): 1053–09.

Kissebah, A. H., N. Vydelingum, R. Murray, D. J. Evans, A. J. Hartz, R. K. Kalkhoff, and P. W. Adams. "Relation of Body Fat Distribution to Metabolic Complications of Obesity." *Journal of Clinical Endocrinology and Metabolism* 54 (1982): 254–60.

Knopp, R. H., J. Ginsberg, J. J. Albers, C. Hoff, J. T. Ogilvie, G. R. Warnick, E. Burrows, B. Retzlaff, M. Poole. "Contrasting Effects of Unmodified and Time-Release Forms of Niacin on Lipoproteins in Hyperlipidemic Subjects: Clues to Mechanism of Action of Niacin." *Metabolism* 34 (1985): 642–50.

Koplan, J. P., C. J. Caspersen, and K. E. Powell. "Physical Activity, Physical Fitness, and Health: Time to Act." *Journal of the American Medical Association* 262 (1989): 2437.

Kromhout, D., E. B. Bosschieter, and C. de L. Coulander. "The Inverse Relation Between Fish Consumption and 20-Year Mortality from Coronary Heart Disease." *New England Journal of Medicine* 312 (1985): 1205–09.

Lacey, H. J. "Anorexia Nervosa and a Bearded Female Saint." *British Journal of Medicine* 285 (1982): 1816–17.

Larsson, B., K. Svardsudd, L. Welin, L. Wilhelmsen, P. Björntorp, and G. Tibblin. "Abdominal Adipose Tissue Distribution, Obesity, and Risk of Cardiovascular Disease and Death: 13-Year Follow-up of Participants in the Study of Men Born in 1913." *British Medical Journal* 288 (1984): 1401–04.

Lawrence, M. S., and J. W. Anderson. "Dietary Fiber Content of Selected Foods." *American Journal of Clinical Nutrition* 47 (1988): 440–47.

Levin, B. E. "Thermogenic Agents as a Treatment of Obesity." In *Recent Advances in Obesity Research: IV,* edited by J. Hirsch and T. B. Van Itallie. London: John Libby, 1985.

Lew, E. A., and L. Garfinkel. "Variations in Mortality by Weight Among 750,000 Men and Women." *Journal of Chronic Disease* 32 (1979): 563–76.

———. "Mortality and Weight: Insured Lives and the American Cancer Society Studies." *Annals of Internal Medicine* 103 (1985): 1024–29.

Lipid Research Clinics Program. "The Lipid Research Clinics Coronary Primary Prevention Trial Results: I. Reduction in Incidence of Coronary Heart Disease." *Journal of the American Medical Association* 251 (1984): 351–64.

———. "The Lipid Research Clinics Coronary Primary Prevention Trial Results: II. The Relationship of Reduction in Incidence of Coronary Heart Disease to Cholesterol Lowering." *Journal of the American Medical Association* 251 (1984): 365–74.

London, S. J., G. A. Colditz, M. J. Stampfer, W. C. Willett, B. Rosner, F. E. Speizer. "Prospective Study of Relative Weight, Height, and Risk of Breast Cancer." *Journal of the American Medical Association* 262 (1989): 2853–58.

Malchow-Moller, A., S. Larsen, H. Hey, K. H. Stokholm, E. Juhl, and F. Quaade. "Ephedrine as an Anorectic: The Story of the Elsinore Pill." *International Journal of Obesity* 5 (1981): 183–87.

Manson, J. E., G. A. Colditz, M. J. Stampfer, W. C. Willett, B. Rosner, R. R. Monson, F. E. Speizer, and C. H. Hennekens. "A Prospective Study of Obesity and Risk of Coronary Heart Disease in Women." *New England Journal of Medicine* 322 (1990): 882–89.

————, M. J. Stampfer, C. H. Hennekens, and W. C. Willett. "Body Weight and Longevity: A Reassessment." *Journal of the American Medical Association* 257 (1987): 353–58.

Martin, M. J., S. B. Hulley, W. S. Browner, L. H. Kuller, and D. Wentworth. "Serum Cholesterol, Blood Pressure, and Mortality: Implications from a Cohort of 361,662 Men." *Lancet* II (1986): 933–36.

McMahon, A. T., L. Gese, J. P. O'Leary, and G. S. M. Cowan, eds. *Surgical Stapling, Volume III: Bariatric Procedures for Morbid Obesity.* St. Paul, Minn.: 3M Health Care, 1989.

Medsger, T. A. Jr. "Tryptophan-Induced Eosinophilia-Myalgia Syndrome." *New England Journal of Medicine* 322 (1990): 926–28.

"Metropolitan Height and Weight Tables." *Statistical Bulletin of the Metropolitan Life Foundation* 64 (1983): 1–9.

Miller, A. B. "Obesity and Cancer." In *Dietary Treatment and Prevention of Obesity,* edited by R. T. Frankle, J. Dwyer, L. Moragne, and A. Owen. London: John Libbey, 1985.

Morton, R. *Phthisiologica, or a Treatise of Consumption.* London: S. Smith and B. Walford, 1694.

The Multiple Risk Factor Intervention Trial Research Group. "Mortality Rates After 10.5 Years for Participants in the Multiple Risk Factor Intervention Trial." *Journal of the American Medical Association* 263 (1990): 1795–1801.

National Center for Health Statistics. *Plan and Operation of the Health and Nutrition Survey, United States 1971–73.* Washington, D.C.: Health Services and Mental Health Administration, 1973. DHEW publication no. (HSM) 73-1310 (Vital and Health Statistics, series 1, no. 10a and 10b).

————. *Plan and Operation of the National Health and Nutrition Examination Survey, 1976–80.* Washington, D.C.: U.S. Public Health Service, 1981. DHHS publication no. (PHS) 81-1317. (Vital and Health Statistics, series 1, no. 15).

Norell, S. E., A. Ahlbom, M. Feychting, and N. L. Pedersen. "Fish

Consumption and Mortality from Coronary Heart Disease." *British Medical Journal* 293 (1986): 426.

Office of Medical Applications of Research, National Institutes of Health. "Lowering Blood Cholesterol to Prevent Heart Disease." *Journal of the American Medical Association* 253 (1985): 2080–86.

Ostlund, R. E., M. Staten, W. M. Kohrt, J. Schultz, and M. M. Malley. "The Ratio of Waist-to-Hip Circumference, Plasma Insulin Level, and Glucose Intolerance as Independent Predictors of the HDL$_2$ Cholesterol Level in Older Adults." *New England Journal of Medicine* 322 (1990): 229–34.

Palumbo, P. J. "Cholesterol Lowering for All: A Closer Look." *Journal of the American Medical Association* 262 (1989): 91–92.

Pasulka, P. S., B. R. Bistrian, P. N. Benotti, and G. L. Blackburn. "The Risks of Surgery in Obese Patients." *Annals of Internal Medicine* 104 (1986): 540–46.

Peiris, A. N., M. S. Sothmann, R. G. Hoffmann, M. I. Hennes, C. R. Wilson, A. B. Gustafson, and A. H. Kissebah. "Adiposity, Fat Distribution, and Cardiovascular Risk." *Annals of Internal Medicine* 110 (1989): 867–72.

Pugliese, M. T., F. Lifshitz, G. Grad, P. Fort, and M. Marks-Katz. "Fear of Obesity: A Cause of Short Stature and Delayed Puberty." *New England Journal of Medicine* 309 (1983): 513–18.

Rabkin, S. W., F. A. Mathewson, and P. H. Hsu. "Relation of Body Weight to Development of Ischemic Heart Disease in a Cohort of Young North American Men after a 26-Year Observation Period: the Manitoba Study." *American Journal of Cardiology* 39 (1977): 452–58.

Ravussin, E., S. Lillioja, W. C. Knowler, L. Christin, D. Freymond, W. G. H. Abbott, V. Boyce, B. V. Howard, and C. Bogardus. "Reduced Rate of Energy Expenditure as a Risk Factor for Body-Weight Gain." *New England Journal of Medicine* 318 (1988): 467–72.

Roberts, S. B., J. Savage, W. A. Coward, B. Chew, and A. Lucas. "Energy Expenditure and Intake in Infants Born to Lean and Overweight Mothers." *New England Journal of Medicine* 318 (1988): 461–66.

Rodin, J. "Weight Change Following Smoking Cessation: The Role of Food Intake and Exercise." *Journal of Addictive Behavior* 12 (1987): 303–17.

Schachter, S., and L. P. Gross. "Manipulated Time and Eating Behaviors." *Journal of Personality and Social Psychology* 10 (1968): 98–106.

Schwartz, H. *Never Satisfied: A Cultural History of Diets, Fantasies, and Fat*. New York: The Free Press, 1986.

Shekelle, R. B., L. V. Missell, O. Paul, A. M. Shyrock, and J. Stamler. "Fish Consumption and Mortality from Coronary Heart Disease." *New England Journal of Medicine* 313 (1985): 820.

Sheldon, W. H. *Atlas of Men*. New York: Harper & Brothers, 1954.

Shimokata, H., D. C. Muller, and R. Andres. "Studies in the Distribution of Body Fat: III. Effects of Cigarette Smoking." *Journal of the American Medical Association* 261 (1989): 1169–73.

Silverstone, T. "Appetite Suppressant Drugs in the Management of Obesity: The Current View." *International Journal of Obesity* 11 (1987): 135–40.

Sims, E. A. H. "Destiny Rides Again As Twins Overeat." *New England Journal of Medicine* 322 (1990): 1522–24.

Stallones, L., W. H. Meuller, and B. L. Christensen. "Blood Pressure, Fatness, and Fat Patterning Among USA Adolescents from Two Ethnic Groups." *Hypertension* 4 (1982): 483–86.

Stamler, J., E. Farinaro, L. M. Mojonnier, Y. Hall, D. Moss, and R. Stamler. "Prevention and Control of Hypertension by Nutritional-Hygienic Means: Long-Term Experience of the Chicago Coronary Prevention Evaluation Program." *Journal of the American Medical Association* 243 (1980): 1819–23.

Stern, M. J., and S. M. Haffner. "Body Fat Distribution and Hyperinsulinemia as Risk Factors for Diabetes and Cardiovascular Disease." *Arteriosclerosis* 6 (1986): 123–30.

Stifler, L. T. P., L. G. Schwarz, and E. McFadden. *The HMR Calorie System*. Boston: Health Management Resources Corp., 1987.

Stuart, R. B. "Behavioral Control of Overeating." *Behavioral Research and Therapy* 5 (1967): 357–65.

Stuart, R. B. *Act Thin, Stay Thin: New Ways to Lose Weight and Keep It Off*. New York: W. W. Norton & Co., 1978.

Stunkard, A. J., J. R. Harris, N. L. Pedersen, and G. McClearn. "The Body-Mass Index of Twins Who Have Been Reared Apart." *New England Journal of Medicine* 322 (1990): 1483–87.

Theander, S. "Anorexia Nervosa: A Psychiatric Investigation of Ninety-four Female Patients." *Acta Psychiatrica Scandinavica Supplementum,* 214 (1970): 1–194.

U.S. Dept. of Health and Human Services. *The Surgeon General's Report on Nutrition and Health*. Public Health Service, DHHS (PHS) Publication No. 88-50210. 1988.

Vague, J. "The Degree of Masculine Differentiation of Obesities: A Factor Determining Predisposition to Diabetes, Atherosclerosis, Gout, and Uric Calculous Disease." *American Journal of Clinical Nutrition* 4 (1956): 20–34.

Van Itallie, T. B. "The Perils of Obesity in Middle-Aged Women." *New England Journal of Medicine* 322 (1990): 928–29.

Wadden, T. A., and A. J. Stunkard. "Social and Psychological Consequences of Obesity." *Annals of Internal Medicine* 103 (1985): 1062–67.

———, and K. D. Brownell. "Very-Low-Calorie Diets: Their Efficacy, Safety, and Future." *Annals of Internal Medicine* 99 (1983): 675–84.

———, T. B. Van Itallie, and G. A. Blackburn. "Responsible and Irresponsible Use of Very-Low-Calorie Diets in the Treatment of Obesity." *Journal of the American Medical Association* 263 (1990): 83–85.

Welin, L., K. Svardsudd, L. Wilhelmsen, B. Larsson, and G. Tibblin. "Analysis of Risk Factors for Stroke in a Cohort of Men Born in 1913." *New England Journal of Medicine* 317 (1987): 521–26.

West, K. M. *Epidemiology of Diabetes and its Vascular Lesions.* New York: Elsevier, 1978.

Wilber, J. F. "Neuropeptides, Appetite Regulation, and Obesity." In *The Endocrine Society 41st Postgraduate Annual Assembly Syllabus.* Bethesda, Md.: The Endocrine Society, 1989.

Wilson, P. W. F., J. C. Christiansen, K. M. Anderson, and W. B. Kannel. "Impact of National Guidelines for Cholesterol Risk Factor Screening: The Framingham Offspring Study." *Journal of the American Medical Association* 262 (1989): 41–44.

Wilt, T. J., R. P. Lofgren, K. L. Nichol, A. E. Schorer, L. Crespin, D. Downes, and J. Eckfeldt. "Fish Oil Supplementation Does Not Lower Plasma Cholesterol in Men with Hypercholesterolemia: Results of a Randomized, Placebo-Controlled Crossover Study." *Annals of Internal Medicine* 111 (1989): 900–05.

Wood, P. D., M. L. Stefanick, D. M. Dreon, B. Frey-Hewitt, S. C. Garay, P. T. Williams, H. R. Superko, S. P. Fortmann, J. J. Albers, K. M. Vranzian, N. M. Ellsworth, R. B. Terry, and W. L. Haskell. "Changes in Plasma Lipids and Lipoproteins in Overweight Men During Weight Loss Through Dieting as Compared with Exercise." *New England Journal of Medicine* 319 (1988): 1173–79.

Wooley, W., and S. Wooley. "Feeling Fat in a Thin Society." *Glamour* (February, 1984): 198–259.

Wurtman, J. J., and R. J. Wurtman. "Suppression of Carbohydrate Consumption as Snacks and at Mealtime by dl-Fenfluramine or Tryptophan." In *Anorectic Agents: Mechanisms of Action and Tolerance,* edited by S. Garratini and R. Samanian. New York: Raven Press, 1981.

Young, R. L., R. J. Fuchs, and H. J. Woltjen. "Chorionic Gonadotropin in Weight Control: A Double-Blind Crossover Study." *Journal of the American Medical Association* 236 (1976): 2495–97.

About the Authors

Lynn J. Bennion, M.D., is a practicing physician who specializes in endocrinology and metabolism and teaches at Stanford University School of Medicine as an Associate Clinical Professor. Prior to entering private practice, he did full-time research in obesity and cholesterol metabolism for five years at the National Institutes of Health. His research is published in leading scientific medical journals such as the *Journal of Clinical Investigation* and the *New England Journal of Medicine*. He is the author of a book for the lay public on low blood sugar, entitled *Hypoglycemia: Fact or Fad?*

Edwin L. Bierman, M.D., is Professor of Medicine at the University of Washington Medical School, and Head of the Division of Metabolism, Endocrinology and Nutrition. He is the author of more than 250 scientific research articles and textbook chapters, and is an internationally recognized authority on the subject of fat and cholesterol metabolism. He has contributed treatises on obesity to widely used textbooks of medicine and endocrinology.

James M. Ferguson, M.D., is a psychiatrist who helped pioneer behavior modification as a means of treating obesity, and who has written handbooks for teachers and patients on that subject. In his private practice he treats many patients with eating disorders, including anorexia and bulimia, and he has written articles for doctors and medical students on the modern treatment of these problems.

Index